Nanocarrier-based Drug Delivery for the Management of Fatty Liver Disease

Edited by

Anjali Sharma
Department of Pharmaceutics
Guru Gobind Singh College of Pharmacy
Yamunanagar, Haryana, India

Devkant Sharma
Department of Pharmaceutics
Ch. DeviLal College of Pharmacy
Jagadhri, Haryana, India

Ajmer Singh Grewal
Department of Pharmaceutical Chemistry
Guru Gobind Singh College of Pharmacy
Yamunanagar, Haryana, India

Geeta Deswal
Department of Pharmacognosy
Guru Gobind Singh College of Pharmacy
Yamunanagar, Haryana, India

&

Ganga Reddy Velma
Department of Pharmacology & Toxicology
R. Ken Coit College of Pharmacy, University of Arizona
Tucson, Arizona, United States

Nanocarrier-based Drug Delivery for the Management of Fatty Liver Disease

Editors: Anjali Sharma, Devkant Sharma, Ajmer Singh Grewal,

Geeta Deswal and Ganga Reddy Velma

ISBN (Online): 979-8-89881-567-7

ISBN (Print): 979-8-89881-568-4

ISBN (Paperback): 979-8-89881-569-1

Published by Bentham Science Publishers Pte. Ltd. Singapore,

in collaboration with Eureka Conferences, USA.

First published in 2026.

need for a court order if at any point you breach any terms of this License Agreement. In no event will any delay or failure by Bentham Science Publishers in enforcing your compliance with this License Agreement constitute a waiver of any of its rights.

3. You acknowledge that you have read this License Agreement, and agree to be bound by its terms and conditions. To the extent that any other terms and conditions presented on any website of Bentham Science Publishers conflict with, or are inconsistent with, the terms and conditions set out in this License Agreement, you acknowledge that the terms and conditions set out in this License Agreement shall prevail.

Bentham Science Publishers Pte. Ltd.
No. 9 Raffles Place
Office No. 26-01
Singapore 048619
Singapore
Email: subscriptions@benthamscience.net

BENTHAM SCIENCE

CONTENTS

FOREWORD i

PREFACE ii

LIST OF CONTRIBUTORS iv

CHAPTER 1 INTRODUCTION TO FATTY LIVER DISEASE 1

Vishnu Mittal, Anjali Sharma and *Dinesh Mishra*

INTRODUCTION 2
Overview of Fatty Liver Disease 2
Epidemiology and Global Burden 2
CLASSIFICATION OF FATTY LIVER DISEASE 3
Non-Alcoholic Fatty Liver Disease (NAFLD) 3
Alcoholic Fatty Liver Disease (AFLD) 4
PATHOPHYSIOLOGY OF FATTY LIVER DISEASE 4
Mechanisms of Hepatic Lipid Accumulation 5
Role of Inflammation and Oxidative Stress 6
Progression to Non-Alcoholic Steatohepatitis (NASH), Fibrosis, and Cirrhosis 6
RISK FACTORS AND CAUSES 7
Genetic Predisposition 7
Metabolic Disorders (Obesity, Diabetes, and Dyslipidemia) 7
Dietary and Lifestyle Factors 7
Alcohol Consumption and Liver Health 7
CLINICAL MANIFESTATIONS AND DIAGNOSIS 8
Symptoms and Stages of Fatty Liver Disease 8
Biomarkers and Laboratory Tests 9
Clinical Features 9
Common Biomarkers 9
Novel Biomarkers 10
Panels of Markers 10
Imaging Techniques (Ultrasound, MRI, and FibroScan) 10
Magnetic Resonance Imaging (MRI) and Proton Magnetic Resonance Spectroscopy (MRS) 11
Transient Elastography 11
Histology 11
LIFESTYLE MODIFICATIONS (DIET, EXERCISE) 11
Pharmacological Approaches 11
Limitations of Conventional Therapies 12
ROLE OF NANOTECHNOLOGY IN FATTY LIVER DISEASE MANAGEMENT 12
Nanocarrier-based Drug Delivery: A Patent Perspective 12
Types of Nanocarriers Used 13
Liposomes 13
Solid Lipid Nanoparticles (SLNs) 14
Polymeric Nanoparticles 15
FUTURE PERSPECTIVES AND CHALLENGES 17
Advancements in Nanomedicine for Fatty Liver Disease 17
Regulatory and Safety Concerns 18
Potential for Clinical Translation 18
CONCLUSION 18
LIST OF ABBREVIATIONS 18
REFERENCES 19

CHAPTER 2 NON-ALCOHOLIC FATTY LIVER DISEASE: A METABOLIC THREAT 25
Kalpana Garg, Sakshi Bajaj, Lakhveer Singh, Abhishek and *Aniket*
INTRODUCTION 25
TYPES OF NAFLD 26
Non-alcoholic Fatty Liver (Simple Steatosis) 26
Non-alcoholic Steatohepatitis without Fibrosis 27
Non-alcoholic Steatohepatitis with Fibrosis 27
EPIDEMIOLOGY OF NAFLD 28
PATHOPHYSIOLOGY OF NAFLD 29
CLINICAL PRESENTATION OF NAFLD 29
CURRENT DIAGNOSTIC MODALITIES 30
LIFESTYLE INTERVENTIONS AND THEIR ROLE IN DISEASE MANAGEMENT 31
CHALLENGES IN THE MANAGEMENT OF NAFLD 32
REGULATORY AND SAFETY CONCERNS 33
FUTURE PERSPECTIVES FOR FATTY LIVER DISEASE MANAGEMENT 34
CONCLUSION 34
LIST OF ABBREVIATIONS 35
REFERENCES 35

CHAPTER 3 OVERVIEW OF NANOCARRIER-BASED DRUG DELIVERY SYSTEMS 40
Himani Bajaj, Mayank Yadav, Mukesh Maithani, Abhay Mishra and *Navin Chandra Pant*
INTRODUCTION 40
NPS AS DRUG-DELIVERY SYSTEMS 42
Lipid Nanosystems 42
Polymeric NPs 45
Inorganic NPs 45
Nanogels 45
Dendrimers 46
Nanoemulsion 46
Exosomes 47
BIOLOGICAL, PHYSICOCHEMICAL, AND TOXICOLOGICAL CONSIDERATIONS WHEN DESIGNING A DRUG-DELIVERY SYSTEM 47
Biodistribution 47
Cellular Uptake and Biocompatibility 48
NP Kinetics 49
Toxicological Concerns 49
NANOMEDICINE IN NAFLD DIAGNOSIS 50
Nanomedicine for NAFLD Therapeutics 50
FUTURE PERSPECTIVE 50
CONCLUSION 51
LIST OF ABBREVIATIONS 52
REFERENCES 53

CHAPTER 4 LIVER TARGETING STRATEGIES WITH NANOCARRIERS 59
Afreen Usmani, Mohd Aftab Siddiqui, Mohd Nazam Ansari and *Rania I.M. Almoselhy*
INTRODUCTION 60
Fatty Liver Disease 60
Limitations of Conventional Therapies 61
NANOCARRIERS IN DRUG DELIVERY FOR LIVER DISEASES 62

Liposomes 64
Polymeric Nanoparticles 64
Solid Lipid Nanoparticles 65
Inorganic Nanoparticles 65
Albumin Nanoparticles 65
Extracellular Vesicles 65
Low-density Lipoprotein 66
Chitosan Nanoparticles 66
Gold Nanoparticles 66
Carbon-based Nanocarriers 67
Dendrimers 67
Micelles 67
Metal-organic Frameworks 68
Nanostructured Lipid Carriers (NLCs) 68
Carbon Quantum Dots (CQDs) 68
Nanosuspensions 68
Nanogels 69
LIVER-TARGETING STRATEGIES 69
Active Targeting 70
Passive Targeting 70
Synergistic Potential 70
Receptor-mediated Targeting Strategies 70
Stimuli-responsive Nanocarriers 71
INTEGRATION WITH ADVANCED THERAPEUTICS 72
RNA-based and siRNA Delivery 72
CRISPR-Cas9 Delivery 72
Natural Compounds in Nanocarriers 72
Targeting NAFLD and NASH with combination therapies 73
Resveratrol and Astaxanthin 73
Fibrosis and Inflammation 73
RECENT ADVANCES IN PRECLINICAL AND CLINICAL STUDIES 73
Success Stories and Ongoing Trials 73
Emerging Innovations in Nanomedicine for Liver Diseases 74
Lipid Nanoparticles (LNPs) 74
Cell Membrane-coated Nanoparticles (CMNPs) 74
Hybrid Nanocarrier Systems 74
CRISPR and Gene Therapy Delivery Platforms 74
Emerging Nanotechnology-based Pharmacological Agents in Clinical Trials for Liver Targeting 74
BMS-986263 75
ARCT-810 75
SAFETY AND REGULATORY CONSIDERATIONS 75
Safety Considerations 75
Biocompatibility of Nanocarriers 76
Regulatory Challenges in Nanomedicine 76
Standardization of Characterization Protocols 76
Long-term Safety Data 77
Batch-to-batch Consistency and Scalability 77
Risk-benefit Assessment 77
CHALLENGES IN CLINICAL TRANSLATION 77
Optimization of Drug Loading and Release Profiles 77

Immunogenicity and Biocompatibility Issues 78
Manufacturing and Scalability Challenges 78
FUTURE PERSPECTIVES IN NANOCARRIER-BASED THERAPIES 78
CONCLUSION 79
LIST OF ABBREVIATIONS 80
REFERENCES 80

CHAPTER 5 LIPID-BASED NANOCARRIERS FOR FATTY LIVER DISEASE 86
Monika Sharma, Diksha Sharma, Sonia Gupta and *Jasmine Bhatia*
INTRODUCTION TO FATTY LIVER DISEASES 86
CURRENT THERAPEUTIC APPROACHES AND THEIR LIMITATIONS 87
ROLE OF NANOTECHNOLOGY IN THE TREATMENT OF LIVER DISEASE 87
Role of Nanocarriers in the Management of NASH and NAFLD 88
Lipid-based Nano Carriers (LBCs) in the Management of NASH and NAFLD 88
LIVER-TARGETED DRUG DELIVERY SYSTEMS 89
Liver Targeting Mechanisms 89
Passive Targeting 89
Active Targeting 89
Reticuloendothelial System (RES): 90
Effect of Surface Modifications for Enhanced Liver Targeting 90
Folic Acid Conjugation for Targeting 90
OPTIMIZATION AND SCALE-UP STRATEGIES FOR LBC 92
Scale-up Challenges 92
CLINICAL IMPLICATIONS AND CHALLENGES 93
FUTURE DIRECTIONS IN LIPID NANOCARRIER RESEARCH 93
Emerging Trends 93
Challenges and Regulatory Considerations 94
CONCLUSION 94
LIST OF ABBREVIATIONS 94
REFERENCES 94

CHAPTER 6 POLYMERIC NANOCARRIERS FOR FATTY LIVER DISEASE 99
Kshama Srivastava, Deepika Rani, Vinit K Sharma and *Ranjit Singh*
INTRODUCTION 99
Current Therapeutic Challenges 100
Role of Nanotechnology in Liver-targeted Therapy 101
ANATOMY OF THE LIVER 102
PATHOPHYSIOLOGY OF FATTY LIVER DISEASE 103
STRATEGIES FOR HEPATIC-TARGETED DRUG DELIVERY 104
Passive Targeting 104
Active Targeting 105
OVERVIEW OF POLYMERIC NPS 106
Nanospheres 107
Structural Characteristics 107
Drug Release Mechanisms 107
Applications 108
Nanocapsules 108
Structural Characteristics 108
Drug Release Mechanisms 108
Applications 108
PREPARATION OF POLYMERIC NPS 109
Polymer-based NM for Liver Disease Treatment 109

Hepatitis ... 109
HBV Infection ... 110
NASH and Nanomaterial-based Therapeutics ... 111
Liver Fibrosis ... 112
Hepatocellular Carcinoma ... 113
Host-versus-Graft Disease (HVGD) ... 114
The Fate of NPs in the Liver: ... 115
FUTURE PROSPECTS ... 116
CONCLUSION ... 117
LIST OF ABBREVIATIONS ... 117
REFERENCES ... 118

CHAPTER 7 DENDRIMERS AND HYBRID NANOCARRIERS FOR FATTY LIVER DISEASE ... 127
Minky Mukhija, Himanshu Sharma, Jyoti Monga, Ankush Sundriyal and *Jasmine Chaudhary*
INTRODUCTION ... 128
CONVENTIONAL THERAPEUTIC APPROACHES FOR FATTY LIVER DISEASE ... 128
Lifestyle Modifications ... 128
Pharmacological Interventions ... 128
LIMITATIONS OF CONVENTIONAL TREATMENTS ... 129
NANOTECHNOLOGY IN THE TREATMENT OF FATTY LIVER DISEASE ... 130
Advantages of Nanocarriers in Liver Targeting ... 130
Types of Nanocarriers Used for FLD Therapy ... 130
DENDRIMERS IN LIVER DISEASE ... 131
Structure and Properties of Dendrimers ... 131
Mechanisms of Hepatic Targeting Using Dendrimers ... 132
Dendrimer-based drug delivery systems for FLD ... 132
RECENT ADVANCEMENTS IN DENDRIMER-BASED THERAPIES ... 133
HYBRID NANOCARRIERS FOR FATTY LIVER DISEASE ... 134
Types of Hybrid Systems ... 135
ADVANTAGES OF HYBRID NANOCARRIERS OVER TRADITIONAL NANOCARRIERS ... 135
CHALLENGES AND LIMITATIONS ... 136
RECENT DEVELOPMENTS IN HYBRID NANOCARRIERS FOR LIVER-TARGETED DRUG DELIVERY ... 137
FUTURE PERSPECTIVES ... 139
CONCLUSION ... 140
LIST OF ABBREVIATIONS ... 140
REFERENCES ... 141

CHAPTER 8 NOVEL THERAPEUTICS FOR FATTY LIVER DISEASE ... 145
Kirti Goel, Sonia Kamboj and *Rajan Swami*
INTRODUCTION ... 146
PATHOPHYSIOLOGY AND DISEASE PROGRESSION ... 146
CONVENTIONAL THERAPEUTICS: LIMITATIONS AND CHALLENGES ... 149
EXISTING PHARMACOLOGICAL OPTIONS AND THEIR EFFICACY ... 150
Insulin Sensitizers ... 150
Lipid-Lowering Agents ... 150
Antioxidants and Anti-inflammatory Components ... 150

Bile Acid Modulators ... 150
CONS OF CURRENT TREATMENT APPROACHES ... 151
EMERGING PHARMACOLOGICAL INTERVENTIONS ... 151
NANOTECHNOLOGY-BASED DRUG DELIVERY FOR NAFLD/NASH ... 153
GENE THERAPY AND RNA-BASED APPROACHES FOR NAFLD/NASH ... 158
NON-PHARMACOLOGICAL THERAPIES ... 160
Impact of Diet, Exercise, and Lifestyle Interventions ... 160
Microbiome Modulation as a Therapeutic Strategy ... 162
BIOMARKERS AND PRECISION MEDICINE ... 163
CHALLENGES IN TRANSLATIONAL RESEARCH IN NAFLD/NASH ... 164
Barriers to Clinical Adoption of New Therapeutics ... 165
Regulatory and Ethical Implications ... 165
FUTURE DIRECTIONS AND CONCLUSION ... 166
LIST OF ABBREVIATIONS ... 167
REFERENCES ... 168

CHAPTER 9 NANOCARRIER-BASED IMAGING AGENTS FOR FATTY LIVER DISEASE DIAGNOSIS ... 178
Hadi Sardarabadi, Saeedeh Zare Jalise, Piao Yang and *Mohsen Sheykhhasan*
INTRODUCTION ... 179
NANOCARRIERS TO TARGETED DELIVERY OF IMAGING AGENTS ... 182
The Main Physicochemical Properties of Nanocarriers ... 182
Size and Shape ... 183
Surface Characteristics ... 183
In vivo Imaging Capabilities of Biocompatible Targeted Nanocarriers ... 183
NOVEL IMAGING AGENTS FOR MONITORING FATTY LIVER DISEASE STATES 185
Drawbacks of Traditional Imaging Agents and Nanotechnology Approaches ... 185
Optical Imaging ... 185
Ultrasound (US) ... 186
Computed Tomography (CT) ... 187
Magnetic Resonance Imaging (MRI) ... 188
Nanomaterial-based Contrast Agents to Cover the Imaging Limitations ... 188
Iron Nanoparticles ... 189
Nanoemulsion ... 191
Gold Nanoparticles ... 191
Quantum Dots ... 191
Extracellular Vesicles (EVs) ... 192
Nanocomposites ... 193
Polymeric Nanocarriers ... 194
Nano-biosensors for in vitro and in vivo Sensing of Fatty Liver Diseases ... 194
REAL-TIME MONITORING VIA INTEGRATION OF NANOCARRIERS AND ADVANCED IMAGING TECHNIQUES ... 197
CONCLUSION AND FUTURE PERSPECTIVES ... 200
LIST OF ABBREVIATIONS ... 202
REFERENCES ... 203

CHAPTER 10 CLINICAL TRANSLATION OF NANOCARRIER-BASED DRUG DELIVERY SYSTEMS FOR THE TREATMENT OF FATTY LIVER DISEASE ... 210
Pranav J Shah, Priyanka Patil, Divya Gupta, Swati Gupta, Aarti Patel and *J.K Patel*
INTRODUCTION ... 211
EPIDEMIOLOGY OF NAFLD ... 212

THE MOLECULAR PATHOGENESIS OF NAFLD 213
CURRENT PHARMACOLOGIC THERAPIES 215
Diet 215
Exercise 216
Vitamin E (alpha-tocopherol) 216
(PPAR)-γ agonist 216
Lipid-lowering drugs 216
Pentoxifylline 216
Ursodeoxycholic Acid 217
Blockers of angiotensin receptors 217
Probiotics and Synbiotics 217
THR-b (thyroid hormone receptor b) Agonist 217
Obeticholic Acid, or OCA, as an Agonist of the Farnesoid X Receptor (FXR) 217
Bariatric Surgery 218
CHALLENGES IN TREATING FATTY LIVER DISEASE 218
Liver-specific Targeting 218
Hepatotoxicity and Off-target Effects 218
NANO CARRIER-BASED DRUG DELIVERY SYSTEMS 218
NANO MEDICINE FOR FLD THERAPEUTICS 220
Passive Targeting 221
Active Targeting 221
LIMITATIONS OF CURRENT APPROACHES AND CHALLENGES IN CLINICAL TRANSLATION 223
FUTURE PROSPECTS 224
CONCLUSION 224
LIST OF ABBREVIATIONS 224
REFERENCES 225

CHAPTER 11 PHARMACOKINETICS AND PHARMACODYNAMICS OF NANOCARRIER-BASED THERAPEUTICS 231
Akashdeep Singh, Sonu Kumar, Palak Sharma, Sanchit Dhankhar, Thakur Gurjeet Singh and *Samrat Chauhan*
INTRODUCTION 232
Overview of Fatty Liver Disease (FLD) 232
Non-Alcoholic Fatty Liver Disease (NAFLD) 232
Non-alcoholic Steatohepatitis (NASH) 233
OBSTACLES IN CONVECTIONAL THERAPEUTIC STRATEGIES 234
New Drug Development 234
Lifestyle Interventions 234
Diagnostic Challenges 234
Heterogeneity of NAFLD Progression 235
Limited Targeted Therapies 235
ROLE OF ADVANCED DRUG DELIVERY SYSTEMS IN LIVER-TARGETED THERAPY 235
Nanoparticle-based Delivery Systems 236
Lipid Nanoparticles (LNPs)-mediated siRNA Delivery 236
Advanced Drug Delivery Systems (ADDS) in MASH 236
Hepatic Stellate Cell (HSC) Targeting 237
Biomaterials as Drug Delivery Carrier 237
PHARMACOKINETIC AND PHARMACODYNAMIC OF NANO-CARRIER (NC)-BASED THERAPEUTICS 237

Pharmacokinetics of Nanocarriers ... 238
Absorption and Bioavailability ... 238
Distribution to the Liver ... 240
LIVER-SPECIFIC TARGETING MECHANISMS ... 241
Passive Targeting (Permeability and Retention Effect) ... 242
Active Targeting via Surface Ligands ... 242
ROLE OF NANOCARRIER IN LIVER-TARGETED DRUG DELIVERY ... 243
Metabolism and Elimination ... 244
Metabolic Pathways Involved in the Breakdown of Nanocarriers ... 244
Routes of Elimination ... 244
Physicochemical Properties of Nanocarriers and their Impact on Pharmacokinetics ... 246
Size ... 246
Shape ... 247
Surface Charge ... 247
Surface Hydrophobicity ... 248
Target Ligand ... 248
Bio-sensitive NCs ... 249
PHARMACODYNAMICS OF NANOCARRIERS IN FLD ... 249
Nanocarrier-mediated Drug Release Within Liver Cells ... 249
Cellular Uptake Mechanism of Nanocarriers ... 250
Clathrin-dependent Endocytosis ... 251
Caveolin-dependent Endocytosis ... 251
Clathrin/Caveolin-independent Endocytosis ... 252
Macropinocytosis ... 252
Passive Uptake ... 252
Impact of Nanocarriers on Cellular Uptake ... 253
Improve Cellular Uptake ... 253
Targeted Delivery to the Liver ... 253
Overcoming Physiological Obstacles ... 253
Delivery of siRNA ... 253
Targeted Therapeutic Effects in Hepatocytes and other Liver Cells ... 254
Immune Modulation ... 254
Anti-Inflammatory Actions ... 254
CONCLUSION ... 255
LIST OF ABBREVIATIONS ... 255
REFERENCES ... 256

CHAPTER 12 SAFETY AND TOXICITY CONSIDERATIONS OF NANOCARRIER-BASED THERAPEUTICS ... 265
Himanshu Sharma, Akashdeep Singh, Vishnu Mittal and *Pooja Mittal*
INTRODUCTION ... 266
Rising Interest Due to Enhanced Drug Delivery, Targeting, and Bioavailability ... 266
Importance of Safety and Toxicity Evaluation in Clinical Translation ... 266
TYPES OF NANOCARRIERS ... 267
Liposomes ... 267
Polymer Nanoparticles ... 268
Solid Lipid Nanoparticles ... 268
Dendrimers ... 268
Carbon-based Nanocarriers (e.g., Carbon Nanotubes, Graphene Oxide) ... 269
Metallic Nanoparticles (e.g., Gold, Silver) ... 269
MECHANISMS OF NANOCARRIER TOXICITY ... 270

IN VITRO AND *IN VIVO* TOXICITY EVALUATION 270
IMPACT OF SURFACE ON NANOPARTICLE PROPERTIES 271
Particle Size and Surface Charge 271
Hydrophobicity 272
Regulatory and Ethical Considerations 272
• *Implications for Ethics* 272
• *Safety Concerns* 272
• *Effect on the Environment* 272
• *Analysing and Assessing Risks* 273
• *Optimisations of Formulation and Materials* 273
• *Social and Moral Factors* 273
STRATEGIES TO IMPROVE SAFETY 273
CASE STUDIES AND CLINICAL TRANSLATION 273
FUTURE DIRECTIONS AND CHALLENGES 275
CONCLUSION 275
LIST OF ABBREVIATIONS 276
REFERENCES 276

CHAPTER 13 CASE STUDIES: NANOCARRIERS BASED DRUG DELIVERY IN FATTY LIVER DISEASE 281
Rakesh Sindhu, Gagandeep Kaur, Parul Sood, Soumya Banerjee, Nitin Jangra and *Aanandita Thakur*
INTRODUCTION 281
CASE STUDIES ON NANOCARRIER-BASED APPROACHES TO FATTY LIVER DISEASE 283
Case Study 1 284
Case Study 2 284
Case Study 3 284
Case Study 4 285
Case Study 5 285
Case Study 6 285
Case Study 7 286
Case Study 8 286
Case Study 9 286
Case Study 10 287
Case Study 11 287
Case Study 12 287
Case Study 13 288
Case Study 14 288
Case Study 15 289
Case Study 16 289
Case Study 17 289
Case Study 18 290
Case Study 19 290
Case Study 20 290
CONCLUSION 291
LIST OF ABBREVIATIONS 292
REFERENCES 292

CHAPTER 14 CHALLENGES AND OPPORTUNITIES IN NANOCARRIER-BASED DRUG DELIVERY FOR FATTY LIVER DISEASE 296

Saksham Sharma, Shushank Mahajan, Sanchit Dhankhar, Sabina Yasmin, Monika Saini and *Samrat Chauhan*
INTRODUCTION 297
PATHOPHYSIOLOGY OF FATTY LIVER DISEASE 298
NANOCARRIERS IN DRUG DELIVERY 299
APPLICATION OF NANOCARRIERS IN FLD MANAGEMENT 302
CHALLENGES IN NANOCARRIER-BASED FLD THERAPY 303
Biological Barriers in Liver Targeting 303
Impact of Disease-related Liver Architecture 304
Stability and Toxicity Concerns 304
Manufacturing Scalability Challenges 305
STRATEGIES TO OVERCOME CHALLENGES 305
RECENT ADVANCES IN NANOCARRIER-BASED DRUG DELIVERY FOR FATTY LIVER DISEASE 307
REGULATORY AND COMMERCIALIZATION ASPECTS 310
MECHANISTIC CHALLENGES AND TRANSLATIONAL OPPORTUNITIES IN NANOCARRIER-BASED THERAPY FOR FATTY LIVER DISEASE 311
Lipotoxicity 312
Inflammatory Microenvironment 312
Fibrotic Progression 312
Clinical Translation Opportunities 312
FUTURE PERSPECTIVES AND OPPORTUNITIES 313
DISCUSSION 314
CONCLUSION 315
LIST OF ABBREVIATIONS 316
REFERENCES 317

CHAPTER 15 EMERGING TRENDS AND FUTURE PERSPECTIVES FOR FATTY LIVER DISEASE MANAGEMENT 324
Vinod Kumar Gauttam, Kavita Munjal, Arushi, Sheelu Singh and *Kunal Nepali*
INTRODUCTION 325
Overview of Fatty Liver Disease 325
Types of Fatty Liver Diseases 326
Simple Fatty Liver Disease: 327
NAFL Disease: 327
Steatosis 327
Alcoholic Fatty Liver Disease: 327
PATHOPHYSIOLOGY OF HEPATIC STEATOSIS 327
NAFLD Involves the Gut-Liver Axis 328
Fibrosis and Inflammation in Fatty Livers 328
Hepatic Fibrosis as a Bad Prognosis for NASH 328
Genetics 329
The Study of Epigenetics 329
RNAs that Do Not Code 329
EMERGING TRENDS IN THE MANAGEMENT OF FATTY LIVER DISEASE 330
Personalized Medicines 330
with Reference to the Patient's Sex 330
With the Help of Computer Models 330
With Reference to Drug Metabolism 331
Imaging Biomarker 331
Liver Fat Indicators Based on Ultrasound 332

Liver Fat Indicators Based on Magnetic Resonance Spectroscopy 332
Lifestyle Interventions 332
PRACTICAL USAGE: CASES IN VARIOUS PATIENTS 333
Examples and Trial Data 334
Dietary and Physical Activity Interventions 334
Exercise Training and Liver Fat 334
Intrahepatic fat Reductions through Dietary (Mediterranean / Green Mediterranean) means 334
Combinations Diet + Exercise + Fibre in Pre-diabetic/NAFLD: 334
Combining Gut-liver and Lifestyle Approaches to Achieve Optimal Results: 335
Clinical Trial and Meta-Analysis Evidence 335
The Gut-Liver Axis and Its Role in Liver Fat Accumulation 336
Probiotics, Prebiotics, and Synbiotics in Reducing Fat in the Liver 336
Probiotics, Synbiotics, and Microbiome Interventions 337
Trial on synbiotic yogurt in adults with NAFLD: 337
Synbiotic Supplementation in Lean NAFLD 337
Synbiotics for NAFLD: A Meta-analysis Review: 337
Probiotics in Children/adolescents: 337
Meta-analyses of Probiotics and Synbiotics: 338
Digital Health Technologies 338
NEW DRUG DEVELOPMENT AND CLINICAL TRIALS 338
FUTURE PERSPECTIVES ON FATTY LIVER DISEASE MANAGEMENT 339
CONCLUSION 341
LIST OF ABBREVIATIONS 341
REFERENCES 341

SUBJECT INDEX 349

FOREWORD

The field of nanomedicine has revolutionized modern therapeutics by enabling precise, targeted, and efficient delivery systems for drugs. Among the many diseases that demand innovative treatment strategies, **Fatty Liver Disease (FLD)**—both alcoholic and non-alcoholic—stands out as a global health challenge, affecting millions worldwide. The complexity of its pathophysiology necessitates advanced approaches that transcend conventional pharmacotherapy.

This book, "*Nanocarrier-based Drug Delivery for the Management of Fatty Liver Disease*," provides a comprehensive and insightful exploration of the potential of nanotechnology to address this pressing medical concern. From the fundamentals of fatty liver disease to sophisticated nanocarrier-based therapeutic and diagnostic approaches, the book integrates scientific innovation with clinical relevance.

Each chapter, authored by distinguished experts in the field, delves into critical aspects such as liver-targeting nanocarriers, lipid- and polymer-based systems, pharmacokinetic considerations, safety profiles, and translational perspectives. This book is expected to serve as a valuable resource for researchers, academicians, clinicians, and pharmaceutical scientists seeking to leverage nanotechnology for the management of liver diseases. It is a commendable initiative that bridges the gap between nanoscience and hepatology, paving the way for future advancements in precision medicine.

I extend my heartfelt congratulations to the authors for their dedicated efforts in bringing this comprehensive and insightful book to fruition.

Bhawna Chopra
Guru Gobind Singh College of Pharmacy, Yamuna Nagar
Haryana, India

Preface

Fatty liver disease has become a serious public health problem due to the rise in instances of obesity, diabetes, and associated metabolic diseases worldwide. Effective therapy remains difficult to achieve, even as advances in medical science have improved diagnosis and management. Numerous current treatments have drawbacks, including low medication absorption, insufficient liver tissue targeting, and unfavorable side effects. These difficulties highlight the need for creative therapeutic approaches.

With benefits, such as improved drug absorption, site-specific distribution, and reduced systemic toxicity, nanocarrier-based drug delivery systems have become a viable alternative. These technologies offer the opportunity to improve treatment outcomes for individuals with fatty liver disease by addressing the drawbacks of traditional approaches.

This book offers a thorough analysis of nanocarrier technologies and their potential for treating fatty liver disease. It provides readers with a comprehensive understanding of the potential impact of nanotechnology in this field by examining key concepts, therapeutic applications, and current research. The material bridges the gap between theoretical understanding and real-world application, covering everything from fundamental scientific concepts to the latest developments.

The book is intended as a useful resource for medical researchers, healthcare practitioners, and those in the pharmaceutical sector. It supports upcoming research projects in the field of drug delivery systems, fosters multidisciplinary collaboration, and stimulates new ideas.

We express our heartfelt gratitude to all of the writers and specialists who gave their time and expertise to this collection. In addition to offering clarification and direction, we hope that our work encourages further research and development in the management of fatty liver disease.

Anjali Sharma
Department of Pharmaceutics
Guru Gobind Singh College of Pharmacy
Yamunanagar, Haryana
India

Devkant Sharma
Department of Pharmaceutics
Ch. DeviLal College of Pharmacy
Jagadhri, Haryana
India

Ajmer Singh Grewal
Department of Pharmaceutical Chemistry
Guru Gobind Singh College of Pharmacy
Yamunanagar, Haryana
India

Geeta Deswal
Department of Pharmacognosy
Guru Gobind Singh College of Pharmacy
Yamunanagar, Haryana
India

&

Ganga Reddy Velma
Department of Pharmacology & Toxicology
R. Ken Coit College of Pharmacy
University of Arizona, Tucson
Arizona, United States

List of Contributors

Abhay Mishra	Department of Pharmaceutical Technology, Faculty of Pharmaceutical Sciences, Naresuan University, Phitsanulok, Thailand
Afreen Usmani	Department of Pharmacology, MESCO Institute of Pharmacy, Amroha, Uttar Pradesh, India
Ankush Sundriyal	Department of Pharmacognosy, School of Pharmaceutical Sciences, Sardar Bhagwan Singh Post Graduate Institute of Biomedical Sciences and Research, Dehradun, Uttarakhand, India
Aarti Patel	Faculty of Pharmacy, Sigma University, Vadodara, Gujarat, India
Akashdeep Singh	Chitkara College of Pharmacy, Chitkara University, Rajpura, Punjab, India
Aanandita Thakur	School of Pharmacy, Chitkara University, Solan, Himachal Pradesh, India
Arushi	RIMS Split Campus, Motherhood University, Roorkee, Uttarakhand, India
Deepika Rani	Department of Pharmaceutics, School of Pharmacy and Emerging Sciences, Baddi University of Emerging Sciences and Technology, Baddi, Himachal Pradesh, India
Divya Gupta	Faculty of Pharmacy, Sigma University, Vadodara, Gujarat, India
Diksha Sharma	Swami Devi Dyal Institute of Pharmacy, Panchkula, Haryana, India
Gagandeep Kaur	School of Pharmacy, Chitkara University, Solan, Himachal Pradesh, India
Hina Sharif	SINA Health, Education & Welfare Trust, Karachi, Pakistan
Himani Bajaj	Adarsh Vijendra Institute of Pharmaceutical Sciences, Shobhit University, Gangoh, Saharanpur, Uttar Pradesh, India
Hadi Sardarabadi	Department of Pharmacology and Medical Physics, Faculty of Medicine, Qom University of Medical Sciences, Qom, Iran
Himanshu Sharma	Chitkara College of Pharmacy, Chitkara University, Rajpura, Punjab, India
Jasmine Bhatia	Swami Devi Dyal Institute of Pharmacy, Panchkula, Haryana, India
Jyoti Monga	Department of Pharmacognosy, Ch. Devi Lal College of Pharmacy, Jagadhri, Haryana, India
Jasmine Chaudhary	Department of Pharmaceutical Chemistry, Maharishi Markandeshwar (Deemed to be University), Mullana, Haryana, India
J.K Patel	Viesain Pharma LLC, Atlanta, Georgia, USA
Kshama Srivastava	Department of Pharmaceutics, School of Pharmaceutical Sciences, Maharishi University of Information Technology, Noida, Uttar Pradesh, India
Kirti Goel	Department of Pharmaceutics, Lala Ami Chand College of Pharmacy, Ambala, Haryana, India
Kavita Munjal	Amity Institute of Pharmacy, Amity University, Noida, Uttar Pradesh, India
Kunal Nepali	School of Pharmacy, Taipei Medical University, Taipei, Taiwan
Mayank Yadav	Adarsh Vijendra Institute of Pharmaceutical Sciences, Shobhit University, Gangoh, Saharanpur, Uttar Pradesh, India

Mukesh Maithani	Department of Pharmaceutical Sciences, Hemvati Nandan Bahuguna Garhwal University, Chaurus Campus, Srinagar Garhwal, Uttarakhand, India
Mohd Aftab Siddiqui	Faculty of Pharmacy, Integral University, Lucknow, Uttar Pradesh, India
Mohd Nazam Ansari	Department of Pharmacology and Toxicology, College of Pharmacy, Prince Sattam Bin Abdulaziz University, Alkharj, Saudi Arabia
Monika Saini	MM College of Pharmacy, Maharishi Markandeshwar (Deemed to be University), Mullana, Haryana, India
Minky Mukhija	Department of Pharmacognosy, Ch. Devi Lal College of Pharmacy, Jagadhri, Haryana, India
Monika Sharma	Bharat Institute of Pharmacy, Kurukshetra, Haryana, India
Mohsen Sheykhhasan	Cellular and Molecular Research Center, Qom University of Medical Sciences, Qom, Iran
Navin Chandra Pant	Faculty of Pharmaceutical Sciences, Amrapali University, Haldwani, Uttarakhand, India
Nitin Jangra	School of Pharmacy, Chitkara University, Solan, Himachal Pradesh, India
Piao Yang	Department of Molecular Genetics, College of Arts and Sciences, The Ohio State University, Columbus, OH, USA
Pranav J Shah	Maliba Pharmacy College, UKA Tarsadia University, Surat, Gujarat, India
Priyanka Patil	Faculty of Pharmacy, Sigma University, Vadodara, Gujarat, India
Palak Sharma	Chitkara College of Pharmacy, Chitkara University, Rajpura, Punjab, India
Pooja Mittal	GITAM School of Pharmacy, GITAM (Deemed to be University), Sangareddy, Telangana, India
Parul Sood	School of Pharmacy, Chitkara University, Solan, Himachal Pradesh, India
Rania I.M. Almoselhy	Oils and Fats Research Department, Food Technology Research Institute, Agricultural Research Center, Giza, Egypt
Ranjit Singh	Department of Pharmaceutics, Adarsh Vijendra Institute of Pharmaceutical Sciences, Shobhit University, Gangoh, Uttar Pradesh, India
Rajan Swami	Department of Pharmaceutics, Chitkara College of Pharmacy, Chitkara University, Rajpura, Punjab, India
Rakesh Sindhu	School of Pharmacy, Sharda University, Noida, Uttar Pradesh, India
Sheikh Mohd Saleem	EMTCT, UNICEF, New Delhi, India
Shah Sumaya Jan	Department of Anatomy, Government Medical College, Srinagar, Jammu & Kashmir, India
Sonia Gupta	Swami Devi Dyal Institute of Pharmacy, Panchkula, Haryana, India
Sonia Kamboj	Department of Pharmaceutical Chemistry, Ch. Devi Lal College of Pharmacy, Jagadhri, Haryana, India
Saeedeh Zare Jalise	Department of Tissue Engineering and Applied Cell Sciences, School of Medicine, Qom University of Medical Sciences, Qom, Iran
Swati Gupta	Faculty of Pharmacy, Sigma University, Vadodara, Gujarat, India

Sonu Kumar	Department of Pharmaceutical Sciences and Drug Research, Punjabi University, Patiala, Punjab, India
Sanchit Dhankhar	Chitkara College of Pharmacy, Chitkara University, Rajpura, Punjab, India
Soumya Banerjee	School of Pharmacy, Chitkara University, Solan, Himachal Pradesh, India
Saksham Sharma	Chitkara College of Pharmacy, Chitkara University, Rajpura, Punjab, India
Shushank Mahajan	Chitkara College of Pharmacy, Chitkara University, Rajpura, Punjab, India
Sanchit Dhankhar	Chitkara College of Pharmacy, Chitkara University, Rajpura, Punjab, India
Sabina Yasmin	Department of Pharmaceutical Chemistry, College of Pharmacy, King Khalid University, Abha, Saudi Arabia
Sheelu Singh	IES Institute of Pharmacy, IES University, Bhopal, Madhya Pradesh, India
Thakur Gurjeet Singh	Chitkara College of Pharmacy, Chitkara University, Rajpura, Punjab, India
Vishnu Mittal	Department of Pharmaceutics, Adesh Institute of Pharmacy and Biomedical Sciences, Adesh University, Bathinda, Punjab, India
Vinod Kumar Gauttam	SGT College of Pharmacy, SGT University, Gurugram, Haryana, India
Vinit K Sharma	Department of Pharmacology, Adarsh Vijendra Institute of Pharmaceutical Sciences, Shobhit University, Gangoh, Uttar Pradesh, India

CHAPTER 1

Introduction to Fatty Liver Disease

Vishnu Mittal[1], **Anjali Sharma**[2] and **Dinesh Mishra**[3,*]

[1] *Department of Pharmaceutics, Adesh Institute of Pharmacy and Biomedical Sciences, Adesh University, Bathinda, Punjab, India*

[2] *Department of Pharmaceutics, Guru Gobind Singh College of Pharmacy, Yamunanagar, Haryana, India*

[3] *Department of Pharmaceutics, Guru Ghasidas Vishwavidyalaya, Bilaspur, Chhattisgarh, India*

Abstract: Fatty liver disease, encompassing non-alcoholic fatty liver disease and alcoholic fatty liver disease, is a growing global health concern characterized by excessive fat accumulation in liver cells. It is associated with metabolic disorders, obesity, and lifestyle factors, often progressing to severe conditions like non-alcoholic steatohepatitis, fibrosis, cirrhosis, or hepatocellular carcinoma. The objective of this chapter is to provide an overview of fatty liver disease, its pathophysiology, risk factors, and current therapeutic challenges, while introducing the potential of nanocarrier-based drug delivery systems for its management. This chapter reviews the current literature on the etiology, progression, and treatment strategies for fatty liver disease. The chapter also explores various nanocarrier systems, including liposomes, solid lipid nanoparticles, and polymeric nanoparticles, highlighting their advantages in enhancing drug solubility, targeting, and therapeutic efficacy. Nanocarrier-based drug delivery systems have demonstrated significant potential in improving the bioavailability and liver-specific delivery of therapeutic agents. Studies indicate that these systems can reduce hepatic fat accumulation, modulate inflammatory pathways, and prevent disease progression, with fewer side effects than conventional therapies. The integration of nanotechnology into the management of fatty liver disease represents a promising frontier in hepatology. By addressing the limitations of traditional treatments, nanocarriers offer a targeted, efficient, and safer approach to treating this prevalent condition.

Keywords: Disease, Fatty liver, Metabolism, Nanotechnology, Non-alcoholic, Targeting, Therapeutic efficacy.

* **Corresponding author Dinesh Mishra:** Department of Pharmaceutics, Guru Ghasidas Vishwavidyalaya, Bilaspur, Chhattisgarh, India; E-mail: dineshdops@gmail.com

Anjali Sharma, Devkant Sharma, Ajmer Singh Grewal, Geeta Deswal & Ganga Reddy Velma (Eds.)

INTRODUCTION

Fatty liver and non-alcoholic fatty liver diseases are characterized by alterations in the macrovesicular fat accumulation that are not caused by excessive alcohol use and do not include lobular inflammation or inflammation (steatosis) [1]. The two primary forms are Non-Alcoholic Steatohepatitis (NASH) and Non-Alcoholic Fatty Liver (NAFL), sometimes referred to as steatosis. NAFL is hepatic steatosis without hepatocyte edema or other indications of liver injury [2 - 4]. High cholesterol, diabetes, obesity, and metabolic syndrome are often linked to non-alcoholic fatty liver disease (NAFLD). Approximately 80% of people with metabolic syndrome have NAFLD. Moreover, several reasons have been proposed for why fat might build up in the liver [5, 6].

Overview of Fatty Liver Disease

In 1986, Schaffner coined the phrase "non-alcoholic fatty liver disease" (NAFLD) [7]. It is characterized by abnormal buildup of liver fat, insulin resistance, and histological evidence of steatosis in more than 5% of hepatocytes. NAFLD is diagnosed after excluding other clear-cut factors, such as excessive alcohol use, viral hepatitis, and drugs that change fat that might cause steatosis or change the liver profile [8]. Non-invasive techniques, such as computed tomography [CT], ultrasonography [US], and magnetic resonance imaging (MRI), are used to detect hepatic fat accumulation in the liver [9]. Fatty liver is the term used to describe an excess of fat in the liver. It is common, especially in those with diabetes and obesity. Even without symptoms, it may cause serious health problems [10]. There are two kinds:

- **Simple fatty liver**, characterized by liver fat with little to no inflammation or damage to liver cells.
- **Nonalcoholic steatohepatitis (NASH)**, which is characterized by inflammation, loss of liver cells, and liver fat [11].

The development of fatty liver disease is associated with reduced beta-oxidation of mitochondrial fatty acids, increased endogenous fatty acid production or increased supply of fatty acids to the liver, and inadequate absorption or release of triglycerides as very low-density lipoprotein (VLDL) [12 - 14].

Epidemiology and Global Burden

The frequency of NAFLD varies significantly across cohorts. In the general population, the prevalence of NAFLD is estimated to be between 11.5% and 46%, whereas in the US, it is 20%. NASH, on the other hand, accounts for 2% to 3% of the cases [15]. The average age at diagnosis is 50, with a range of 16–80. It is more common in white people than in black people, and it is more common in Hispanic individuals than in white people [16].

Nonalcoholic fatty liver disease (NAFLD) is one of the main causes of liver disease worldwide. With an estimated 47 cases per 1,000 people globally, NAFLD occurs more frequently in men than in women [17]. It is estimated that 32% of people globally are expected to have NAFLD, with males more likely to be affected by it (40%) than females (26%). The worldwide incidence of NAFLD has increased over time, from 26% in studies conducted before 2005 to 38% in studies conducted after 2016 [18].

CLASSIFICATION OF FATTY LIVER DISEASE

Fatty liver disease is primarily classified into two major types:

Non-Alcoholic Fatty Liver Disease (NAFLD)

Nonalcoholic fatty liver disease (NAFLD) is characterized by an excessive buildup of fat in the liver (≥5% of cells) in individuals who drink little or no alcohol. It is the most common chronic liver disease in the world [19]. NAFLD may be further divided into the following categories:

- A benign condition with a low risk of progressing to fibrosis, non-alcoholic fatty liver (NAFL) is characterized by hepatic fat accumulation without significant inflammation or damage to liver cells [20].
- Its prevalence is estimated at 25-30% of the world's population.
- Hepatocellular carcinoma (HCC), liver failure, and cirrhosis are possible outcomes.
- Globally, the prevalence ranges from 2 to 6%.

Risk Factors for NAFLD

- **Obesity:** Present in 60-90% of NAFLD cases.
- **Type 2 Diabetes Mellitus:** 70% of people with diabetes develop NAFLD.
- **Dyslipidemia:** High triglycerides and low HDL cholesterol.
- **Hypertension:** Common in NAFLD patients.
- **Genetic Predisposition:** PNPLA3 and TM6SF2 gene variants.
- **Sedentary Lifestyle and Poor Diet:** High fructose and fat intake.

Alcoholic Fatty Liver Disease (AFLD)

Increased alcohol consumption causes hepatic fat to accumulate, which ultimately results in AFLD. The quantity and duration of alcohol use influence the development of AFLD.

Excessive alcohol use causes the early-stage, treatable condition known as alcoholic fatty liver (AFL). Table **1** compares Non-Alcoholic Fatty Liver Disease [NAFLD] and Alcoholic Fatty Liver Disease [AFLD] based on etiology, risk factors, clinical features, and diagnostic criteria.

Risk Factors for AFLD

- **Chronic Alcohol Consumption:** 60-80g/day for men, >20-40g/day for women, for 10+ years increases risk.
- **Genetic Factors:** ADH and ALDH enzyme polymorphisms.
- **Gender Differences:** Women are more susceptible due to lower alcohol metabolism.
- **Malnutrition:** Deficiencies in vitamins (B_1, B_6, folate) aggravate liver damage.
- **Hepatitis Co-infection:** Higher risk of cirrhosis in individuals with Hepatitis B or C.

Table 1. Comparison of NAFLD *vs.* AFLD.

Feature	NAFLD	AFLD
Cause	Metabolic dysfunction, obesity, and insulin resistance	Chronic excessive alcohol intake
Fat Accumulation	Yes	Yes
Inflammation	Possible (in NASH)	Yes (alcoholic hepatitis)
Progression to Cirrhosis	Possible	Common in chronic alcohol users
Reversibility	Yes, with lifestyle changes	Yes, with alcohol abstinence (early stage)
Treatment	Lifestyle modification, weight loss, and insulin sensitizers	Alcohol cessation, nutritional support, and corticosteroids in severe cases

PATHOPHYSIOLOGY OF FATTY LIVER DISEASE

The complexity and variety of biology of nonalcoholic fatty liver disease (NAFLD) are already demonstrated by the fact that its clinical spectrum ranges from simple steatosis to cirrhosis as the final stage of liver disease [21]. Hepatic stellate cells and other inflammatory mediators are activated as NASH worsens due to increased inflammation and oxidative stress, which may eventually lead to cirrhosis and fibrosis [22]. Fig. (**1**) shows the comparison of normal liver and fatty liver disease.

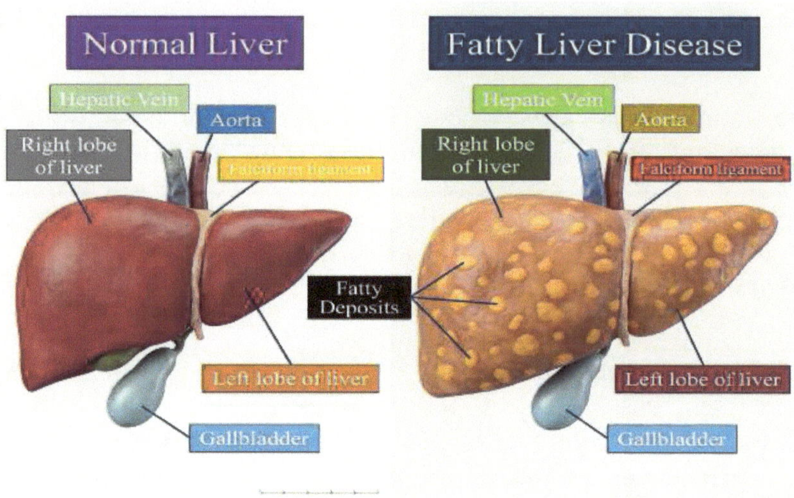

Fig. (1). Comparison of normal liver and fatty liver disease.

The most commonly recognized explanations for this second damage include oxidative stress, lipopolysaccharides, and certain cytokines, although the precise source is unclear. Hepatic fibrosis may develop over time as a consequence of stellate cell activation triggered by chronic liver damage. The diagnosis of NASH can only be verified by a liver biopsy [23].

Mechanisms of Hepatic Lipid Accumulation

Due to enhanced fatty acid uptake and DNL, NAFLD enhances hepatic lipid absorption even in the context of steatosis. Long-term prevention of the growing intrahepatic fat buildup is impossible, despite possible increases in lipid elimination [24]. Hepatic lipid accumulation results from an imbalance between lipid intake and excretion, leading to excessive fat deposition in the liver. Another important factor is the increased intake of free fatty acids (FFAs) from adipose tissue due to insulin resistance-induced lipolysis, which leads to accumulation of FFAs in the liver [25].

- **Increased absorption of fatty acids:** The liver may readily absorb excess fat, particularly saturated fat, via transporters like CD36, which contributes to lipid accumulation [26].

Role of Inflammation and Oxidative Stress

The two main causes of fatty liver disease are inflammation and oxidative stress. Excessive fat accumulation in hepatocytes leads to lipotoxicity, triggering an inflammatory response. These factors cause increased reactive stress, mitochondrial dysfunction, and hepatocyte death. Hepatic fat buildup, which leads to lipotoxicity, is associated with changes in lipid metabolism, ER stress, and disruption of the autophagy system at the cellular level.

Lipotoxin: By producing damage-associated molecular patterns (DAMPs), which in turn trigger inflammatory responses, excess fat in hepatocytes may cause direct cell damage.

Activation of Kupffer cells: Liver-resident macrophages, also known as Kupffer cells, are activated by fat buildup and release pro-inflammatory cytokines, including TNF-alpha and IL-6, which worsen inflammation.

Mitochondrial dysfunction: Oxidative stress is induced by hepatocytes with damaged mitochondria, which produce more reactive oxygen species (ROS).

Liver stellate cell activation: Oxidative stress and inflammatory signals may turn liver stellate cells into myofibroblasts, which create extracellular matrix proteins that cause fibrosis.

Progression to Non-Alcoholic Steatohepatitis (NASH), Fibrosis, and Cirrhosis

When fat accumulation results in persistent inflammation and hepatocyte injury, simple liver steatosis (NAFL) may develop into non-alcoholic steatohepatitis (NASH) [27]. Widespread fibrosis, portal hypertension, and hepatic dysfunction are all linked to cirrhosis, and these conditions significantly raise the risk of hepatocellular carcinoma (HCC) and liver failure [28].

Insulin resistance: Excessive insulin may exacerbate inflammation and increase hepatic fat accumulation [29].

Adipokines: Leptin and adiponectin, two adipokines produced by adipose tissue, may influence inflammation of the liver [25].

Dysbiosis of the gut microbiome: Changes in gut flora may increase the amount of bacterial products that enter the liver and induce inflammation [30].

RISK FACTORS AND CAUSES

Fatty liver disease may result from a confluence of dietary, lifestyle, metabolic, and hereditary factors [31].

Genetic Predisposition

Genetics has a significant role in determining an individual's vulnerability to fatty liver disease. Variations in certain genes, such as TM6SF2 and PNPLA3, have been strongly linked to non-alcoholic fatty liver disease (NAFLD), its progression to non-alcoholic steatohepatitis (NASH), and cirrhosis [32]. The PNPLA3 I148M polymorphism has been linked to increased liver fat storage and fibrosis severity, independent of metabolic risk variables.

Metabolic Disorders (Obesity, Diabetes, and Dyslipidemia)

Metabolic complications are one of the primary risk factors for fatty liver disease, especially NAFLD. By increasing the release of free fatty acids (FFA) from adipose tissue, obesity, especially abdominal obesity, contributes to insulin resistance and the formation of hepatic fat [33].

Dietary and Lifestyle Factors

Sedentary lifestyles and poor eating habits are common causes of fatty liver disease. Liver fat is promoted by diets rich in fatty lipids, refined carbohydrates, and high fructose corn syrup because they increase lipogenesis and interfere with insulin signaling [34].

Alcohol Consumption and Liver Health

Excessive alcohol usage is known to induce alcoholic fatty liver disease (AFLD). The breakdown of alcohol in the liver results in the production of acetaldehyde and reactive oxygen species (ROS), which lead to oxidative stress, mitochondrial damage, and hepatocyte injury [35, 36].

CLINICAL MANIFESTATIONS AND DIAGNOSIS

Symptoms and Stages of Fatty Liver Disease

Fatty liver disease has different stages, and symptoms vary depending on the stage.

Early stages

- Non-alcoholic fatty liver disease, or NAFLD
- There are often no symptoms in the early stages. Conversely, some people suffer from exhaustion, persistent sleepiness, and mental haze.

Advanced stages

- **NASH:** A more severe kind of NAFLD that may lead to inflammation of the liver and toxic stress.
- **Fibrosis:** Scar tissue forms in the liver.
- **Cirrhosis**: Cirrhosis, in which scar tissue replaces good liver tissue, is the most severe kind of fatty liver disease. The clinical presentation and diagnostic approaches for fatty liver disease are summarized in Table **2**.

Table 2. Symptoms, causes, and diagnosis of fatty liver disease.

Sr. No.	Parameter	Description
1	Jaundice	Yellowing of skin and eyes due to increased bilirubin levels indicating liver dysfunction.
2	Itchy skin	Caused by bile salt accumulation, leading to persistent skin irritation and discomfort.
3	Swelling (Edema)	Fluid accumulation in legs, ankles, feet, or abdomen due to impaired liver and blood vessel function.
4	Weakness	General fatigue and reduced energy are commonly experienced with chronic liver conditions.
5	Loss of appetite	Decreased desire to eat, often leading to unintended weight loss in liver disease patients.
6	Nausea	Sensation of stomach discomfort, especially after eating fatty or heavy meals.
7	Abdominal distension	Swelling due to fluid buildup (ascites) as a result of portal hypertension.
8	Mental confusion	Signs of hepatic encephalopathy caused by toxin accumulation affecting brain function.

(Table 2) cont.....

Sr. No.	Parameter	Description
9	GI bleeding	Often due to variceal rupture or coagulopathy in advanced liver disease stages.
10	Shortness of breath	Due to pressure on the diaphragm from ascites or anemia-related fatigue.
11	Causes	Includes excessive alcohol consumption, obesity, unhealthy diet, insulin resistance, and T2DM.
12	Liver function tests	Blood tests like ALT and AST to assess liver enzyme levels and detect hepatic injury.
13	Ultrasound imaging	Non-invasive tool to visualize fatty infiltration and liver size changes.
14	FibroScan	Measures liver stiffness to evaluate fibrosis and potential progression to cirrhosis.
15	CT/MRI scans	Advanced imaging techniques for quantifying liver fat and structural assessment [36, 37].

Biomarkers and Laboratory Tests

Fatty liver disease is diagnosed by a combination of imaging methods, blood tests, and sometimes liver biopsies. Although elevated liver tests are often used as indications, they may sometimes stay normal [38]. Imaging methods, including ultrasound, MRI-based proton density fat fraction, and FibroScan, may be used to measure the volume and stiffness of liver fat. The most reliable method for proving NASH and fibrosis in advanced patients is still liver biopsy.

Clinical Features

The majority of people with a NAFLD diagnosis remain asymptomatic. When present, physical evidence and clinical indications in people with NAFLD are vague and imprecise, making it difficult to assess the severity of the condition [39].

Common Biomarkers

Moderately raised blood aminotransferase levels are the main issue in patients with non-alcoholic fatty liver disease (NAFLD); up to 78% of these people may have regular liver tests. Furthermore, the whole histological spectrum of non-alcoholic fatty liver disease (NAFLD) may be present in people with normal alanine aminotransferase (ALT) levels.

Novel Biomarkers

Some researchers have suggested measuring other novel biomarkers to help diagnose NAFLD. However, these studies have been limited by their lack of repeatability or their inability to reliably differentiate between basic steatosis and more advanced inflammation and fibrosis [40].

Panels of Markers

To replace invasive conventional liver biopsy, several studies have been conducted to develop benign diagnostic panels and scoring systems that may aid in diagnosing NASH, assessing the degree of fibrosis, and identifying hepatic steatosis.

Imaging Techniques (Ultrasound, MRI, and FibroScan)

Non-invasive imaging methods are crucial for identifying and measuring fatty liver disease. The most popular technique is ultrasonography, which has a higher echogenicity and is thus more successful in identifying liver fat buildup but less accurate for moderate steatosis [41]. It provides highly accurate measurements of liver fibrosis and fat. Several MRI methods have been tested in individuals with NAFLD, with the primary goal of evaluating liver fat [42].

Ultrasonography (US)

The most popular technique for screening asymptomatic individuals with elevated liver tests and potential NAFLD is now the US [43]. Hepatomegaly, vascular blunting, and broad elevations in the liver tissue's echogenicity are US indicators of fatty liver. The sensitivity, specificity, PPV, and NPV for detecting at least 30% steatosis in 235 patients undergoing liver biopsy and US were 91%, 93%, 89%, and 94%, respectively, according to recent research [44].

Computed Tomography (CT)

By quantifying liver attenuation in Hounsfield units (HU), CT offers a more quantitative assessment than US; however, radiologists' documentation of liver attenuation data varies [45].

Magnetic Resonance Imaging (MRI) and Proton Magnetic Resonance Spectroscopy (MRS)

There is a strong correlation between histology, MRI, and US in patients with NAFLD [46]. MRI has been shown to be the most accurate of these techniques for identifying less steatosis than CT and US.

Transient Elastography

A non-invasive technique for evaluating liver fibrosis is transient elastography, which may be performed at a patient's bedside or in an outpatient setting [47]. It uses ultrasound-based technologies to measure liver stiffness.

Histology

Among the liver tissue changes associated with NAFLD are simple steatosis, steatohepatitis, fibrosis, and cirrhosis. The gold standard for detection is liver biopsy, which also has the added advantage of allowing differentiation between NASH and simple steatosis [48].

LIFESTYLE MODIFICATIONS (DIET, EXERCISE)

The Mediterranean diet, rich in whole grains, nuts, olive oil, and vegetables, has been shown to reduce liver fat and inflammation. Regular exercise, such as lifting weights and aerobic activities like running, brisk walking, or cycling, improves insulin sensitivity and promotes fat burning, both of which help prevent liver fat from building up.

Pharmacological Approaches

Insulin sensitizers like metformin and thiazolidinediones (pioglitazone, rosiglitazone) have shown varying degrees of efficacy in altering liver histology, despite concerns about side effects, including weight gain and cardiovascular risks [23]. Antioxidants, especially vitamin E, have shown benefits in reducing inflammation in non-diabetic NASH patients, despite ongoing long-term safety concerns. Examples of lipid-lowering drugs that raise metabolic parameters but have not been well studied for their effects on liver tissue include statins and ezetimibe [49].

Limitations of Conventional Therapies

Despite improvements in the area, traditional treatments for fatty liver disease have some drawbacks. Despite being very successful, lifestyle changes need consistent commitment, and many patients find it difficult to continue regular exercise and weight loss [50].

ROLE OF NANOTECHNOLOGY IN FATTY LIVER DISEASE MANAGEMENT

Nanotechnology plays an important role in the management of fatty liver disease by enabling targeted drug delivery to the liver through nanocarrier systems, which can significantly increase the effectiveness of therapeutic agents while minimizing systemic side effects by concentrating the medication at the disease site. Since there are presently limited therapy alternatives for NAFLD, this strategy shows particular promise [51, 52].

Nanocarrier-based Drug Delivery: A Patent Perspective

Nanocarriers, ranging in size from 1 to 1000 nm, have emerged as promising systems for enhancing solubility, stability, and targeted delivery of therapeutic agents to diseased liver cells. These nanoscale carriers encapsulate drugs, protect them from degradation, and enable controlled release at the intended site of action [53]. Recent patents, summarized in Table **3**, showcase diverse nanocarrier platforms, including lipid nanoparticles, polymeric nanoparticles, liposomes, and solid lipid nanoparticles designed to improve therapeutic efficacy and safety in the treatment of fatty liver disease.

Table 3. Patents related to nanocarrier-based drug delivery systems for the management of fatty liver disease.

Patent Number	Title	Short Description	Ref
US20210007997A1	Nanoparticle-Based Liver-Targeting Therapy	Describes a nanoparticle-based therapy designed to specifically target liver cells	[54]
US20190381035A1	Lipid Nanoparticle Compositions for Delivery of Therapeutic Agents	Covers lipid nanoparticle compositions optimized for delivering therapeutic agents to the liver, aiming to treat conditions, such as non-alcoholic steatohepatitis (NASH).	[55]
US20180078430A1	Nanoparticle Compositions for Treatment of Liver Fibrosis	Focuses on nanoparticle formulations intended to deliver antifibrotic agents directly to the liver to address liver fibrosis associated with fatty liver disease.	[56]

(Table 3) cont.....

Patent Number	Title	Short Description	Ref
US20170216258A1	Targeted Nanoparticle Delivery System for Liver Diseases	Introduces a targeted nanoparticle delivery system engineered to transport therapeutic compounds specifically to liver tissues, aiming to treat various liver diseases, including fatty liver disease.	[57]
US20160128952A1	Polymeric Nanoparticles for Treatment of Metabolic Disorders	Describes polymeric nanoparticles designed to deliver therapeutic agents by improving drug solubility and bioavailability.	[58]
US20150209432A1	Liposome-Based Drug Delivery for Liver Conditions	Covers liposome-based drug delivery systems tailored for targeting liver conditions, including NAFLD, to enhance therapeutic efficacy and reduce side effects.	[59]
US20140161854A1	Solid Lipid Nanoparticles for Hepatic Drug Delivery	Focuses on solid lipid nanoparticles formulated to deliver drugs to the liver effectively, aiming to treat hepatic diseases, such as fatty liver disease.	[60]
US20130266656A1	Nanoparticle-Based Therapeutics for Liver Inflammation	Describes nanoparticle-based therapeutic compositions targeting liver inflammation, a common feature in the progression of fatty liver disease.	[61]
US20120263745A1	Targeted Polymeric Nanoparticles for Liver Disease Treatment	Introduces targeted polymeric nanoparticles designed by enhancing drug targeting and minimizing systemic exposure.	[62]
US20110293529A1	Nanoparticle Compositions for Reducing Liver Lipid Accumulation	Covers nanoparticle compositions aimed at reducing lipid accumulation in the liver, addressing a key aspect of fatty liver disease pathology.	[63]

Types of Nanocarriers Used

Liposomes

Hydrophilic and lipophilic drugs can be encapsulated in phospholipid spheres known as liposomes, which improves their stability and liver transport [64]. Their surfaces may be modified with specific ligands, such as glycyrrhizin or lactobionic acid, to improve liver absorption.

- **Crucial information on liposomes in fatty liver disease:**

Targeted delivery: Liposomes can be designed to target liver cells specifically by adding ligands to their surface that bind to receptors on liver cells [64], such as

Kupffer cells (liver macrophages), which are crucial players in the inflammatory process associated with NAFLD.

Drug encapsulation: By encapsulating medications in liposomes, researchers can improve their delivery to the liver and, in turn, increase the effectiveness of treatment for NAFLD [65].

- **Potential benefits:**

Reduced inflammation: The characteristic inflammatory response in NASH, a more severe form of NAFLD, may be reduced by liposomes' ability to deliver anti-inflammatory agents to the liver [66].

Better lipid metabolism: By altering lipid intake, synthesis, and release in the liver, liposomal treatments may reduce hepatic fat accumulation.

Increased bioavailability: Liposomes have the potential to improve the bioavailability and absorption of poorly soluble drugs, potentially expanding their use in the treatment of NAFLD.

- **Liposome-based therapies for fatty liver disease include:**

Liposomes loaded with silibinin: Research indicates that adding silibinin, a naturally occurring substance with anti-inflammatory and antioxidant properties, to liposomes may significantly improve their ability to treat NAFLD by increasing their transport to the liver and reducing hepatic inflammation.

Curcumin-loaded liposomes: Similar to silibinin, curcumin-loaded liposomes have the ability to deliver powerful antioxidants to the liver, where they may reduce oxidative stress and inflammation linked to NAFLD.

Solid Lipid Nanoparticles (SLNs)

Lipid-based carriers, or SLNs, provide a controlled release feature together with a reliable and secure drug delivery system. They lessen systemic effects while increasing hepatic drug accumulation [67]. This improves treatment efficacy while reducing adverse effects on other organs. Important details about SLNs in fatty liver disease are as follows:

Targeted distribution: The lipid composition of SLNs causes them to concentrate in the liver, which facilitates the direct delivery of medications to the injured tissue in fatty liver disease.

Better drug solubility: SLNs can contain both hydrophilic and hydrophobic drugs, which is particularly useful for poorly soluble drugs that may be difficult to administer when treating fatty liver.

Controlled release: The medication may be released from SLNs at a controlled rate by altering the composition of the solid lipid matrix.

Safety and biocompatibility: SLNs are often considered harmless and disposable, reducing the potential risks associated with pharmaceutical transportation methods.

- **SLNs' possible use in fatty liver disease:**

Lipids, insulin resistance, and oxidative stress are major risk factors for NAFLD, and SLNs include drugs that address these issues.

Management of hepatic fibrosis: Antifibrotic medications included in SLNs may target and reduce liver fibrosis associated with advanced stages of fatty liver disease.

Antioxidant delivery: SLNs may help reduce oxidative damage in fatty liver diseases by delivering antioxidants, such as vitamin E or curcumin, to the liver.

Polymeric Nanoparticles

Polymeric nanoparticles provide extended drug release and may be tailored for targeted distribution. They are both biocompatible and biodegradable. To improve drug stability and liver absorption, polymers like chitosan and PLGA (poly(lactic-co-glycolic acid)) are often used [68, 69]. These nanoparticles could provide better therapeutic outcomes and fewer adverse effects than conventional therapies.

- **Polymeric nanoparticles and fatty liver disease [70]:**

Targeted delivery: Polymeric nanoparticles have a unique structure that allows them to accumulate in the liver due to their size and surface properties, ensuring that the drug reaches the injured area efficiently.

Enhanced bioavailability: By improving the body's absorption of poorly soluble drugs, polymeric nanoparticles can maximize therapeutic efficacy.

Sustained release: The polymer matrix may control the release of the encapsulated medication over an extended period, leading to fewer dosing intervals and longer-lasting therapeutic effects.

Decreased toxicity: Well-made nanoparticles may lessen systemic adverse effects and the chance of damage to other organs by precisely delivering the medicine to the liver [71].

- **Polymeric nanoparticles may be used to treat fatty liver disease in the following ways:**

Antioxidant delivery: To combat oxidative stress associated with fatty liver disease, antioxidants like vitamin E or silymarin may be encapsulated [72].

Reducing inflammation: Nanoparticles laden with anti-inflammatory drugs could target the inflammatory response in the liver.

Modifying lipid metabolism: Medications that promote fat burning or inhibit fat synthesis may help reduce the quantity of lipids that accumulate in the liver.

Fibrosis treatment: To prevent the progression of liver fibrosis in advanced stages of fatty liver disease, antifibrotic medications may be administered via nanoparticles.

- **Preclinical and Clinical Studies on Nanocarrier Systems**

The efficacy of nanocarrier-based therapies for NAFLD and NASH has been the subject of several clinical and experimental investigations. Preclinical research using animal models of non-alcoholic fatty liver disease has shown that nanoparticles are superior to conventional formulations in improving liver drug accumulation, reducing fat accumulation, and regulating inflammatory responses.

- **Advantages of Nanocarrier Systems**

The following are the benefits of using nanocarriers for drug delivery in the treatment of fatty liver disease:

Improved bioavailability makes poorly water-soluble drugs more soluble and easier to absorb, thereby enabling effective targeting of the liver.

Targeted drug delivery: Surface modifications that target liver cells, particularly, help prevent systemic side effects.

Controlled and sustained release: By ensuring sustained pharmaceutical effect, this reduces dosage frequency and improves patient compliance.

Reduced toxicity: Minimizes adverse effects by preventing medication accumulation in organs not the intended target.

Improved therapeutic efficacy: Facilitates the co-administration of multiple drugs, thereby improving the outcomes of NAFLD/NASH treatment [73].

FUTURE PERSPECTIVES AND CHALLENGES

The future of treating fatty liver disease depends on developments in nanomedicine, which enable tailored drug delivery, enhanced absorption, and reduced toxicity [74 - 78]. Novel advancements, such as multifunctional nanoplatforms, stimuli-responsive nanoparticles, and gene-editing nanocarriers, may lead to more customized and effective treatments. It is necessary to address clinical evidence, large-scale production, long-term harm, and other safety and legal issues. Fatty liver disease, which encompasses non-alcoholic steatohepatitis (NASH) and non-alcoholic fatty liver disease (NAFLD), has few effective pharmacological treatments. Since traditional medications have shortcomings, such as poor absorption, systemic toxicity, and lack of liver-specific targeting, nanotechnology-based therapeutic techniques are necessary [79]. Several studies have discussed nanocarrier-based drug delivery techniques that have shown significant promise in improving drug solubility, liver-specific targeting, and prolonged drug release [80]. Numerous experimental and clinical studies are now underway to examine lipid nanoparticles, siRNA treatments, and antisense drugs targeting key pathways implicated in NAFLD (including BMS-986263, ARO-HSD, and HU6) [81].

Advancements in Nanomedicine for Fatty Liver Disease

With the development of next-generation drug delivery methods for the treatment of fatty liver disease, nanomedicine is rapidly evolving [82]. Stimulus-responsive nanoparticle developments enable regulated drug release in response to liver-specific factors, including pH, oxidative stress, and enzyme activity. Researchers are exploring the use of CRISPR/Cas9-loaded nanoparticles to alter genes linked to NAFLD development, potentially providing a solution rather than just treating its symptoms [83].

Regulatory and Safety Concerns

Despite the potential of nanocarrier-based medicines, safety and regulatory concerns continue to impede clinical translation. The long-term effects of nanoparticles on liver metabolism, clearance mechanisms, and potential toxicity must be thoroughly evaluated [84].

Potential for Clinical Translation

To be used effectively in the treatment of fatty liver disease, nanocarrier-based medicines must demonstrate significant therapeutic benefits with few side effects in large-scale human studies [85]. Current problems include lowering production costs, ensuring repeatability, and improving nanocarrier formulas [86].

CONCLUSION

Fatty liver disease, which encompasses AFLD and NAFLD, is a growing global health problem that significantly affects metabolic health and liver function. Research into drug transport systems based on nanocarriers is needed due to the limitations of existing treatment options. There are several examples of nanocarriers that have shown significant promise in improving drug absorption, targeting liver cells, and lowering systemic toxicity. Advances in nanomedicine, including CRISPR-based treatments, multifunctional nanoparticles, and gene-editing methods, further emphasize the promise of precision medicine in hepatology. However, regulatory barriers, safety concerns, and challenges with large-scale production must be addressed before nanocarrier-based drugs can be fully integrated into clinical practice. Ongoing clinical and experimental research is paving the way for a better, more focused, and more efficient treatment of fatty liver disease. With more collaborative research, corporate engagement, and technological breakthroughs, nanotechnology has the potential to revolutionize the treatment of fatty liver disease.

LIST OF ABBREVIATIONS

NAFLD	Non-Alcoholic Fatty Liver Disease
NASH	Non-Alcoholic Steatohepatitis
MRI	Magnetic Resonance Imaging
TG	Triglyceride
HDL	High-Density Lipoprotein
LDL	Low-Density Lipoprotein
VLDL	Very-Low-Density Lipoprotein
ROS	Reactive Oxygen Species

MDA	Malondialdehyde
PUFAs	Polyunsaturated Fatty Acids
SFA	Saturated Fatty Acid
LCPUFA	Long-Chain Polyunsaturated Fatty Acids
CYP2E1	Cytochrome P450 2E1
TNF-α	Tumor Necrosis Factor-alpha
IL-6	Interleukin-6
ALT	Alanine Aminotransferase
AST	Aspartate Aminotransferase
HOMA-IR	Homeostatic Model Assessment of Insulin Resistance
FFA	Free Fatty Acid
DNL	De Novo Lipogenesis
HSC	Hepatic Stellate Cell
PNPLA3	Patatin-Like Phospholipase Domain-Containing 3
SREBP	Sterol Regulatory Element-Binding Protein
FXR	Farnesoid X Receptor
PPAR	Peroxisome Proliferator-Activated Receptor
AMPK	AMP-Activated Protein Kinase
T2DM	Type 2 Diabetes Mellitus
MetS	Metabolic Syndrome
GLP-1	Glucagon-Like Peptide-1
MRI-PDFF	Magnetic Resonance Imaging Proton Density Fat Fraction
ER	Endoplasmic Reticulum
DILI	Drug-Induced Liver Injury

REFERENCES

[1] Brown GT, Kleiner DE. Histopathology of nonalcoholic fatty liver disease and nonalcoholic steatohepatitis. Metabolism 2016; 65(8): 1080-6. [http://dx.doi.org/10.1016/j.metabol.2015.11.008] [PMID: 26775559]

[2] Giashuddin S, Alawad M. Histopathological diagnosis of nonalcoholic steatohepatitis (NASH). In: Non-Alcoholic Steatohepatitis: Methods in Molecular Biology. New York: Springer; 2022. p. 1–18.

[3] Mlaga SM. Magnitude of liver diseases discovered during medico legal autopsies at Muhimbili National Hospital. Dar-Es-Salaam, Tanzania: Muhimbili University of Health and Allied Sciences 2019.

[4] Koch LK, Yeh MM. Nonalcoholic fatty liver disease (NAFLD): Diagnosis, pitfalls, and staging. Ann Diagn Pathol 2018; 37: 83-90. [http://dx.doi.org/10.1016/j.anndiagpath.2018.09.009] [PMID: 30312882]

[5] Paschos P, Paletas K. Non alcoholic fatty liver disease and metabolic syndrome. Hippokratia 2009; 13(1): 9-19.

[PMID: 19240815]

[6] Salsamendi J, Pereira K, Kang K, Fan J. Minimally invasive percutaneous endovascular therapies in the management of complications of non-alcoholic fatty liver disease (NAFLD): A case report. J Radiol Case Rep 2015; 9(9): 36-43. [http://dx.doi.org/10.3941/jrcr.v9i9.2557] [PMID: 26629307]

[7] Méndez-Sánchez N, Díaz-Orozco LE. International consensus recommendations to replace the terminology of non-alcoholic fatty liver disease (NAFLD) with metabolic-associated fatty liver disease (MAFLD). Med Sci Monit 2021; 27: e933860-1. [http://dx.doi.org/10.12659/MSM.933860] [PMID: 34248137]

[8] Jorge ASB, Jorge GCB, Crespo TS. Non-alcoholic fatty liver disease: clinical, laboratory and imaging diagnostic methods. In: Hepatic Steatosis. 2014. p. 23.

[9] Clinical and Molecular Hepatology. 2023;29(Suppl). Available from: https://www.e-cmh.org/upload/pdf/cmh_v29nSuppl_full.pdf

[10] Corey KE, Kaplan LM. Obesity and liver disease: the epidemic of the twenty-first century. Clin Liver Dis 2014; 18(1): 1-18. [http://dx.doi.org/10.1016/j.cld.2013.09.019] [PMID: 24274861]

[11] Koyama Y, Brenner DA. Liver inflammation and fibrosis. J Clin Invest 2017; 127(1): 55-64. [http://dx.doi.org/10.1172/JCI88881] [PMID: 28045404]

[12] Panov AV, Mayorov VI, Dikalov SI. Role of fatty acids β-oxidation in the metabolic interactions between organs. Int J Mol Sci 2024; 25(23): 12740. [http://dx.doi.org/10.3390/ijms252312740] [PMID: 39684455]

[13] Tripodi A, Fracanzani AL, Primignani M, *et al.* Procoagulant imbalance in patients with non-alcoholic fatty liver disease. J Hepatol 2014; 61(1): 148-54. [http://dx.doi.org/10.1016/j.jhep.2014.03.013] [PMID: 24657400]

[14] Martínez-Uña M, López-Mancheño Y, Diéguez C, Fernández-Rojo MA, Novelle MG. Unraveling the role of leptin in liver function and its relationship with liver diseases. Int J Mol Sci 2020; 21(24): 9368. [http://dx.doi.org/10.3390/ijms21249368] [PMID: 33316927]

[15] Younossi Z, Stepanova M, Ong JP, *et al.* Nonalcoholic steatohepatitis is the fastest growing cause of hepatocellular carcinoma in liver transplant candidates. Clinical gastroenterology and hepatology. 2019; 17(4): 748-55. e3. [http://dx.doi.org/10.1016/j.cgh.2018.05.057]

[16] Huang DQ, El-Serag HB, Loomba R. Global epidemiology of NAFLD-related HCC: trends, predictions, risk factors and prevention. Nat Rev Gastroenterol Hepatol 2021; 18(4): 223-38. [http://dx.doi.org/10.1038/s41575-020-00381-6] [PMID: 33349658]

[17] Teng MLP, Ng CH, Huang DQ, *et al.* Global incidence and prevalence of nonalcoholic fatty liver disease. Clin Mol Hepatol 2023; 29 (Suppl.): S32-42. [http://dx.doi.org/10.3350/cmh.2022.0365] [PMID: 36517002]

[18] Henry L, Paik J, Younossi ZM. Review article: the epidemiologic burden of non-alcoholic fatty liver disease across the world. Aliment Pharmacol Ther 2022; 56(6): 942-56. [http://dx.doi.org/10.1111/apt.17158] [PMID: 35880713]

[19] Han SK, Baik SK, Kim MY. Non-alcoholic fatty liver disease: Definition and subtypes. Clin Mol Hepatol 2023; 29 (Suppl.): S5-S16. [http://dx.doi.org/10.3350/cmh.2022.0424] [PMID: 36577427]

[20] De A, Panigrahi M, Duseja A, Singh SP. Metabolic-dysfunction associated steatotic liver disease (MASLD) Hepatology. Elsevier 2025; pp. 861-88.

[21] Karkucinska-Wieckowska A, Simoes ICM, Kalinowski P, *et al.* Mitochondria, oxidative stress and nonalcoholic fatty liver disease: A complex relationship. Eur J Clin Invest 2022; 52(3): e13622.

[http://dx.doi.org/10.1111/eci.13622] [PMID: 34050922]

[22] Sharma S, Sharma A, Gupta P, *et al.* The green path to liver health: Herbal solutions for non-alcoholic steatohepatitis. Cardiovasc Hematol Disord Drug Targets 2025; 25(3): 168-92.
[http://dx.doi.org/10.2174/011871529X360903250211101856] [PMID: 40108906]

[23] Tacke F, Weiskirchen R. Non-alcoholic fatty liver disease (NAFLD)/non-alcoholic steatohepatitis (NASH)-related liver fibrosis: mechanisms, treatment and prevention. Ann Transl Med 2021; 9(8): 729.
[http://dx.doi.org/10.21037/atm-20-4354] [PMID: 33987427]

[24] Di Ciaula A, Passarella S, Shanmugam H, *et al.* Nonalcoholic fatty liver disease (NAFLD). Mitochondria as players and targets of therapies? Int J Mol Sci 2021; 22(10): 5375.
[http://dx.doi.org/10.3390/ijms22105375] [PMID: 34065331]

[25] Ren Y, Zhao H, Yin C, *et al.* Adipokines, hepatokines and myokines: focus on their role and molecular mechanisms in adipose tissue inflammation. Front Endocrinol (Lausanne) 2022; 13: 873699.
[http://dx.doi.org/10.3389/fendo.2022.873699] [PMID: 35909571]

[26] Abumrad NA, Nassi F, Marcus A. Digestion and absorption of dietary fat, carbohydrate, and protein. In: Feldman M, Friedman LS, Brandt LJ, Eds. Sleisenger and Fordtran's Gastrointestinal and Liver Disease. 10th ed. Philadelphia: Elsevier; 2016

[27] Jou J, Choi SS, Diehl AM, Eds. Mechanisms of disease progression in nonalcoholic fatty liver disease. 2008.
[http://dx.doi.org/10.1055/s-0028-1091981]

[28] Li H. Angiogenesis in the progression from liver fibrosis to cirrhosis and hepatocelluar carcinoma. Expert Rev Gastroenterol Hepatol 2021; 15(3): 217-33.
[http://dx.doi.org/10.1080/17474124.2021.1842732] [PMID: 33131349]

[29] Yki-Järvinen H. Fat in the liver and insulin resistance. Ann Med 2005; 37(5): 347-56.
[http://dx.doi.org/10.1080/07853890510037383] [PMID: 16179270]

[30] Belizário JE, Faintuch J, Garay-Malpartida M. Gut microbiome dysbiosis and immunometabolism: new frontiers for treatment of metabolic diseases. Mediators Inflamm 2018; 2018(1): 1-12.
[http://dx.doi.org/10.1155/2018/2037838] [PMID: 30622429]

[31] Iacob S, Beckebaum S, Iacob R, *et al.* Genetic and life style risk factors for recurrent non-alcoholic fatty liver disease following liver transplantation. Front Nutr 2022; 8: 787430.
[http://dx.doi.org/10.3389/fnut.2021.787430] [PMID: 35096933]

[32] Sookoian S, Pirola CJ, Valenti L, Davidson NO. Genetic pathways in nonalcoholic fatty liver disease: insights from systems biology. Hepatology 2020; 72(1): 330-46.
[http://dx.doi.org/10.1002/hep.31229] [PMID: 32170962]

[33] Bugianesi E, Moscatiello S, Ciaravella MF, Marchesini G. Insulin resistance in nonalcoholic fatty liver disease. Curr Pharm Des 2010; 16(17): 1941-51.
[http://dx.doi.org/10.2174/138161210791208875] [PMID: 20370677]

[34] Verma MK, Tripathi M, Singh BK. Dietary determinants of metabolic syndrome: focus on the obesity and metabolic dysfunction-associated steatotic liver disease (MASLD). Metabolic Syndrome-Lifestyle and Biological Risk Factors: IntechOpen; 2024.

[35] Galicia-Moreno M, Gutiérrez-Reyes G. The role of oxidative stress in the development of alcoholic liver disease. Rev Gastroenterol Mex 2014; 79(2): 135-44.
[http://dx.doi.org/10.1016/j.rgmx.2014.03.001] [PMID: 24861526]

[36] Iwaki M, Kobayashi T, Nogami A, Saito S, Nakajima A, Yoneda M. Impact of sarcopenia on non-alcoholic fatty liver disease. Nutrients 2023; 15(4): 891.
[http://dx.doi.org/10.3390/nu15040891] [PMID: 36839249]

[37] Heidelbaugh JJ, Bruderly M. Cirrhosis and chronic liver failure: part I. Diagnosis and evaluation. Am

Fam Physician 2006; 74(5): 756-62.
[PMID: 16970019]

[38] Obika M, Noguchi H. Diagnosis and evaluation of nonalcoholic fatty liver disease. Exp Diabetes Res 2012; 2012(1): 1-12.
[http://dx.doi.org/10.1155/2012/145754] [PMID: 22110476]

[39] Wang D, Zhou BY, Xiang L, Chen XY, Feng JX. Alanine aminotransferase as a risk marker for new-onset metabolic dysfunction-associated fatty liver disease. World J Gastroenterol 2024; 30(25): 3132-9.
[http://dx.doi.org/10.3748/wjg.v30.i25.3132] [PMID: 39006380]

[40] Zhang H, Ma Y, Cheng X, *et al.* Targeting epigenetically maladapted vascular niche alleviates liver fibrosis in nonalcoholic steatohepatitis. Sci Transl Med 2021; 13(614): eabd1206.
[http://dx.doi.org/10.1126/scitranslmed.abd1206] [PMID: 34613814]

[41] Madrazo BL. Diagnosis of nonalcoholic steatohepatitis without liver biopsy. Gastroenterol Hepatol (N Y) 2017; 13(6): 378-80.
[PMID: 28690456]

[42] Zhang YN, Fowler KJ, Hamilton G, *et al.* Liver fat imaging—a clinical overview of ultrasound, CT, and MR imaging. Br J Radiol 2018; 91(1089): 20170959.
[http://dx.doi.org/10.1259/bjr.20170959] [PMID: 29722568]

[43] Curtis PJ, van der Velpen V, Berends L, *et al.* Blueberries improve biomarkers of cardiometabolic function in participants with metabolic syndrome—results from a 6-month, double-blind, randomized controlled trial. Am J Clin Nutr 2019; 109(6): 1535-45.
[http://dx.doi.org/10.1093/ajcn/nqy380] [PMID: 31136659]

[44] Stern C, Castera L. Non-invasive diagnosis of hepatic steatosis. Hepatol Int 2017; 11(1): 70-8.
[http://dx.doi.org/10.1007/s12072-016-9772-z] [PMID: 27783208]

[45] Lietz P, Brüntgens M, Wang-Leandro A, Volk HA, Meller S, Merhof K. Virtual non-contrast images of detector-based spectral computed tomography in dogs: a promising alternative to true non-contrast images in veterinary medicine. Front Vet Sci 2023; 10: 1251535.
[http://dx.doi.org/10.3389/fvets.2023.1251535] [PMID: 38105773]

[46] Deibert P, Lazaro A, Schaffner D, *et al.* Comprehensive lifestyle intervention *vs* soy protein-based meal regimen in non-alcoholic steatohepatitis. World J Gastroenterol 2019; 25(9): 1116-31.
[http://dx.doi.org/10.3748/wjg.v25.i9.1116] [PMID: 30862999]

[47] Nguyen-Khac E, Capron D. Noninvasive diagnosis of liver fibrosis by ultrasonic transient elastography (Fibroscan). Eur J Gastroenterol Hepatol 2006; 18(12): 1321-5.
[http://dx.doi.org/10.1097/01.meg.0000243884.55562.37] [PMID: 17099382]

[48] Lu YC, Chang CC, Wang CP, *et al.* Circulating fatty acid-binding protein 1 (FABP1) and nonalcoholic fatty liver disease in patients with type 2 diabetes mellitus. Int J Med Sci 2020; 17(2): 182-90.
[http://dx.doi.org/10.7150/ijms.40417] [PMID: 32038102]

[49] Polyzos SA, Goulis DG, Giouleme O, Germanidis GS, Goulas A. Anti-obesity medications for the management of nonalcoholic fatty liver disease. Curr Obes Rep 2022; 11(3): 166-79.
[http://dx.doi.org/10.1007/s13679-022-00474-0] [PMID: 35501557]

[50] Raza S, Rajak S, Upadhyay A, Tewari A, Anthony Sinha R. Current treatment paradigms and emerging therapies for NAFLD/NASH. Front Biosci 2021; 26(2): 206-37.
[http://dx.doi.org/10.2741/4892] [PMID: 33049668]

[51] Moghtadaie A, Mahboobi H, Fatemizadeh S, Kamal MA. Emerging role of nanotechnology in treatment of non-alcoholic fatty liver disease (NAFLD). EXCLI J 2023; 22: 946-74.
[PMID: 38023570]

[52] Chávez-López LM, Carballo-López GI, Lugo-Ibarra KC, Castro-Ceseña AB. A comprehensive

framework for managing metabolic dysfunction-associated steatotic liver disease: analyzing novel risk factors and advances in nanotechnology-based treatments and diagnosis. RSC Med Chem 2024; 15(8): 2622-42.
[http://dx.doi.org/10.1039/D4MD00420E] [PMID: 39149095]

[53] Bhatia S. Nanoparticles: types, classification, characterization, fabrication methods and drug delivery applications. In: Poletto M, editor. Natural Polymer Drug Delivery Systems. Cham: Springer; 2016. p. 33–58.
[http://dx.doi.org/10.1007/978-3-319-41129-3_2]

[54] US Patent US20210007997A1. Nanoparticle-based liver-targeting therapy. 2021.

[55] US Patent US20190381035A1. Lipid nanoparticle compositions for delivery of therapeutic agents. 2019.

[56] US Patent US20180078430A1. Nanoparticle compositions for treatment of liver fibrosis. 2018.

[57] US Patent US20170216258A1. Targeted nanoparticle delivery system for liver diseases. 2017.

[58] US Patent US20160128952A1. Polymeric nanoparticles for treatment of metabolic disorders. 2016.

[59] US Patent US20150209432A1. Liposome-based drug delivery for liver conditions. 2015.

[60] US Patent US20140161854A1. Solid lipid nanoparticles for hepatic drug delivery. 2014.

[61] US Patent US20130266656A1. Nanoparticle-based therapeutics for liver inflammation. 2013.

[62] US Patent US20120263745A1. Targeted polymeric nanoparticles for liver disease treatment. 2012.

[63] US Patent US20110293529A1. Nanoparticle compositions for reducing liver lipid accumulation. 2011.

[64] Lestini BJ. Surface modification of liposomes for targeted intravascular drug delivery. PhD dissertation. Cleveland (OH): Case Western Reserve University; 2002.

[65] Teng W, Zhao L, Yang S, *et al.* The hepatic-targeted, resveratrol loaded nanoparticles for relief of high fat diet-induced nonalcoholic fatty liver disease. J Control Release 2019; 307: 139-49.
[http://dx.doi.org/10.1016/j.jconrel.2019.06.023] [PMID: 31233775]

[66] Tang R, Li R, Li H, *et al.* Design of hepatic targeted drug delivery systems for natural products: insights into nomenclature revision of nonalcoholic fatty liver disease. ACS Nano 2021; 15(11): 17016-46.
[http://dx.doi.org/10.1021/acsnano.1c02158] [PMID: 34705426]

[67] Kesharwani P. Combination drug delivery approach as an effective therapy for various diseases. Academic Press 2022.

[68] Elmowafy EM, Tiboni M, Soliman ME. Biocompatibility, biodegradation and biomedical applications of poly(lactic acid)/poly(lactic-co-glycolic acid) micro and nanoparticles. J Pharm Investig 2019; 49(4): 347-80.
[http://dx.doi.org/10.1007/s40005-019-00439-x]

[69] Li L, Wang H, Ong ZY, *et al.* Polymer- and lipid-based nanoparticle therapeutics for the treatment of liver diseases. Nano Today 2010; 5(4): 296-312.
[http://dx.doi.org/10.1016/j.nantod.2010.06.007]

[70] Athanasopoulou F, Manolakakis M, Vernia S, Kamaly N. Nanodrug delivery systems for metabolic chronic liver diseases: advances and perspectives. Nanomedicine (Lond) 2023; 18(1): 67-84.
[http://dx.doi.org/10.2217/nnm-2022-0261] [PMID: 36896958]

[71] Gao F, Feng X, Li X. Recent advances in polymeric nanoparticles for the treatment of hepatic diseases. Front Pharmacol 2025; 16: 1528752.
[http://dx.doi.org/10.3389/fphar.2025.1528752] [PMID: 39925843]

[72] Ashok A, Andrabi SS, Mansoor S, Kuang Y, Kwon BK, Labhasetwar V. Antioxidant therapy in oxidative stress-induced neurodegenerative diseases: Role of nanoparticle-based drug delivery systems

in clinical translation. Antioxidants 2022; 11(2): 408.
[http://dx.doi.org/10.3390/antiox11020408] [PMID: 35204290]

[73] Ashqar HM, Shaikh Omar AM, El Hamidy SM. The Potential Therapeutic Advantages of Using Nanotechnology in the Treatment of Liver Fibrosis: A Review. Egypt Acad J Biol Sci B Zool 2025; 17(1): 55-86.
[http://dx.doi.org/10.21608/eajbsz.2025.410264]

[74] Mahzari AMA. Repurposing matrine for the treatment of non-alcoholic fatty liver disease. PhD dissertation. Melbourne (VIC): RMIT University; 2018.

[75] Singh S, Sharma N, Shukla S, *et al.* Understanding the potential role of nanotechnology in liver fibrosis: a paradigm in therapeutics. Molecules 2023; 28(6): 2811.
[http://dx.doi.org/10.3390/molecules28062811] [PMID: 36985782]

[76] Chen L, Guo W, Mao C, Shen J, Wan M. Liver fibrosis: pathological features, clinical treatment and application of therapeutic nanoagents. J Mater Chem B Mater Biol Med 2024; 12(6): 1446-66.
[http://dx.doi.org/10.1039/D3TB02790B] [PMID: 38265305]

[77] Abou Assi R, Abdulbaqi IM, Siok Yee C. The evaluation of drug delivery nanocarrier development and pharmacological briefing for metabolic-associated fatty liver disease (MAFLD): an update. Pharmaceuticals (Basel) 2021; 14(3): 215.
[http://dx.doi.org/10.3390/ph14030215] [PMID: 33806527]

[78] AbouSamra MM. Liposomal nano-carriers mediated targeting of liver disorders: mechanisms and applications. J Liposome Res 2024; 34(4): 728-43.
[http://dx.doi.org/10.1080/08982104.2024.2377085] [PMID: 38988127]

[79] Alhalmi A, Beg S, Kohli K, Waris M, Singh T. Nanotechnology based approach for hepatocellular carcinoma targeting. Curr Drug Targets 2021; 22(7): 779-92.
[http://dx.doi.org/10.2174/18735592MTEycMjQp3] [PMID: 33302831]

[80] Xue L, Ding J, Liu Y, *et al.* Strategies and methods of nanocrystal technology for targeting drug delivery. J Nanopart Res 2024; 26(6): 114.
[http://dx.doi.org/10.1007/s11051-024-06025-z]

[81] Goga A, Stoffel M. Therapeutic RNA-silencing oligonucleotides in metabolic diseases. Nat Rev Drug Discov 2022; 21(6): 417-39.
[http://dx.doi.org/10.1038/s41573-022-00407-5] [PMID: 35210608]

[82] Munaweera I, Yapa P. Principles and applications of nanotherapeutics. CRC Press 2024.
[http://dx.doi.org/10.1201/9781003442202]

[83] Gándara Z, Rubio N, Castillo RR. Delivery of therapeutic biopolymers employing silica-based nanosystems. Pharmaceutics 2023; 15(2): 351.
[http://dx.doi.org/10.3390/pharmaceutics15020351] [PMID: 36839672]

[84] Mousa SA, Bawa R, Audette GF. editors. The Road from Nanomedicine to Precision Medicine: Part A. 1st ed. Boca Raton: Jenny Stanford Publishing; 2020. Available from:
[http://dx.doi.org/10.1201/9781003027010]

[85] Kumar S, Fayaz F, Pottoo FH, Bajaj S, Manchanda S, Bansal H. Nanophytomedicine based novel therapeutic strategies in liver cancer. Curr Top Med Chem 2020; 20(22): 1999-2024.
[http://dx.doi.org/10.2174/1568026619666191114113048] [PMID: 31724500]

[86] Liu Y, Wu Y, Li Z, Wan D, Pan J. Targeted drug delivery strategies for the treatment of hepatocellular carcinoma. Molecules 2024; 29(18): 4405.
[http://dx.doi.org/10.3390/molecules29184405] [PMID: 39339402]

CHAPTER 2

Non-Alcoholic Fatty Liver Disease: A Metabolic Threat

Kalpana Garg[1], **Sakshi Bajaj**[1], **Lakhveer Singh**[2,*], **Abhishek**[1] and **Aniket**[1]

[1] *Department of Pharmacognosy, Ch. Devilal College of Pharmacy, Jagadhri, Haryana, India*

[2] *Department of Pharmacology, Gurugram University, Gurugram, Haryana, India*

Abstract: Non-alcoholic fatty liver disease (NAFLD) has emerged as the typical long-term liver disease disorder worldwide, affecting a significant portion of people. This condition includes various hepatic abnormalities, starting with basic steatosis, which can progress to more severe liver disease. NASH may result in fibrosis, cirrhosis, or hepatocellular cancer. NAFLD's pathophysiology is complex, with an intricate interplay among genetic factors, physiological dysregulation, and environmental factors. Central to its development is insulin resistance, which drives lipid accumulation in hepatocytes and triggers inflammatory and fibrotic pathways. In recent years, NAFLD has gained recognition not only as a hepatic condition but also as a systemic disorder intricately linked to being obese, type 2 diabetes, hyperlipidaemia, or heart disease, collectively referred to as metabolic syndrome. Despite its increasing prevalence, NAFLD remains underdiagnosed and undertreated, highlighting the urgent need for non-invasive diagnostic tools and effective therapeutic strategies.

Keywords: Nonalcoholic fatty liver disease, Nanocarriers, Liver targeting strategies, NASH, NAFLD.

INTRODUCTION

NAFLD has been recognized as an extremely chronic ongoing liver condition during the past four decades, impacting approximately 25 percent of the older generation globally [1], and is recognized as having a two-way relationship that includes the elements of metabolic syndrome [2]. While fewer than ten percent of those with NAFLD suffer issues with their livers, determining which patients are particularly at risk within the large number of patients suffering from NAFLD is hard. Due to its growing incidence, NAFLD is currently the most significant contributing factor to liver-related disease globally [3] and is becoming a key

* **Corresponding author Lakhveer Singh:** Department of Pharmacology, Gurugram University, Gurugram, Haryana, India; E-mail: lakhveer.singh52@gmail.com

reason for advanced hepatic disorders [4]. Furthermore, liver transplantation places a substantial financial burden on the healthcare system [5]. Despite growing concern, NAFLD is not widely recognized as a severe chronic condition [6]. Few governmental programs or policies address NAFLD. It represents a group of disorders that induce metabolic abnormalities. Severe fatty hepatitis resulting in fibrosis was described more than twenty years ago [7]. Ludwig and colleagues coined the term "non-alcoholic steatohepatitis" (NASH) in 1980 [8]. NAFLD is diagnosed by the presence of steatosis in more than five percent of the liver in conjunction with biochemical risk factors (especially overweight or type 2 diabetes), along with the absence of significant alcohol consumption (≥30 g per day in men or ≥20 g per day in women) and other ongoing liver diseases [9]. Conventional terminology defines NAFLD as a diagnosis made by excluding other causes of liver disease rather than as a distinct pathological entity; nevertheless, there is ongoing debate regarding the adequacy and clarity of the current terminology and diagnostic criteria [10]. In 2020, a global panel of experts proposed the concept of MAFLD to emphasize the role of cardiovascular risk factors in the development and progression of liver disease, including among patients with other hepatic disorders [11]. Nevertheless, neither the American Association for the Study of Liver Diseases (AASLD) nor the European Association for the Study of the Liver (EASL) has officially adopted the term MAFLD in their clinical guidelines or research publications. The comparison between a healthy and a fatty liver is shown in Fig. (**1**).

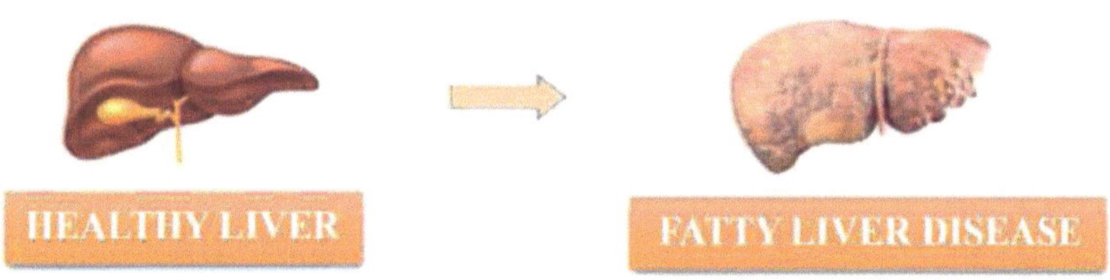

Fig. (1). Healthy liver and fatty liver.

TYPES OF NAFLD

- NAFLD (simple steatosis)
- Non-alcoholic steatohepatitis without fibrosis
- Non-alcoholic steatohepatitis with fibrosis

Non-alcoholic Fatty Liver (Simple Steatosis)

Hepatocellular steatosis is a key feature of NAFLD, with a diagnostic threshold of over 5% fat accumulation [12 - 14]. It is classified into macrovesicular and microvesicular forms. Although macrovesicular steatosis is more common in NAFLD, approximately 10% of cases may present with microvesicular steatosis [15, 16]. Initial studies portrayed NAFLD as a relatively harmless condition, with a slower progression to cirrhosis compared to NASH [17, 18]. However, recent evidence challenges this view, revealing that about 25% of NAFLD patients may experience fibrosis development [19]. Longitudinal studies involving repeated biopsies of NAFLD patients found that 64% of individuals with simple steatosis progressed to NASH within 3.7 years [20]. Furthermore, the extent of steatosis is linked to lobular inflammation, fibrosis in zone 3, and the presence of steatohepatitis [21]. A meta-analysis highlighted comparable rates of liver fibrosis progression in both NAFLD and NASH patients (39.1% *vs.* 34.5%) [22]. In summary, 30-40% of NAFLD patients show fibrosis progression over time, underscoring the importance of monitoring even in the absence of inflammation.

Non-alcoholic Steatohepatitis without Fibrosis

Non-alcoholic steatohepatitis (NASH) without fibrosis is a form of non-alcoholic fatty liver disease (NAFLD) characterized by liver inflammation and fat accumulation without the presence of significant fibrosis (scarring). NASH represents a stage within a spectrum of liver damage, ranging from simple steatosis (fatty liver) to more severe forms, including cirrhosis. In NASH, liver inflammation can damage hepatocytes, leading to potential progression to fibrosis and cirrhosis if not managed. However, in the absence of fibrosis, NASH may not cause significant long-term liver damage but requires close monitoring to prevent progression [23]. The primary risk factors for NASH without fibrosis include obesity, insulin resistance, type 2 diabetes, and dyslipidemia. The condition is often asymptomatic, and individuals may not be aware of their liver abnormalities until routine blood tests reveal elevated liver enzymes or imaging studies, such as ultrasound, detect fatty liver changes. Symptoms, when present, may include mild fatigue or discomfort in the upper abdomen [24]. Management focuses on lifestyle modifications, including weight loss through a healthy diet and regular exercise. These changes can help reduce liver fat, improve insulin sensitivity, and reduce inflammation. While no specific pharmacological treatments have been approved for NASH without fibrosis, managing underlying conditions like diabetes and hyperlipidemia is crucial to prevent disease progression [25].

Non-alcoholic Steatohepatitis with Fibrosis

Non-alcoholic steatohepatitis (NASH) with fibrosis is a more advanced stage of NAFLD, characterized by liver inflammation and accumulation of fat, or the development of fibrosis, or scarring, within the liver tissue. NASH is a progressive condition, and when fibrosis develops, it signifies that liver damage has occurred over time. The severity of fibrosis can range from mild to severe, with advanced fibrosis potentially leading to cirrhosis and increasing the risk of liver failure and liver cancer [26]. The pathogenesis of NASH with fibrosis involves multiple factors, including insulin resistance, obesity, metabolic syndrome, and dyslipidemia. These factors contribute to liver fat accumulation, leading to oxidative stress and inflammation. Chronic liver inflammation can cause hepatocyte injury, leading to fibrosis as the liver attempts to repair itself. Fibrosis in NASH typically develops over years and may not be detected until liver function becomes significantly impaired. Patients with NASH with fibrosis may present with mild to moderate symptoms, including fatigue, right upper quadrant discomfort, and elevated liver enzymes. Moreover, the condition is frequently asymptomatic until significant liver damage occurs. Diagnosis is generally by liver biopsy or by sophisticated imaging techniques, such as elastography, which may detect liver stiffness and the extent of fibrosis [27]. The pre-diagnosis stage is crucial to avoid progression to cirrhosis and its complications. The management of NASH with fibrosis entails addressing the underlying metabolic risk factors like obesity, type 2 diabetes, and hyperlipidemia. Weight loss, a balanced diet, and regular physical activity are important for improving liver health and preventing disease progression. Although there are no FDA-approved pharmacologic treatments specifically for NASH with fibrosis, agents aimed at improving insulin sensitivity and reducing liver inflammation are being explored in clinical trials [28].

EPIDEMIOLOGY OF NAFLD

Non-alcoholic fatty liver disease (NAFLD) has become one of the most common liver disorders worldwide, with significant public health implications. It is characterized by an excessive accumulation of fat in the liver in the absence of high alcohol consumption. The prevalence of NAFLD has been rising due to increasing rates of obesity, diabetes, and metabolic syndrome worldwide [29].

- **Global prevalence**: NAFLD affects roughly 25-30% of the global population, with some regions, such as the Middle East or South America, experiencing even higher rates (up to 40%). In North America and Europe, the prevalence remains around 25% [30].
- **Risk factors**: Common risk factors for NAFLD include obesity, particularly central obesity, insulin resistance, type 2 DM, hyperlipidemia, and hypertension. These factors are common in metabolic syndrome, which predisposes individuals to NAFLD [31].
- **Age and gender**: NAFLD is more prevalent in middle-aged people, namely those aged 40 to 60. NAFLD is more common in men than in premenopausal women, but the risk in women increases after menopause, leading to a similar incidence between sexes in later life [32].

- **Comorbidities**: NAFLD is frequently associated with metabolic disorders, such as type 2 diabetes, hypertension, and cardiovascular disease. This is associated with an increased risk of hepatitis, liver cancer, or other consequences related to liver malfunction [33].

PATHOPHYSIOLOGY OF NAFLD

The pathophysiology of NAFLD is complex and multifaceted, combining genetic, environmental, and metabolic factors [34]. Main mechanisms that contribute to the development and progression of NAFLD include:

- **Insulin resistance**: Insulin resistance is a key factor in the progression of NAFLD. It increases the entry of saturated fats into the liver while decreasing fatty acid degradation. This triggers triglyceride synthesis in hepatocytes (liver cells) [35].
- **Lipotoxicity**: Excessive fat accumulation in the liver produces harmful intermediates like ceramides and free fatty acids, which harm liver cells. This promotes inflammation and hepatocyte damage [36].
- **Inflammation**: NAFLD is associated with low-grade chronic inflammation. Inflammatory cytokines like TNF-α and interleukins play a critical role in promoting liver damage and the progression from fatty liver disease to NASH, which can lead to fibrosis or cirrhosis [37].
- **Oxidative stress:** Oxidative stress occurs when there is an imbalance between the production of reactive oxygen species (ROS) and the body's antioxidant defenses. This damage accelerates liver injury or contributes to fibrosis [38].
- **Genetic factors**: Certain genetic variations, including those in the PNPLA3 gene, have been linked to an increased risk of NAFLD. These genetic factors influence how the liver processes and stores fats, making some individuals more prone to liver fat accumulation [39].

CLINICAL PRESENTATION OF NAFLD

The clinical presentation of NAFLD can range from asymptomatic to severe liver disease. Many individuals with NAFLD are unaware of their condition until advanced stages, and the stages of NAFLD are shown in Fig. (**2**) [40]. Key aspects of the clinical presentation include:

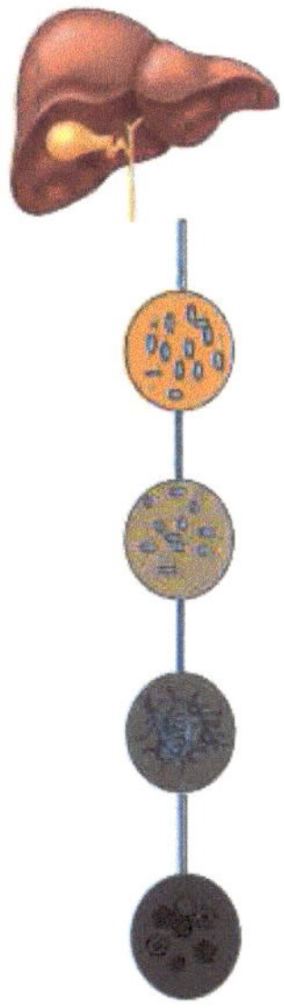

Fig. (2). Stages of NAFLD.

- **Asymptomatic in early stages**: In many cases, NAFLD is discovered incidentally during imaging tests or routine blood tests. Most individuals in the early stages of the disease do not exhibit symptoms [41].
- **Fatigue**: One of the most common and vital subjective symptoms reported by patients with NAFLD is fatigue, which is often nonspecific [42].
- **Right upper quadrant pain**: Some individuals may experience mild pain or dull soreness in the upper right quadrant of the abdomen, near the liver. This pain is often related to hepatomegaly (enlargement of the liver) [43].
- **Progression to NASH**: As the condition develops into NASH, patients may experience more pronounced symptoms, such as jaundice (yellowing of the skin or eyes), ascites (abdominal fluid accumulation), and signs of liver dysfunction, including easy bruising or bleeding [44].
- **Complications of advanced disease**: As NAFLD advances to cirrhosis, patients may have complications such as variceal hemorrhage, encephalopathy, and liver failure. Advanced liver disease greatly decreases quality of life and increases mortality [45].

CURRENT DIAGNOSTIC MODALITIES

NAFLD is diagnosed using a combination of clinical examination, laboratory testing, imaging modalities, and occasionally liver biopsy [46]. The diagnostic process includes:

- **Clinical evaluation**: The first step in diagnosing is a comprehensive medical history and physical examination that rules out other symptoms of liver disease, like alcohol addiction or viral hepatitis [47].
- **Blood tests:** Alanine aminotransferase (ALT) and Aspartate aminotransferase (AST). Routine LFTs are commonly mildly elevated in NAFLD, and the levels of liver enzymes and the severity of disease do not often correlate. High levels of triglycerides, cholesterol, and glucose could indicate the presence of a metabolic disorder [48].
- **Imaging studies:** Sonography is performed (to check whether they are well-meaning), and an edgy liver is noted. Other imaging techniques, such as MRI or controlled attenuation parameter (CAP) examination, can better quantify liver fat content [49].
- **Liver biopsy**: Liver biopsy is still considered a highly dependable approach for detecting and staging NAFLD. It helps differentiate between simple steatosis and NASH, while also assessing the extent of fibrosis. Despite its accuracy, the procedure is invasive and associated with potential risks, making it unsuitable for routine use in all patients [50].
- **Non-invasive tests**: Several non-invasive scoring systems (*e.g.*, the NAFLD fibrosis score and FIB-4) and elastography (ultrasound or MRI) are increasingly used to assess liver stiffness, which correlates with fibrosis and cirrhosis. These tests are less invasive and more widely available than liver biopsy [51].

LIFESTYLE INTERVENTIONS AND THEIR ROLE IN DISEASE MANAGEMENT

The cornerstone of managing NAFLD is lifestyle modification. Evidence overwhelmingly supports the role of diet, exercise, and weight management in improving liver health and preventing disease progression [52]. Key lifestyle interventions include

- **Dietary modifications**
    - **Caloric restriction and Mediterranean diet**: Reducing calorie intake can help achieve weight loss, which is the most effective intervention for lowering liver fat. A 5-10% reduction in body weight has been found to improve liver histology and lessen the risk of NASH progression [53]. A diet rich in healthy fats (*e.g.*, olive oil), fruits, vegetables, whole grains, and lean proteins has been shown to reduce liver fat and inflammation [54].
    - **Low-carb and low-sugar diets**: Reducing refined carbohydrate and sugar intake, particularly fructose (often found in sugary drinks), can improve insulin sensitivity and reduce liver fat accumulation [55].
    - **Physical activity**: Regular exercise, particularly aerobic activity, has been

shown to decrease liver fat content, improve insulin sensitivity, and reduce the risk of NASH. A combination of aerobic exercise (such as walking, cycling, or swimming) and resistance training is ideal for weight loss and improving liver health [56].

- **Weight loss:** Diet-induced weight loss of 5-10% of body weight is the most important factor in reversing fatty liver and enhancing long-term liver health. Even a moderate weight reduction can decrease liver fat, inflammation, and fibrosis [57].
- **Treatment of comorbid conditions:** Comorbid conditions like diabetes and overweight or hyperlipidemia are some associated diseases to be managed along with lifestyle modification. Some drugs, such as metformin and statins, may be considered in certain health conditions, but no specific pharmacotherapy has been shown to be effective for NAFLD [58].
- **Behavioural interventions:** Psychological interventions to support individuals in making and maintaining lifestyle changes can enhance their efficacy. This could involve counselling, weight loss programmes, or psychological help to tackle barriers like food addiction or emotional eating [59].

CHALLENGES IN THE MANAGEMENT OF NAFLD

NAFLD presents a complex challenge in modern healthcare due to its rising prevalence and close association with metabolic disorders, including obesity, diabetes (especially type 2 diabetes), and heart disease. Among the key difficulties in managing NAFLD is its typically asymptomatic nature in the early stages. Many patients remain undiagnosed until significant liver damage has occurred, making early intervention challenging. Furthermore, the disease exhibits a highly variable progression. While some individuals may live for decades with simple steatosis, others progress rapidly to non-alcoholic steatohepatitis (NASH), fibrosis, and even cirrhosis. Currently, there are no approved pharmacological treatments specifically targeting NAFLD or NASH, and management relies heavily on lifestyle interventions, which require long-term patient adherence and are difficult to sustain [60]. Given these challenges, prevention remains the most effective strategy against NAFLD. Lifestyle modification is central to prevention efforts. A healthy, balanced diet, particularly the Mediterranean diet, combined with regular physical activity and sustained weight loss of at least 7–10%, can significantly improve liver function and reduce disease progression. Screening should be targeted toward high-risk populations, especially individuals with obesity, insulin resistance, or type 2 diabetes. Tools such as the FibroScore or NAFLD Fibrosis Score can help identify patients who may require further evaluation [61]. Managing associated metabolic risk factors is equally important.

Reasonable glycaemic control in people with diabetes, lipid-lowering therapies like statins, and the management of hypertension all contribute to reducing liver and cardiovascular risk. Public health measures also play a vital role. Increasing awareness through education campaigns and implementing policies to reduce the consumption of processed and high-sugar foods can support healthier lifestyles at a population level. Finally, long-term surveillance of patients diagnosed with NAFLD is essential to monitor for progression and adjust interventions accordingly [62]. In summary, NAFLD management is hindered by diagnostic, therapeutic, and systemic challenges. A comprehensive strategy that integrates prevention, early detection, lifestyle interventions, and metabolic control is key to reducing the individual and societal burden of this increasingly common liver disease.

REGULATORY AND SAFETY CONCERNS

The regulatory and safety concerns surrounding non-alcoholic fatty liver disease (NAFLD) management are multifaceted, reflecting the absence of standardized therapeutic options and the growing reliance on experimental approaches. Since there are no FDA- or EMA-approved drugs specifically targeting NAFLD or NASH, most therapeutic strategies currently fall under off-label use of antidiabetic, lipid-lowering, or anti-obesity medications. This regulatory gap raises challenges in ensuring consistent clinical outcomes, patient safety, and long-term efficacy. Safety concerns also extend to the use of investigational drugs under clinical trials, where hepatotoxicity, metabolic disturbances, and unforeseen systemic effects may occur [63]. Additionally, dietary supplements and herbal remedies, which are often promoted as supportive interventions for fatty liver, remain poorly regulated and may pose risks due to variability in composition, contamination, or unverified claims of efficacy. From a public health perspective, the lack of globally harmonized guidelines for screening, early detection, and long-term monitoring of NAFLD further complicates patient management, especially in populations with high prevalence but limited healthcare infrastructure [64]. Ethical considerations also arise in clinical research, particularly regarding informed consent, trial transparency, and the inclusion of vulnerable groups, such as children and elderly patients. To address these concerns, regulatory bodies are increasingly emphasizing pharmacovigilance, robust clinical trial design, and post-marketing surveillance to safeguard patients. Collaborative frameworks among researchers, clinicians, and policymakers are essential to establish evidence-based regulatory standards that balance innovation with patient safety, ultimately paving the way for the approval of effective, safe therapies for NAFLD [65, 66].

FUTURE PERSPECTIVES FOR FATTY LIVER DISEASE MANAGEMENT

Pharmacological strategies, genetic applications, and lifestyle changes are promising approaches for the management of meta-associated steatohepatitis (MAS) in the future. Promising drugs also include GLP-1 receptor agonists, such as semaglutide, which appear to reduce liver fat and inflammation, and FGF21 analogues, such as efruxifermin, which show promise in reversing fibrosis. The thyroid hormone receptor beta agonist resmetirom, for example, has recently been approved for non-cirrhotic NASH, and agonists, including lanifibranor, are in phase III development for lipid metabolism and inflammation. Novel genetic and molecular therapies, including RNA interference (*e.g.*, aro-hsd) and antifibrotic agents (*e.g.*, bms-986263), are being developed to influence the liver disease continuum. Lifestyle interventions, such as the Mediterranean diet and physical activity, remain crucial. The convergence of combination medicines, new diagnostics, and personalized medicine is likely to revolutionize MASLD therapy, improving long-term patient outcomes.

CONCLUSION

Non-alcoholic fatty liver disease (NAFLD) has become the most prevalent chronic liver ailment in the world, and it is closely connected to the rise in obesity, metabolic syndrome, and diabetes type 2 diabetes. This chapter has highlighted the multifaceted nature of NAFLD, beginning with its increasing epidemiological burden and the complex pathophysiological mechanisms involving insulin resistance, lipid accumulation, inflammation, and fibrosis. The clinical presentation of NAFLD is often asymptomatic in early stages, making early diagnosis a challenge. Although several diagnostic modalities exist, including imaging and liver biopsy, there remains a need for non-invasive, cost-effective tools with higher sensitivity and specificity. Lifestyle modification, primarily diet, physical activity, and weight loss, remains the cornerstone of NAFLD management. Despite their proven benefits, adherence to these interventions poses a significant challenge in real-world settings. Furthermore, the absence of approved pharmacological therapies specifically targeting NAFLD underscores the urgent need for novel therapeutic strategies. Current research is focused on understanding disease heterogeneity and developing personalized treatment approaches. Future perspectives in NAFLD management include improved risk stratification, early identification of at-risk individuals, and the integration of emerging therapies targeting specific molecular pathways. Collaborative efforts among clinicians, researchers, and public health policymakers are essential to reduce the growing burden of NAFLD and its associated complications. Continued advancements in both diagnostics and therapeutics are crucial to transforming NAFLD from a silent epidemic into a manageable clinical entity.

LIST OF ABBREVIATIONS

NAFLD Non-Alcoholic Fatty Liver Disease

MAFLD Metabolic Dysfunction-Associated Fatty Liver Disease

NASH Non-Alcoholic Steatohepatitis

FGF21 Fibroblast Growth Factor 21

EMA European Medicines Agency

FDA Food and Drug Administration

TNF Tumour Necrosis Factor

REFERENCES

[1] Younossi ZM, Koenig AB, Abdelatif D, Fazel Y, Henry L, Wymer M. Global epidemiology of nonalcoholic fatty liver disease—Meta□analytic assessment of prevalence, incidence, and outcomes. Hepatology 2016; 64(1): 73-84.
[http://dx.doi.org/10.1002/hep.28431] [PMID: 26707365]

[2] Younossi Z, Anstee QM, Marietti M, et al., Global burden of NAFLD and NASH: trends, predictions, risk factors and prevention. Nat Rev Gastroenterol Hepatol. 2018; 15(1): 11–20.
[http://dx.doi.org/10.1038/nrgastro.2017.109]

[3] Paik JM, Golabi P, Younossi Y, Mishra A, Younossi ZM. Paik jm, golabi p, younossi y, mishra a, younossi zm. Changes in the global burden of chronic liver diseases from 2012 to 2017: the growing impact of NAFLD. Hepatology 2020; 72(5): 1605-16.
[http://dx.doi.org/10.1002/hep.31173] [PMID: 32043613]

[4] Estes C, Razavi H, Loomba R, Younossi Z, Sanyal AJ. Modeling the epidemic of nonalcoholic fatty liver disease demonstrates an exponential increase in burden of disease. Hepatology 2018; 67(1): 123-33.
[http://dx.doi.org/10.1002/hep.29466] [PMID: 28802062]

[5] Wong RJ, Cheung R, Ahmed A. Nonalcoholic steatohepatitis is the most rapidly growing indication for liver transplantation in patients with hepatocellular carcinoma in the U.S. Hepatology. 2014;59(6):2188–2195.
[http://dx.doi.org/10.1002/hep.26973]

[6] Alexander M, Loomis AK, Fairburn-beech J, *et al.* Real-world data reveal a diagnostic gap in non-alcoholic fatty liver disease. Bmc med. 2018;16(1):130.

[7] Thaler H. [The fatty liver and its pathogenetic relation to liver cirrhosis]. Virchows Arch Pathol Anat Physiol Klin Med 1962; 335(2): 180-210.
[http://dx.doi.org/10.1007/BF02438705] [PMID: 13920484]

[8] Ludwig J, Viggiano TR, McGILL DB, Ott BJ. Nonalcoholic steatohepatitis: Mayo Clinic experiences with a hitherto unnamed disease. Mayo Clin Proc 1980; 55(7): 434-8.
[http://dx.doi.org/10.1016/S0025-6196(24)00530-5] [PMID: 7382552]

[9] European Association for the Study of the Liver (EASL); European Association for the Study of Diabetes (EASD); European Association for the Study of Obesity (EASO). EASL–EASD–EASO clinical practice guidelines for the management of non-alcoholic fatty liver disease. J Hepatol 2016;

64(6): 1388-402.
[http://dx.doi.org/10.1016/j.jhep.2015.11.004] [PMID: 27062661]

[10] Eslam M, Newsome PN, Sarin SK, *et al.* A new definition for metabolic dysfunction-associated fatty liver disease: an international expert consensus statement. J hepatol. 2020; 73(1): 202–9.

[11] Younossi ZM, Rinella ME, Sanyal A, *et al.* From NAFLD to MAFLD: implications of a premature change in terminology. Hepatology. 2020; published online june 16.

[12] Brunt EM. Histopathology of non-alcoholic fatty liver disease. Clin Liver Dis 2009; 13(4): 533-44.
[http://dx.doi.org/10.1016/j.cld.2009.07.008] [PMID: 19818303]

[13] Yeh MM, Brunt EM. Pathology of nonalcoholic fatty liver disease. Am J Clin Pathol 2007; 128(5): 837-47.
[http://dx.doi.org/10.1309/RTPM1PY6YGBL2G2R] [PMID: 17951208]

[14] Bondini S, Kleiner DE, Goodman ZD, Gramlich T, Younossi ZM. Pathologic assessment of non-alcoholic fatty liver disease. Clin Liver Dis 2007; 11(1): 17-23, vii.
[http://dx.doi.org/10.1016/j.cld.2007.02.002] [PMID: 17544969]

[15] Sharma S, Sharma A, Gupta P, *et al.* The green path to liver health: Herbal solutions for non-alcoholic steatohepatitis. Cardiovasc Hematol Disord Drug Targets 2025; 25(3): 168-92.
[http://dx.doi.org/10.2174/011871529X360903250211101856] [PMID: 40108906]

[16] Ikejima K, Kon K, Yamashina S. Nonalcoholic fatty liver disease and alcohol-related liver disease: From clinical aspects to pathophysiological insights. Clin Mol Hepatol 2020; 26(4): 728-35.
[http://dx.doi.org/10.3350/cmh.2020.0202] [PMID: 33053942]

[17] Teli MR, James OFW, Burt AD, Bennett MK, Day CP. The natural history of nonalcoholic fatty liver: A follow-up study. Hepatology 1995; 22(6): 1714-9.
[http://dx.doi.org/10.1002/hep.1840220616] [PMID: 7489979]

[18] Ekstedt M, Hagström H, Nasr P, Fredrikson M, Stål P, Kechagias S, *et al.* Fibrosis stage is the strongest predictor for disease-specific mortality in NAFLD after up to 33 years of follow-up. Hepatology. 2015; 61(5): 1547-54.

[19] Mazzolini G, Sowa JP, Atorrasagasti C, Kücükoglu Ö, Syn WK, Canbay A. Significance of simple steatosis: an update on the clinical and molecular evidence. Cells 2020; 9(11): 2458.
[http://dx.doi.org/10.3390/cells9112458] [PMID: 33187255]

[20] Pais R, Charlotte F, Fedchuk L, *et al.* Lido study group. A systematic review of follow-up biopsies reveals disease progression in patients with non-alcoholic fatty liver. J hepatol. 2013; 59(3): 550-6.

[21] Chalasani N, Wilson L, Kleiner DE, Cummings OW, Brunt EM, Ünalp A. Relationship of steatosis grade and zonal location to histological features of steatohepatitis in adult patients with non-alcoholic fatty liver disease. J Hepatol 2008; 48(5): 829-34.
[http://dx.doi.org/10.1016/j.jhep.2008.01.016]

[22] Singh S, Allen AM, Wang Z, Prokop LJ, Murad MH, Loomba R. Fibrosis progression in nonalcoholic fatty liver *vs* nonalcoholic steatohepatitis: a systematic review and meta-analysis of paired-biopsy studies. Clin gastroenterol hepatol. 2015; 13:643-54. E1-9; quiz e39-40.

[23] Zhang X, Zhang F, Li H. Non-alcoholic steatohepatitis without fibrosis: a review of current knowledge and therapeutic options. World J Gastroenterol 2016; 22(19): 4732-40.
[PMID: 27217704]

[24] Chalasani N, Younossi Z, Lavine JE, *et al.* The diagnosis and management of non-alcoholic fatty liver disease: practice guidance from the American Association for the Study of Liver Diseases. Hepatology. 2018;67(1):328–357.
[http://dx.doi.org/10.1002/hep.29367]

[25] Bellentani S. The epidemiology of non-alcoholic fatty liver disease. Liver Int 2017; 37(Suppl 1): 718-27.

[26] Lemoinne S, Housset C, Lemoine M. Fibrosis progression in non-alcoholic steatohepatitis: a complex pathophysiological process. J Hepatol 2018; 68(2): 216-29.

[27] Mazzella G, Meroni M, Malvestiti F. The role of liver stiffness measurement in the diagnosis of non-alcoholic steatohepatitis with fibrosis. J Gastroenterol Hepatol 2020; 35(10): 1713-20.

[28] Younossi ZM, Anstee QM, Marietti M, *et al.* Global burden of NAFLD and NASH: trends, predictions, risk factors, and prevention. Nat rev gastroenterol hepatol. 2018; 15(1): 11-20.

[29] Lazo M, Clark JM., *et al.* The epidemiology of nonalcoholic fatty liver disease: a global perspective. Semin Liver Dis. 2008;28(4):339–350.
[http://dx.doi.org/10.1055/s-0028-1091978] [PMID: 18956290]

[30] Younossi Zobair M, Koenig Aaron B, Abdelatif Deena, Fazel Yousef, Henry Linda, Wymer Mark. Global epidemiology of nonalcoholic fatty liver disease—meta-analytic assessment of prevalence, incidence, and outcomes. Hepatology 2016; 64(1): 73-84.[http://dx.doi.org/10.1002/hep.28431]

[31] Estes Chad, Anstee Quentin M, Arias-Loste Maria T, *et al.* Modeling NAFLD disease burden across countries. J Hepatol 2018; 69(4): 896-904.
[http://dx.doi.org/10.1016/j.jhep.2018.05.036]

[32] Lonardo Amedeo, Nascimbeni Francesca, Ballestri Stefano, *et al.* Sex differences in NAFLD. Hepatology 2019; 70(4): 1457-69.
[http://dx.doi.org/10.1002/hep.30626]

[33] Byrne Christopher D, Targher Giovanni. NAFLD: a multisystem disease. J Hepatol 2015; 62(1 Suppl): S47-64.
[http://dx.doi.org/10.1016/j.jhep.2014.12.012]

[34] Buzzetti Elena, Pinzani Massimo, Tsochatzis Emmanuel A. The multiple-hit pathogenesis of NAFLD. Metabolism 2016; 65(8): 1038-48.
[http://dx.doi.org/10.1016/j.metabol.2015.12.012]

[35] Samuel Varman T, Shulman Gerald I. NAFLD as metabolic disease. Cell Metab 2018; 27(1): 22-41.
[http://dx.doi.org/10.1016/j.cmet.2017.08.020]

[36] Musso Giovanni, Gambino Roberto, Cassader Maurizio. Lipotoxicity in NASH. Free Radic Biol Med 2010; 52(5): 1021-30.
[http://dx.doi.org/10.1016/j.freeradbiomed.2011.12.009]

[37] Tilg Herbert, Moschen Alexander R. Inflammation in NAFLD. Hepatology 2010; 52(5): 1836-46.
[http://dx.doi.org/10.1002/hep.24001]

[38] Seki Seishiro, Kitada Toshikazu, Yamada Tetsuya, Sakaguchi Hitoshi, Nakatani Kenji, Wakasa Kazuya. Oxidative stress in NAFLD. J Hepatol 2002; 37(1): 56-62.
[http://dx.doi.org/10.1016/S0168-8278(02)00078-8]

[39] Anstee Quentin M, Seth Dipanjan, Day Christopher P. Genetic factors in NAFLD. Gastroenterology 2016; 150(8): 1728-44.
[http://dx.doi.org/10.1053/j.gastro.2016.02.011]

[40] Chalasani Naga, Younossi Zobair, Lavine Joel E, *et al.* Diagnosis and management of NAFLD. Hepatology 2018; 67(1): 328-57.
[http://dx.doi.org/10.1002/hep.29367]

[41] European Association for the Study of the Liver; European Association for the Study of Diabetes; European Association for the Study of Obesity. Clinical practice guidelines. J Hepatol 2016; 64(6): 1388-402.
[http://dx.doi.org/10.1016/j.jhep.2015.11.004]

[42] Newton Jennifer L. Systemic symptoms in NAFLD. Dig Dis 2010; 28(1): 214-9.
[http://dx.doi.org/10.1159/000282091]

[43] Adams Leon A, Lymp Jeffrey F, St Sauver Jennifer, Sanderson Steven O, Lindor Keith D, Feldstein Ariel E. Natural history of NAFLD. Gastroenterology 2005; 129(1): 113-21. [http://dx.doi.org/10.1053/j.gastro.2005.04.014]

[44] Friedman Scott L, Neuschwander-Tetri Brent A, Rinella Mary, Sanyal Arun J. Mechanisms of NAFLD. Nat Med 2018; 24(7): 908-22. [http://dx.doi.org/10.1038/s41591-018-0104-9]

[45] Angulo Paul. Nonalcoholic fatty liver disease. N Engl J Med 2002; 346(16): 1221-31. [http://dx.doi.org/10.1056/NEJMra011775]

[46] Castera Laurent, Friedrich-Rust Mireen, Loomba Rohit. Noninvasive assessment in NAFLD. Gastroenterology 2019; 156(5): 1264-81. [http://dx.doi.org/10.1053/j.gastro.2018.12.036]

[47] Rinella Mary E. NAFLD: systematic review. JAMA 2015; 313(22): 2263-73. [http://dx.doi.org/10.1001/jama.2015.5370]

[48] McPherson Stuart, Hardy Tim, Henderson Emma, Burt Alastair D, Day Christopher P, Anstee Quentin M. Fibrosis progression. J Hepatol 2015; 62(5): 1148-55. [http://dx.doi.org/10.1016/j.jhep.2014.11.008]

[49] Hernaez R, Lazo M, Bonekamp S, *et al.* Diagnostic Accuracy And Reliability Of Ultrasonography For The Detection Of Fatty Liver: A Meta-Analysis. Hepatology 2011; 54(3): 1082-90. [http://dx.doi.org/10.1002/hep.24452]

[50] Rockey DC, Caldwell SH, Goodman ZD, Nelson RC, Smith AD. American Association for the Study of Liver Diseases. Liver Biopsy. Hepatology 2009; 49(3): 1017-44.

[51] Eddowes Peter J, Sasso Maurizio, Allison Mark, *et al.* FibroScan accuracy. Gastroenterology 2019; 156(6): 1717-30. [http://dx.doi.org/10.1053/j.gastro.2019.01.042]

[52] Promrat Kittichai, Kleiner David E, Niemeier Heather M, *et al.* Weight loss and NASH. Hepatology 2010; 51(1): 121-9. [http://dx.doi.org/10.1002/hep.23276]

[53] Koutoukidis Dimitrios A, Astbury Neil M, Tudor Katy E, *et al.* Calorie restriction. BMJ 2019; 366: l5365. [http://dx.doi.org/10.1136/bmj.l5365]

[54] Ryan Margriet C, Itsiopoulos Catherine, Thodis Thomas, *et al.* Mediterranean diet and NAFLD. J Hepatol 2013; 59(1): 138-43. [http://dx.doi.org/10.1016/j.jhep.2013.02.012]

[55] Kirk EP, Reeds DN, Finck BN, Mayurranjan S. Vojnosanitetski pregled. Vojnosanit Pregl 2018 Jan; 75(1): 1-142. [http://dx.doi.org/10.1016/j.jhep.2013.02.012]

[56] Hayes K. Physical activity and its impact on NAFLD. Exerc Med 2021; 25(2): 200-10.

[57] Bell J. The effect of weight loss on NAFLD progression. Obes Res Clin Pract 2023; 17(6): 1278-89.

[58] Greenfield p. Management of comorbidities in NAFLD patients. Endocrinol metab clin. 2021; 15(1): 61-70.

[59] Mitchell L. Behavioural interventions for NAFLD patients. J Clin Psychol Med Settings 2022; 16(3): 309-20.

[60] Marchesini G, Bugianesi E, Forlani G, *et al.* Nonalcoholic fatty liver, steatohepatitis, and the metabolic syndrome. Hepatology 2003; 37(4): 917-23. [http://dx.doi.org/10.1053/jhep.2003.50161] [PMID: 12668987]

[61] Chalasani N, Younossi Z, Lavine JE, *et al.* The diagnosis and management of non-alcoholic fatty liver

disease: practice guideline by the american association for the study of liver diseases, american college of gastroenterology, and the american gastroenterological association. Hepatology 2012; 55(6): 2005-23.
[http://dx.doi.org/10.1002/hep.25762] [PMID: 22488764]

[62] Athyros VG, Tziomalos K, Gossios TD, *et al.* Safety and efficacy of long-term statin treatment for cardiovascular events in patients with coronary heart disease and abnormal liver tests in the Greek Atorvastatin and Coronary Heart Disease Evaluation (GREACE) Study: a post-hoc analysis. Lancet 2010; 376(9756): 1916-22.
[http://dx.doi.org/10.1016/S0140-6736(10)61272-X] [PMID: 21109302]

[63] Chalasani N, Younossi Z, Lavine JE, *et al.* The diagnosis and management of nonalcoholic fatty liver disease: Practice guidance from the american association for the study of liver diseases. Hepatology 2018; 67(1): 328-57.
[http://dx.doi.org/10.1002/hep.29367] [PMID: 28714183]

[64] Younossi ZM, Rinella ME, Sanyal AJ, *et al.* From NAFLD to MAFLD: implications of a premature change in terminology. Hepatology 2021; 73(3): 1194-8.
[http://dx.doi.org/10.1002/hep.31420] [PMID: 32544255]

[65] Wong VWS, Chitturi S, Wong GLH, Yu J, Chan HLY, Farrell GC. Pathogenesis and novel treatment options for non-alcoholic steatohepatitis. Lancet Gastroenterol Hepatol 2016; 1(1): 56-67.
[http://dx.doi.org/10.1016/S2468-1253(16)30011-5] [PMID: 28404113]

[66] Athyros VG, Mikhailidis DP, Liberopoulos EN, Kakafika AI, Karagiannis A, Papageorgiou AA, Tziomalos K, Ganotakis ES, Elisaf M. Effect of statin treatment on renal function and serum uric acid levels and their relation to vascular events in patients with coronary heart disease and metabolic syndrome: a subgroup analysis of the GREek Atorvastatin and Coronary heart disease Evaluation (GREACE) Study. Nephrol Dial Transplant. 2007 Jan; 22(1): 118-27.
[http://dx.doi.org/10.1016/S0140-6736(10)61272-X] [PMID: 21109302]

CHAPTER 3

Overview of Nanocarrier-based Drug Delivery Systems

Himani Bajaj[1], Mayank Yadav[1], Mukesh Maithani[2,*], Abhay Mishra[3] and **Navin Chandra Pant[4]**

[1] *Adarsh Vijendra Institute of Pharmaceutical Sciences, Shobhit University, Gangoh, Saharanpur, Uttar Pradesh, India*

[2] *Department of Pharmaceutical Sciences, Hemvati Nandan Bahuguna Garhwal University, Chaurus Campus, Srinagar Garhwal, Uttarakhand, India*

[3] *Department of Pharmaceutical Technology, Faculty of Pharmaceutical Sciences, Naresuan University, Phitsanulok, Thailand*

[4] *Faculty of Pharmaceutical Sciences, Amrapali University, Haldwani, Uttarakhand, India*

Abstract: Up to 25% of adults worldwide may suffer from noncommunicable chronic liver disorders, which is a serious and expanding public health concern. These illnesses currently have no known cure or effective treatment. With billions of doses safely administered worldwide, nanomedicines are transforming healthcare. However, there is significant interest in developing new translational techniques to address unmet diagnostic and treatment needs. As a step towards precision medicine, nanoparticle-based techniques present new possibilities for targeted and effective medication delivery to liver cells. Nanocarrier delivery systems offer a tool to address the urgent and unmet clinical needs of metabolic chronic liver diseases, including non-alcoholic fatty liver disease. This chapter emphasizes recent developments in nanomedicine to develop innovative diagnostic and therapeutic tools for non-alcoholic fatty liver disease and associated liver disorders.

Keywords: Chronic liver disease, Nanomedicine, Nanoparticle, Non-alcoholic fatty liver disease.

INTRODUCTION

With an estimated global prevalence of 24% and higher incidence rates in South America and the Middle East, followed by Asia, the United States, and Europe, nonalcoholic fatty liver disease (NAFLD) is the most prevalent noncommunicable

* **Corresponding author Mukesh Maithani:** Department of Pharmaceutical Sciences, Hemvati Nandan Bahuguna Garhwal University, Chaurus Campus, Srinagar Garhwal, Uttarakhand, India; E-mail: mukeshmaithani@gmail.com

Anjali Sharma, Devkant Sharma, Ajmer Singh Grewal, Geeta Deswal & Ganga Reddy Velma (Eds.)

chronic liver disease [1]. As NAFLD poses a major medical and economic burden, it is essential to develop evidence-based strategies for its diagnosis, treatment, and prevention, and to integrate these strategies into healthcare systems and globally accepted clinical guidelines [2]. It is widely acknowledged that underlying irregularities in metabolic health raise the risk of non-alcoholic fatty liver disease (NAFLD) and that it can coexist with other chronic disorders like diabetes and obesity. NAFLD is characterized by significant clinical heterogeneity [3].

The clinical spectrum of NAFLD begins with simple steatosis and can lead to liver cirrhosis, nonalcoholic steatohepatitis (NASH), and ultimately hepatocellular carcinoma (HCC). In the coming years, NASH, a complicated and multifactorial metabolic illness, is predicted to overtake the most common cause of liver transplants in the United States [4, 5]. It is also becoming a global health concern. As the fibrosis stage advances, especially with the prevalence of cirrhosis, the risk of all-cause mortality and the morbidity of NAFLD/NASH increase dramatically [6, 7]. According to estimates, 7–30% of individuals with NAFLD will develop NASH at some point in their lives [8]. Addressing the development of NASH can significantly aid in preventing the progression of NAFLD to more severe stages because liver damage is still reversible at this stage [9]. However, the presence of other comorbidities, such as metabolic syndrome, obesity, hyperglycemia, dyslipidemia, hypertension, insulin resistance, or dysbiosis, as well as lifestyle factors, such as diet, can alter this course [10].

Although age is acknowledged as a significant risk factor for non-alcoholic fatty liver disease (NAFLD), the rising incidence of juvenile obesity is raising concerns for kids and teenagers [11]. Individuals with a childhood onset of NASH may be more susceptible to an early or worse outcome [12]. Insulin sensitization, antioxidant medication, lifestyle changes (weight loss), and bariatric surgery are common therapeutic modalities for chronic metabolic liver disorders [13].

Effective cell-specific drug delivery offers a means to address the challenges and constraints in developing innovative treatments and may improve the efficacy of therapeutic drugs targeting the liver [14]. In this regard, the ability of nanomedicines to target specific cells offers unique opportunities for pharmacological control of the intricate interactions between proinflammatory and pro-resolution signals in chronic metabolic liver diseases. This chapter describes recent developments in nanomedicines and how the characteristics of nanoparticles (NPs) can be leveraged to enhance drug delivery and liver cell targeting, enabling new precision treatments and diagnostics for chronic liver diseases.

NPS AS DRUG-DELIVERY SYSTEMS

The field of nanomedicine is expanding rapidly and has the potential to deliver highly specific and effective treatments [15]. NPs, which are defined as entities up to 100 nm in a single dimension but can also encompass structures up to several hundred nanometers in diameter, are the building blocks of nanomedicines [16]. They can be created via bottom-up or self-assembly techniques, or a top-down process that uses mechanical force to create smaller particles from bigger compartments [17]. The administration of macromolecules and poorly water-soluble medications, combination therapy, tissue- or cell-specific drug delivery, and drug uptake across a variety of epithelial and endothelial barriers can all be facilitated by nanotechnology. By minimizing renal excretion and hepatic degradation, enabling "site-specific" drug delivery, raising the therapeutic index, and consequently lowering toxicity, nanomedicines' superiority over traditional medications enables them to extend the payload's circulation period [18]. The idea of nanomedicine is not limited to a straightforward drug delivery system; under the term "theranostics," a combination of therapeutic and diagnostic entities has been envisioned, establishing a framework for next-generation NPs that will facilitate drug transport, release, and noninvasive diagnostics [19]. Currently, the FDA or EMA has approved over 27 nanomedicines for clinical use [20]. Targeting/surface components, the encapsulated payload, and a core material make up organic, inorganic, or hybrid nanocarrier units employed in nanomedicine applications [21]. Small molecules, proteins, peptides, nucleic acids, and RNA oligonucleotides are just a few of the payloads that may be loaded into these NPs to enable either targeted or nontargeted distribution [22]. Therapeutic and diagnostic agents for a variety of disorders have been delivered using a wide range of nanostructures [23].

The advantages of nanocarriers are depicted in Fig. (**1**). Moreover, various types of nanosystems employed for therapeutic or diagnostic delivery to the liver, along with some of their fundamental characteristics, are briefly discussed in the following discussion.

Lipid Nanosystems

Nanostructured lipid carriers, liposomes, and solid lipid nanoparticles (SLNs) are the three categories of lipid nanosystems [24]. As liposomes can encapsulate medications regardless of their chemical properties and mimic the shape of the cell membrane, they appear to be a near-perfect drug-delivery method. Increased bioavailability, biodistribution, and degradability, together with decreased toxicity and antigenicity, are key benefits for their usage in clinical settings [25]. Lipid-based NPs are the most commonly used NPs in the clinic, ranging from Doxil and

OnpattroR to Pfizer/BioNTech and Moderna COVID-19 vaccines (Table **1**) [26]. By enhancing the distribution of hepatoprotective medications, nanostructured lipid carriers (NLCs) represent a promising nanotechnology for the treatment of fatty liver disease. NLCs reduce systemic toxicity by improving drug solubility and bioavailability, protecting encapsulated compounds from degradation, and enabling targeted delivery to liver tissue. Due to their biocompatibility, high drug-loading capacity, and adjustable release characteristics, they can be used to deliver synthetic medications and phytoconstituents to combat inflammation and oxidative stress that fuel the development of chronic liver illnesses, including nonalcoholic fatty liver disease. Drug concentrations in hepatic tissue can be improved by using NLCs to passively target the liver [27].

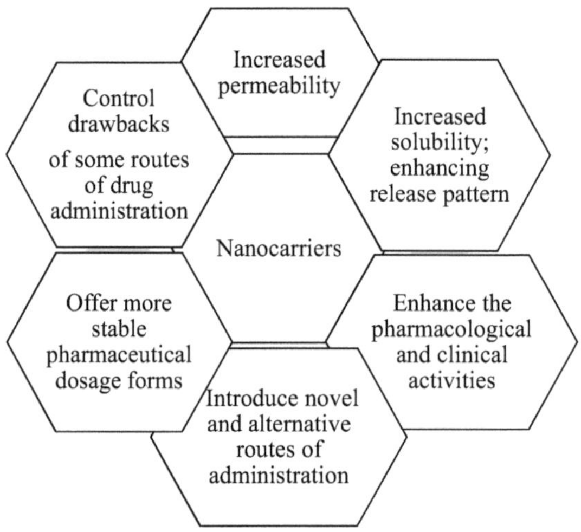

Fig. (1). Advantages of nanocarriers.

Table 1. Different types of NPs for clinical use.

Type of Nanocarriers	Therapeutic Payload	Targeting Mechanism	Key Findings	Reference
Lipid nanosystems	Silybin, polyphenols, lipid-lowering agents, nucleic acids	Interacting with the liver's microarchitecture and binding to serum proteins like Apolipoprotein E (ApoE), which then interact with LDL receptors on liver cells	Doxil and OnpattroR to Pfizer/BioNTech and Moderna COVID-19 vaccines.	[28]

(Table 1) cont.....

Type of Nanocarriers	Therapeutic Payload	Targeting Mechanism	Key Findings	Reference
Polymeric nanoparticles	Antioxidants, anti-inflammatory agents, metabolic modulators, and anti-steatotic compounds	Nanoparticles can be conjugated with ligands, such as lactobionic acid, for hepatocytes to improve liver accumulation.	Polymer-based nanocarriers that show promise for the specific delivery of therapeutic agents to treat HBV infection, NASH, hepatic fibrosis, HCC, and HVGD after LT.	[29]
Dendrimers	Gene therapy components, antioxidants, antifibrotic compounds	Encapsulation	Hydrophobic and hydrophilic drugs can be delivered, such as podophyllotoxin dendrimer conjugates; Demonstrated a significant reduction in liver histopathological changes, inflammatory markers (IL-6, NF-κB), and fibrotic tissue deposition in a preclinical model of liver cancer, which is often linked to chronic inflammation and fibrosis.	[30]
Nanoemulsion	Natural polyphenols (curcumin), plant oil (pomegranate seed oil), fatty acid oxidation promoters (BAM15)	Encapsulation	Enhanced bioavailability, improved delivery to the liver, and exerted antioxidant, anti-inflammatory, and lipid-lowering effects to combat fatty liver disease (NAFLD or MAFLD).	[31]
Exosome-based delivery systems	MicroRNAs (miRNAs, siRNA, DNA))	Exosomes act as messengers, transferring their genetic and protein cargo between liver cells (hepatocytes, Kupffer cells, HSCs, etc.). These cell-derived vesicles exhibit high biocompatibility and low immunogenicity, allowing them to safely reach their target cells without triggering a strong immune response.	Reduce fibrosis and proteins that modulate inflammation and lipid metabolism.	[32]

(Table 1) cont.....

Type of Nanocarriers	Therapeutic Payload	Targeting Mechanism	Key Findings	Reference
Liposomes	Silibinin, astaxanthin, fenofibrate, naringenin, and taurine	Encapsulation	Targeted to liver cells for enhanced efficacy and reduced side effects, showing promise for treating hepatic steatosis, inflammation, and fibrosis associated with fatty liver disease.	[33]

Polymeric NPs

Natural or synthetic polymers can physically or covalently combine to form polymeric nanoparticles. Among them, poly (lactic-co-glycolic acid) (PLGA) is the most widely used material for biomedical applications. Other synthetic polymers that are often used and approved by the FDA and EMA include poly (D, L-lactide) (PLA) and poly (D, L-glycolide) (PLG) [34]. Polymeric nanoparticles have two main advantages: they can promote preferential accumulation at a given site by forming conjugates with tissue-specific ligands, and they favor regulated, sustained drug release to enable functionally tailored administration [35]. Polymeric NPs come in several forms, including dendrimers, chitosan, alginate, polymeric micelles, and polymer–protein or polysaccharide-based NPs [36].

Inorganic NPs

Examples of inorganic NPs include iron oxide (IO), zinc, calcium phosphate, metallic NPs (silver, gold, copper, platinum), carbon nanotubes, quantum dots, cerium oxide, and silica NPs [37]. Due to their small size, they exhibit higher perfusion rates, which make their physical, optical, and chemical features significant for applications, such as tissue imaging and diagnostics, less-hazardous drug delivery in biodegradable inorganic NPs, and reduced drug dosages for cancer treatments [38]. Few inorganic NPs, apart from IO NPs, have received approval for clinical use and are still in the early stages of translation to the clinic [39].

Nanogels

Cross-linked nanostructures, known as nanogels, form a three-dimensional network with swelling and viscoelastic characteristics [40]. They are created from synthetic and/or biopolymer precursors, or they are manufactured by heterogeneous polymerization of monomers, and consist of a core shell with a high capacity for payload and water retention [41].

Dendrimers

As evidenced by galactose-conjugated dendrimers, which effectively transport N-acetyl cysteine to repair liver damage, dendrimers exhibit potential for treating fatty liver disease by serving as nanocarriers for targeted drug delivery, specifically to liver cells. To ensure the therapeutic payload reaches the liver, dendrimers can be modified to carry specific molecules, such as galactose, which bind to receptors on liver cells. Drugs can be encapsulated and protected by their unique three-dimensional structures, which feature interior cavities, thereby increasing their stability and bioavailability. Additionally, medications can be attached to dendrimers to enable regulated, prolonged release, thereby improving treatment efficacy. Research indicates that galactose-conjugated dendrimers may repair acetaminophen-induced liver damage by efficiently delivering NAC to the liver, suggesting the possibility of more widespread liver disease. Dendrimers may provide a means of more precisely targeting and delivering treatments to treat or reverse non-alcoholic fatty liver disease (NAFLD), a leading cause of chronic liver disease. By addressing problems of limited bioavailability and poor water solubility, dendrimers can improve the transport and therapeutic efficacy of natural products, which are frequently used for the treatment of chronic disorders, including those affecting the liver [42].

Nanoemulsion

Nanoemulsions enhance the transport, solubility, and bioavailability of therapeutic compounds to the liver; therefore, they represent a promising nanotechnology for the treatment of fatty liver disease (NAFLD). They may be made to target the liver passively, increasing effectiveness and possibly lowering adverse effects. Due to their nanoscale size, these tiny oil-in-water droplets have a vast surface area, which is advantageous for encapsulating medications and enhancing their release. By mimicking the natural mechanisms of fat absorption, certain nanoemulsion designs can pass through mucous membranes, be absorbed by gastrointestinal epithelial cells, and ultimately accumulate in the liver. They can enhance the therapeutic benefits of natural chemicals with low bioavailability and poor solubility, such as polyphenols, flavonoids, and essential oils, by encapsulating and delivering them. By shielding medicinal substances from gastrointestinal degradation, the nanoemulsion can improve their stability and ensure they reach their intended target. Turmeric extracts and other botanical substances with anti-inflammatory and antioxidant qualities that are helpful in NAFLD can be delivered by nanoemulsions. To enhance targeted liver delivery, scientists are creating “stiff-soft hybrid biomimetic nano-emulsions” that resemble chylomicrons, which are particles involved in fat absorption [43].

Exosomes

Exosomes serve as both therapeutic agents and diagnostic biomarkers for the treatment of non-alcoholic fatty liver disease (NAFLD). Exosomes derived from stem cells may offer a novel treatment option for non-alcoholic fatty liver disease (NAFLD) by promoting fatty acid oxidation, inhibiting fatty acid synthesis, and reducing inflammation. These are potential diagnostic biomarkers because they can transport specific molecules, such as exosomal microRNAs (miRNAs), that reflect the presence and various stages of NAFLD. Better disease monitoring and management are enabled by exosomal miRNAs' ability to distinguish between different stages of NAFLD [44].

Natural extracellular vesicles called exosomes can be altered and manufactured to transport therapeutic payloads, like proteins and RNAs, to specific liver cells. Exosomes produced by stem cells can transport beneficial molecules that support liver tissue regeneration and repair. By upregulating genes involved in fatty acid oxidation and downregulating genes involved in fatty acid synthesis, they can reduce liver damage and prevent fat accumulation. To reduce the inflammatory milieu associated with NAFLD, these exosomes can transport cytokines and anti-inflammatory molecules, including IL-10, to the liver [45].

BIOLOGICAL, PHYSICOCHEMICAL, AND TOXICOLOGICAL CONSIDERATIONS WHEN DESIGNING A DRUG-DELIVERY SYSTEM

Nanomedicine has revolutionized the biomedical field, but it is crucial to remember that experimental therapeutics based on nanotechnology still face obstacles and hurdles before they can be clinically translated for chronic liver diseases. The physicochemical properties of nanocarrier-based delivery systems significantly impact cellular uptake, biodistribution, blood circulation half-life, and activity [46]. Our current understanding of the anatomy, pathophysiology, and molecular etiology of various diseases has provided a framework for identifying the optimal features of potential delivery agents and adjusting NP size, shape, and surface characteristics for specific therapeutic and diagnostic purposes [47].

Biodistribution

The use of nanoscale delivery systems for the diagnosis and treatment of liver diseases appears promising, as evidenced by the empirical observation that injected NPs tend to accumulate to higher levels in the liver than in other tissues [48]. This is explained by the liver's first-pass action and its significant function in the detoxification, metabolism, and excretion of xenobiotics [49]. The portal vein and hepatic artery are the routes by which NPs enter the liver. It has been demonstrated that as NPs travel through the liver sinusoids, their blood velocity decreases, resulting in prolonged interaction with liver cells [50]. The various types of liver cells have been observed to absorb NPs in a hierarchical manner; in fact, the macrophages known as Kupffer cells appear to be the main cells that absorb NPs, followed by hepatic stellate cells (HSCs) and liver sinusoidal endothelial cells (LSECs). However, delivery to hepatocytes is less favorable (see the section on "active liver targeting") [51]. Protein binding at the NPs' surface may significantly impact their retention and, in particular, promote opsonization, which activates the immune system by triggering macrophage recognition. Certain surface modifications have been tested to reduce the recruitment of blood proteins because hydrophobic materials are more likely to opsonize than hydrophilic ones [52].To further lessen opsonization, natural polymers, such as polysaccharides (like chitosan, heparin, or dextran), could be used [53].

Cellular Uptake and Biocompatibility

The cellular uptake of designed NPs is enhanced by multiple mechanisms, such as receptor-mediated endocytosis, pinocytosis, and phagocytosis, which are preferred for large-diameter particles (<500 nm) and depend on particle size and surface modifications [54]. The majority of therapeutic NPs for liver illnesses are smaller than 100 nm to penetrate the 100–200 nm-wide hepatic sinusoidal intravascular space and target hepatocytes, Kupffer cells, LSECs, and HSCs [55]. NPs less than 3 nm can enter hepatocytes from the Disse space, whereas NPs larger than 150 nm are typically taken up by Kupffer cells [56]. All things considered, these investigations highlight how NP size affects the targeting of liver cellular populations. Another important aspect influencing NPs' cellular absorption and biocompatibility is their surface charge. Zeta potential, often known as ζ-potential, is a physical parameter that represents the growing charge at the interface between a solid surface and its liquid surroundings. From a clinical standpoint, NPs are more suitable for testing because of their greater stability at a ζ-potential of ±30 mV [57]. Faster opsonization rates and greater contact with macrophages in vitro are driven by the highly cationic and anionic NPs' propensity to bind substantial amounts of serum proteins and form a protein corona [58]. Macrophage uptake of polymeric NPs appears to increase when the surface charge becomes more positive or negative, according to models of negatively and positively charged polymeric NPs [59]. Therefore, to regulate NPs' excretion rates and biodistribution, their surface charge must be adjusted [60]. When applied to Zedoary turmeric oil (ZTO)- loaded SLNs, the chitosan coating reversed the negative charge of the ZTO-SLNs, enhancing their targeted liver distribution relative to other tissues and increasing their bioavailability [61]. Liver-targeting NPs with negative surface charges are also occasionally explored. The accumulation of cationic GNPs in the liver was much smaller than that of anionic ones, according to research on the biodistribution of intravenously injected 2.8 nm GNPs.The ability of Kupffer and endothelial cells to absorb anionic NPs by binding to scavenger receptors on their membranes may help explain these results. However, NPs with positively charged surfaces are more likely to be absorbed by hepatocytes [62].

NP Kinetics

Random collisions with leukocytes and red blood cells, as well as forces that influence the particle's rotational motion in the bloodstream, affect the behavior and kinetics of NPs *in vivo* [63]. As a result, NP shape is a crucial factor in both their adherence to the target site's endothelium and their margination from the bloodstream to the vessel wall region [64]. NPs of the first generation were spherical, but as materials science and nanotechnology have advanced, it has become possible to manufacture NPs with other geometries and physical properties. Computational techniques have been developed to assess and forecast the uptake and *in vivo* biodistribution of drug carriers in discoidal, cube, rod, ellipsoid, and cylindrical forms [65]. However, several studies further support the idea that elongated NPs often have a long blood circulation half-life [66].

Toxicological Concerns

The surface charge is linked to the possible cytotoxicity of NPs, in addition to its effect on cellular uptake. Despite their improved drug-delivery effectiveness, cationic nanoparticles have been shown to pose a higher risk of membrane damage [67]. Although the resulting cationic formulations of superparamagnetic IO NPs (SPIONs) with their surfaces modified by didodecyldimethyl-ammoniu--bromide (DMAB) were found to be more toxicologically safe than the non-modified SPION controls, a significant increase in the accumulation of SPION-TPGS in the liver *in vivo* was linked to a genotoxicity that was reversible after treatment termination [68]. Conversely, cationic curdlan derivatives, which have been demonstrated to be cytotoxic and unsuitable for *in vivo* research but have a high payload-delivery capacity, may be chemically modified to increase the formulations' biocompatibility while causing the least cell damage. Compared with the control non-PEGylated formulations, positively charged PEGylated 6-amino-6-deoxy-curdlan derivatives demonstrated greater liver accumulation and were more toxicologically safe [69].

NANOMEDICINE IN NAFLD DIAGNOSIS

Since certain clinical characteristics, including inflammation or hepatocyte ballooning, are not effectively captured by imaging techniques, liver biopsy has been the standard for diagnosing and assessing NASH [70]. However, there are now more affordable and noninvasive options available. For diagnostic applications, IO-based magnetic nanoparticles (NPs) smaller than 30 nm, known as SPIONs, are of great interest. New-generation hepatic MRI contrast agents have been developed using SPIONs, such as magnetite (Fe_3O_4) or γ-Fe_2O, which are characterized by significant liver accumulation due to phagocytic Kupffer cells. In the noninvasive assessment of NASH staging and the differentiation of NASH patients from those with NAFLD, SPION-enhanced MRI initially demonstrated encouraging outcomes [71]. Strawberry-like Fe_3O_4-Au NPs were used as CT-MRI dual-modality contrast agents for in vivo testing in fatty and cirrhotic liver and in HCC, and they were found to be highly biocompatible and suitable for future clinical use. In a rat model, NPs conjugated with a cyclic arginine–glycine–aspartic acid octapeptide to target avß34 expressed on activated HSCs, along with a PLGA modification, were used to encapsulate perfluorooctyl bromide and function as an ultrasound contrast agent to diagnose the various stages of liver fibrosis [72].

Nanomedicine for NAFLD Therapeutics

NAFLD and NASH are two types of chronic liver disorders with pressing unmet requirements [73]. As NPs are promising drug delivery systems, some treatment strategies currently in development use them to mediate the inhibition of HSC activation, reduction of inflammation, reversal of scar tissue formation, and interference at key signaling pathways involved in liver pathogenesis. Both passive targeting, which leverages NP physiochemical properties to concentrate in the liver, and active targeting, which employs specific ligands that bind to a favorable cell population [74], can be used to achieve targeted NP delivery. We discuss in more detail later some of the attempts to use these technologies to deliver various payloads to liver cells for the development of innovative therapies for liver disease.

FUTURE PERSPECTIVE

Obesity, Type 2 diabetes, insulin resistance, genetic susceptibility, dietary habits, and physical activity are some of the risk factors that significantly influence the pathophysiology and development of metabolic chronic liver disorders [75].

Recent developments in systemic approaches that combine transcriptomics, proteomics, metabolomics, and epigenetic analyses will aid in identifying new biomarkers and targets, as well as help to unravel the molecular signatures of chronic liver pathologies. This will enable early diagnosis and customized treatments tailored to each patient's unique metabolic profile. The etiology and development of metabolic chronic liver illnesses are greatly influenced by a number of risk factors, including genetic predisposition, insulin resistance, obesity, Type 2 diabetes, dietary practices, and physical activity. In addition to uncovering the molecular signatures of chronic liver pathologies, recent advancements in systemic approaches integrating transcriptomics, proteomics, metabolomics, and epigenetic investigations will also help discover new biomarkers and targets. This will enable early diagnosis and treatment tailored to each patient's metabolic profile [76]. SERS spectra point to a very promising noninvasive method for distinguishing early steatosis from NASH. According to one lipidomic technique, it is feasible and clinically meaningful to distinguish among the various histological classifications in the NAFLD spectrum using a panel of 20 plasma metabolites. Lastly, additional epigenomic research can help us identify risk factors and predict disease course. We believe that cooperation across disciplines will aid the development of next-generation treatments for metabolic chronic diseases. Unlocking the potential of nanomedicines for safer, more effective, and controlled drug delivery, as well as leveraging cutting-edge technologies for targeted identification and selection, may complement current approaches to treating chronic liver diseases and support long-term treatment plans.

CONCLUSION

The key to managing NAFLD is early diagnosis, as there is currently no pharmacological intervention to prevent progression to later stages [77]. To facilitate screening and encourage more patients to participate in clinical trials, future research efforts must develop noninvasive, high-resolution procedures beyond liver biopsy for diagnostic and staging purposes. This can therefore enhance patient care and advance our understanding of disease progression. The intricate pathophysiology and biology underlying metabolic chronic liver disorders contribute to the inadequate effectiveness of conventional, nonspecific therapies. For chronic liver illnesses, current traditional pharmacological treatments necessitate continuous drug delivery to attain high bioavailability, which increases toxicity [78]. Poor solubility, which limits the translational potential of promising therapeutic agents in preclinical studies, is one of the main reasons treatments tested in clinical trials fail to meet the primary endpoints when used as monotherapy for chronic liver diseases. At the end of 2020, the approval of two COVID-19 vaccines, mRNA-1273 and BNT162b, that use lipid NPs to deliver antigen mRNA, highlighted the great value of nanocarriers as a safe and effective drug-delivery method. In numerous preclinical investigations for chronic liver illnesses, various nanocarriers have demonstrated diagnostic and therapeutic potential, indicating a means of bridging the gap between bench and bedside. Phase I clinical trials for liver fibrosis (NCT02227459) and HCC (NCT04682847 and NCT01437007) are used to evaluate nanomedicine formulations; nevertheless, additional testing and optimization are still needed to improve patient outcomes. By providing an alternative pathway for medications to enter cells, nanocarriers overcome the limitations of medicinal substances' limited solubility and achieve a better balance between therapeutic efficacy and toxicity [79]. Designing delivery methods with optimal physicochemical properties to enhance the effectiveness of existing treatments requires an understanding of NP systemic behavior and interactions with hepatic cell populations and the immune system.

LIST OF ABBREVIATIONS

ALT Alanine Transaminase

AE Apolipoprotein E

DMAB Didodecyl dimethylammonium bromide

GNP Gold Nanoparticles

HCV Hepatis C virus

HBV Hepatitis B virus

HSC Hepatic stellate cells

HCC Hepatocellular carcinoma

HVGD Host Versus Graft Disease

IO Iron oxide

LEEC Liver sinusoidal endothelial cells

LTLD Lyso-thermosensitive liposomal doxorubicin

LT Liver Transplantation

MAFLD Metabolic Dysfunction-Associated Fatty Liver Disease

NAFLD Non-alcoholic fatty liver disease

NASH Non-alcoholic steatohepatitis

NP Nanoparticles

ROS Reactive Oxygen Species

ZTO Zedoary turmeric oil

REFERENCES

[1] Younossi Z, Anstee QM, Marietti M, *et al.* Global burden of NAFLD and NASH: trends, predictions, risk factors and prevention. Nat Rev Gastroenterol Hepatol 2018; 15(1): 11-20. [http://dx.doi.org/10.1038/nrgastro.2017.109] [PMID: 28930295]

[2] Lazarus JV, Mark HE, Anstee QM, *et al.* Advancing the global public health agenda for NAFLD: a consensus statement. Nat Rev Gastroenterol Hepatol 2022; 19(1): 60-78. [http://dx.doi.org/10.1038/s41575-021-00523-4] [PMID: 34707258]

[3] Adams LA, Anstee QM, Tilg H, Targher G. Non-alcoholic fatty liver disease and its relationship with cardiovascular disease and other extrahepatic diseases. Gut 2017; 66(6): 1138-53. [http://dx.doi.org/10.1136/gutjnl-2017-313884] [PMID: 28314735]

[4] Sharma S, Sharma A, Gupta P, *et al.* The Green Path to Liver Health: Herbal Solutions for Non-alcoholic Steatohepatitis. Cardiovasc Hematol Disord Drug Targets 2025; 25(3): 168-92. [http://dx.doi.org/10.2174/011871529X360903250211101856] [PMID: 40108906]

[5] Wong RJ, Aguilar M, Cheung R, *et al.* Nonalcoholic steatohepatitis is the second leading etiology of liver disease among adults awaiting liver transplantation in the United States. Gastroenterology 2015; 148(3): 547-55. [http://dx.doi.org/10.1053/j.gastro.2014.11.039] [PMID: 25461851]

[6] Goldberg D, Ditah IC, Saeian K, Lalehzari M, Aronsohn A, Gorospe EC, Charlton M. Changes in the Prevalence of Hepatitis C Virus Infection, Nonalcoholic Steatohepatitis, and Alcoholic Liver Disease Among Patients With Cirrhosis or Liver Failure on the Waitlist for Liver Transplantation. Gastroenterology. 2017 Apr;152(5):1090-1099.

[7] Schuppan D, Surabattula R, Wang XY. Determinants of fibrosis progression and regression in NASH. J Hepatol 2018; 68(2): 238-50. [http://dx.doi.org/10.1016/j.jhep.2017.11.012] [PMID: 29154966]

[8] Cotter TG, Rinella M. Nonalcoholic fatty liver disease 2020: the state of the disease. Gastroenterology 2020; 158(7): 1851-64. [http://dx.doi.org/10.1053/j.gastro.2020.01.052] [PMID: 32061595]

[9] Wattacheril J, Issa D, Sanyal A. Nonalcoholic steatohepatitis (NASH) and hepatic fibrosis: emerging therapies. Annu Rev Pharmacol Toxicol 2018; 58(1): 649-62. [http://dx.doi.org/10.1146/annurev-pharmtox-010617-052545] [PMID: 29058997]

[10] Eslam M, Valenti L, Romeo S. Genetics and epigenetics of NAFLD and NASH: Clinical impact. J Hepatol 2018; 68(2): 268-79. [http://dx.doi.org/10.1016/j.jhep.2017.09.003] [PMID: 29122391]

[11] Vilar-Gomez E, Martinez-Perez Y, Calzadilla-Bertot L, *et al.* Weight loss through lifestyle modification significantly reduces features of nonalcoholic steatohepatitis. Gastroenterology 2015; 149(2): 367-378.e5. [http://dx.doi.org/10.1053/j.gastro.2015.04.005] [PMID: 25865049]

[12] Friedman SL, Neuschwander-Tetri BA, Rinella M, Sanyal AJ. Mechanisms of NAFLD development and therapeutic strategies. Nat Med 2018; 24(7): 908-22. [http://dx.doi.org/10.1038/s41591-018-0104-9] [PMID: 29967350]

[13] Buzzetti E, Pinzani M, Tsochatzis EA. The multiple-hit pathogenesis of non-alcoholic fatty liver disease (NAFLD). Metabolism 2016; 65(8): 1038-48. [http://dx.doi.org/10.1016/j.metabol.2015.12.012] [PMID: 26823198]

[14] BasuRay S, Smagris E, Cohen JC, Hobbs HH. The PNPLA3 variant associated with fatty liver disease (I148M) accumulates on lipid droplets by evading ubiquitylation. Hepatology 2017; 66(4): 1111-24. [http://dx.doi.org/10.1002/hep.29273] [PMID: 28520213]

[15] Abul-Husn NS, Cheng X, Li AH, *et al.* A protein-truncating HSD17B13 variant and protection from chronic liver disease. N Engl J Med 2018; 378(12): 1096-106.

[http://dx.doi.org/10.1056/NEJMoa1712191] [PMID: 29562163]

[16] Danford CJ, Yao ZM, Jiang ZG. Non-alcoholic fatty liver disease: a narrative review of genetics. J Biomed Res 2018; 32(5): 389-400.
[PMID: 30355853]

[17] Daryani NE, Daryani NE, Alavian SM, *et al.* Non-alcoholic steatohepatitis and influence of age and gender on histopathologic findings. World J Gastroenterol 2010; 16(33): 4169-75.
[http://dx.doi.org/10.3748/wjg.v16.i33.4169] [PMID: 20806434]

[18] Della Corte C, Alisi A, Saccari A, De Vito R, Vania A, Nobili V. Nonalcoholic fatty liver in children and adolescents: an overview. J Adolesc Health 2012; 51(4): 305-12.
[http://dx.doi.org/10.1016/j.jadohealth.2012.01.010] [PMID: 22999829]

[19] Temple J, Cordero P, Li J, Nguyen V, Oben J. A guide to non-alcoholic fatty liver disease in childhood and adolescence. Int J Mol Sci 2016; 17(6): 947.
[http://dx.doi.org/10.3390/ijms17060947] [PMID: 27314342]

[20] Stengel JZ, Harrison SA. Nonalcoholic steatohepatitis: clinical presentation, diagnosis, and treatment. Gastroenterol Hepatol (N Y) 2006; 2(6): 440-9.
[PMID: 28316519]

[21] Ferguson D, Finck BN. Emerging therapeutic approaches for the treatment of NAFLD and type 2 diabetes mellitus. Nat Rev Endocrinol 2021; 17(8): 484-95.
[http://dx.doi.org/10.1038/s41574-021-00507-z] [PMID: 34131333]

[22] Kang JH, Toita R, Murata M. Liver cell-targeted delivery of therapeutic molecules. Crit Rev Biotechnol 2016; 36(1): 132-43.
[http://dx.doi.org/10.3109/07388551.2014.930017] [PMID: 25025274]

[23] Patra JK, Das G, Fraceto LF, *et al.* Nano based drug delivery systems: recent developments and future prospects. J Nanobiotechnology 2018; 16(1): 71.
[http://dx.doi.org/10.1186/s12951-018-0392-8] [PMID: 30231877]

[24] Farokhzad OC, Langer R. Impact of nanotechnology on drug delivery. ACS Nano 2009; 3(1): 16-20.
[http://dx.doi.org/10.1021/nn900002m] [PMID: 19206243]

[25] Kumar R, Dalvi SV, Siril PF. Nanoparticle-based drugs and formulations: current status and emerging applications. ACS Appl Nano Mater 2020; 3(6): 4944-61.
[http://dx.doi.org/10.1021/acsanm.0c00606]

[26] Rizzo LY, Theek B, Storm G, Kiessling F, Lammers T. Recent progress in nanomedicine: therapeutic, diagnostic and theranostic applications. Curr Opin Biotechnol 2013; 24(6): 1159-66.
[http://dx.doi.org/10.1016/j.copbio.2013.02.020] [PMID: 23578464]

[27] Lammers T, Aime S, Hennink WE, Storm G, Kiessling F. Theranostic Nanomedicine. Acc Chem Res 2011; 44(10): 1029-38.
[http://dx.doi.org/10.1021/ar200019c] [PMID: 21545096]

[28] Anselmo AC, Mitragotri S. Nanoparticles in the clinic: An update. Bioeng Transl Med 2019; 4(3): e10143.
[http://dx.doi.org/10.1002/btm2.10143] [PMID: 31572799]

[29] Jabr-Milane L, van Vlerken L, Devalapally H, *et al.* Multi-functional nanocarriers for targeted delivery of drugs and genes. J Control Release 2008; 130(2): 121-8.
[http://dx.doi.org/10.1016/j.jconrel.2008.04.016] [PMID: 18538887]

[30] Ross KA, Brenza TM, Binnebose AM, *et al.* Nano-enabled delivery of diverse payloads across complex biological barriers. J Control Release 2015; 219: 548-59.
[http://dx.doi.org/10.1016/j.jconrel.2015.08.039] [PMID: 26315817]

[31] Chamundeeswari M, Jeslin J, Verma ML. Nanocarriers for drug delivery applications. Environ Chem Lett 2019; 17(2): 849-65.

[http://dx.doi.org/10.1007/s10311-018-00841-1]

[32] Onoue S, Yamada S, Chan K. Nanodrugs: pharmacokinetics and safety. Int J Nanomedicine 2014; 9: 1025-37.
[http://dx.doi.org/10.2147/IJN.S38378] [PMID: 24591825]

[33] Bozzuto G, Molinari A. Liposomes as nanomedical devices. Int J Nanomedicine 2015; 10: 975-99.
[http://dx.doi.org/10.2147/IJN.S68861] [PMID: 25678787]

[34] Thi TTH, Suys EJA, Lee JS, Nguyen DH, Park KD, Truong NP. Lipid-based nanoparticles in the clinic and clinical trials: from cancer nanomedicine to COVID-19 vaccines. Vaccines (Basel) 2021; 9(4): 359.
[http://dx.doi.org/10.3390/vaccines9040359] [PMID: 33918072]

[35] Schoenmaker L, Witzigmann D, Kulkarni JA, *et al.* mRNA-lipid nanoparticle COVID-19 vaccines: Structure and stability. Int J Pharm 2021; 601: 120586.
[http://dx.doi.org/10.1016/j.ijpharm.2021.120586] [PMID: 33839230]

[36] Gagliardi A, Giuliano E, Venkateswararao E, *et al.* Biodegradable polymeric nanoparticles for drug delivery to solid tumors. Front Pharmacol 2021; 12: 601626.
[http://dx.doi.org/10.3389/fphar.2021.601626] [PMID: 33613290]

[37] Bennet D, Kim S. Polymer nanoparticles for smart drug delivery. Application of nanotechnology in drug delivery. 2014 Jul 25; 8.
[http://dx.doi.org/10.5772/58422]

[38] Aula S, Lakkireddy S, Jamil K, Kapley A, Swamy AVN, Lakkireddy HR. Biophysical, biopharmaceutical and toxicological significance of biomedical nanoparticles. RSC Advances 2015; 5(59): 47830-59.
[http://dx.doi.org/10.1039/C5RA05889A]

[39] Paul W, Sharma CP. Inorganic nanoparticles for targeted drug delivery. Biointegration of medical implant materials. 2020 Jan 1:333-73.
[http://dx.doi.org/10.1016/B978-0-08-102680-9.00013-5]

[40] Mitchell MJ, Billingsley MM, Haley RM, Wechsler ME, Peppas NA, Langer R. Engineering precision nanoparticles for drug delivery. Nat Rev Drug Discov 2021; 20(2): 101-24.
[http://dx.doi.org/10.1038/s41573-020-0090-8] [PMID: 33277608]

[41] Suhail M, Rosenholm JM, Minhas MU, *et al.* Nanogels as drug-delivery systems: a comprehensive overview. Ther Deliv 2019; 10(11): 697-717.
[http://dx.doi.org/10.4155/tde-2019-0010] [PMID: 31789106]

[42] Dhapte V, Pokharkar V. Nanosystems for drug delivery: Design, engineering, and applications. InGreen Synthesis, Characterization and Applications of Nanoparticles 2019 Jan 1 (pp. 321-345). Elsevier.

[43] Mahajan HS, Patil PH. Gel-based delivery of neurotherapeutics via naso-brain pathways. In: Direct Nose-to-Brain Drug Delivery. Academic Press; 2021:225–245.
[http://dx.doi.org/10.1016/B978-0-12-822522-6.00026-6]

[44] Soares S, Sousa J, Pais A, Vitorino C. Nanomedicine: principles, properties, and regulatory issues. Front Chem 2018; 6: 360.
[http://dx.doi.org/10.3389/fchem.2018.00360] [PMID: 30177965]

[45] Kamaly N, He JC, Ausiello DA, Farokhzad OC. Nanomedicines for renal disease: current status and future applications. Nat Rev Nephrol 2016; 12(12): 738-53.
[http://dx.doi.org/10.1038/nrneph.2016.156] [PMID: 27795549]

[46] Hoshyar N, Gray S, Han H, Bao G. The effect of nanoparticle size on in vivo pharmacokinetics and cellular interaction. Nanomedicine (Lond) 2016; 11(6): 673-92.
[http://dx.doi.org/10.2217/nnm.16.5] [PMID: 27003448]

[47] Park JK, Utsumi T, Seo YE, *et al.* Cellular distribution of injected PLGA-nanoparticles in the liver. Nanomedicine 2016; 12(5): 1365-74.
[http://dx.doi.org/10.1016/j.nano.2016.01.013] [PMID: 26961463]

[48] Poelstra K, Prakash J, Beljaars L. Drug targeting to the diseased liver. J Control Release 2012; 161(2): 188-97.
[http://dx.doi.org/10.1016/j.jconrel.2012.02.011] [PMID: 22370583]

[49] Tsoi KM, MacParland SA, Ma XZ, *et al.* Mechanism of hard-nanomaterial clearance by the liver. Nat Mater 2016; 15(11): 1212-21.
[http://dx.doi.org/10.1038/nmat4718] [PMID: 27525571]

[50] Ngo W, Ahmed S, Blackadar C, *et al.* Why nanoparticles prefer liver macrophage cell uptake in vivo. Adv Drug Deliv Rev 2022; 185: 114238.
[http://dx.doi.org/10.1016/j.addr.2022.114238] [PMID: 35367524]

[51] Weaver JL, Tobin GA, Ingle T, *et al.* Evaluating the potential of gold, silver, and silica nanoparticles to saturate mononuclear phagocytic system tissues under repeat dosing conditions. Part Fibre Toxicol 2017; 14(1): 25.
[http://dx.doi.org/10.1186/s12989-017-0206-4] [PMID: 28716104]

[52] Ezhilarasan D. Advantages and challenges in nanomedicines for chronic liver diseases: A hepatologist's perspectives. Eur J Pharmacol 2021; 893: 173832.
[http://dx.doi.org/10.1016/j.ejphar.2020.173832] [PMID: 33359144]

[53] Baboci L, Capolla S, Di Cintio F, *et al.* The dual role of the liver in nanomedicine as an actor in the elimination of nanostructures or a therapeutic target. J Oncol 2020; 2020(1): 1-15.
[http://dx.doi.org/10.1155/2020/4638192] [PMID: 32184825]

[54] Nguyen VH, Lee BJ. Protein corona: a new approach for nanomedicine design. Int J Nanomedicine 2017; 12: 3137-51.
[http://dx.doi.org/10.2147/IJN.S129300] [PMID: 28458536]

[55] Adabi M, Naghibzadeh M, Adabi M, *et al.* Biocompatibility and nanostructured materials: applications in nanomedicine. Artif Cells Nanomed Biotechnol 2017; 45(4): 833-42.
[http://dx.doi.org/10.1080/21691401.2016.1178134] [PMID: 27247194]

[56] Fattal E, Tsapis N. Nanomedicine technology: current achievements and new trends. Clin Transl Imaging 2014; 2(1): 77-87.
[http://dx.doi.org/10.1007/s40336-014-0053-3]

[57] Li SD, Huang L. Nanoparticles evading the reticuloendothelial system: Role of the supported bilayer. Biochim Biophys Acta Biomembr 2009; 1788(10): 2259-66.
[http://dx.doi.org/10.1016/j.bbamem.2009.06.022] [PMID: 19595666]

[58] Patlolla AK, Shinde AK, Tchounwou PB. A comparison of poly-ethylene-glycol-coated and uncoated gold nanoparticle-mediated hepatotoxicity and oxidative stress in Sprague Dawley rats. Int J Nanomedicine 2019; 14: 639-47.
[http://dx.doi.org/10.2147/IJN.S185574] [PMID: 30697047]

[59] Zhang S, Gao H, Bao G. Physical principles of nanoparticle cellular endocytosis. ACS Nano 2015; 9(9): 8655-71.
[http://dx.doi.org/10.1021/acsnano.5b03184] [PMID: 26256227]

[60] Zhao J, Stenzel MH. Entry of nanoparticles into cells: the importance of nanoparticle properties. Polym Chem 2018; 9(3): 259-72.
[http://dx.doi.org/10.1039/C7PY01603D]

[61] Wang HX, Xiong MH, Wang YC, Zhu J, Wang J. N-acetylgalactosamine functionalized mixed micellar nanoparticles for targeted delivery of siRNA to liver. J Control Release 2013; 166(2): 106-14.
[http://dx.doi.org/10.1016/j.jconrel.2012.12.017] [PMID: 23266452]

[62] Li L, Wang H, Ong ZY, *et al.* Polymer- and lipid-based nanoparticle therapeutics for the treatment of liver diseases. Nano Today 2010; 5(4): 296-312. [http://dx.doi.org/10.1016/j.nantod.2010.06.007]

[63] Zhang YN, Poon W, Tavares AJ, McGilvray ID, Chan WCW. Nanoparticle–liver interactions: Cellular uptake and hepatobiliary elimination. J Control Release 2016; 240: 332-48. [http://dx.doi.org/10.1016/j.jconrel.2016.01.020] [PMID: 26774224]

[64] Ibrahim KE, Al-Mutary MG, Bakhiet AO, Khan HA. Histopathology of the liver, kidney, and spleen of mice exposed to gold nanoparticles. Molecules 2018; 23(8): 1848. [http://dx.doi.org/10.3390/molecules23081848] [PMID: 30044410]

[65] Qi L, Xu Z, Chen M. *In vitro* and *in vivo* suppression of hepatocellular carcinoma growth by chitosan nanoparticles. Eur J Cancer 2007; 43(1): 184-93. [http://dx.doi.org/10.1016/j.ejca.2006.08.029] [PMID: 17049839]

[66] Huang J, Bu L, Xie J, *et al.* Effects of nanoparticle size on cellular uptake and liver MRI with polyvinylpyrrolidone-coated iron oxide nanoparticles. ACS Nano 2010; 4(12): 7151-60. [http://dx.doi.org/10.1021/nn101643u] [PMID: 21043459]

[67] Branda F, Silvestri B, Costantini A, Luciani G. Effect of exposure to growth media on size and surface charge of silica based Stöber nanoparticles: a DLS and ζ-potential study. J Sol-Gel Sci Technol 2015; 73(1): 54-61. [http://dx.doi.org/10.1007/s10971-014-3494-2]

[68] Joseph E, Singhvi G. Multifunctional nanocrystals for cancer therapy: a potential nanocarrier. Nanomaterials for drug delivery and therapy. 2019 Jan 1:91-116. [http://dx.doi.org/10.1016/B978-0-12-816505-8.00007-2]

[69] He C, Hu Y, Yin L, Tang C, Yin C. Effects of particle size and surface charge on cellular uptake and biodistribution of polymeric nanoparticles. Biomaterials 2010; 31(13): 3657-66. [http://dx.doi.org/10.1016/j.biomaterials.2010.01.065] [PMID: 20138662]

[70] Xiao K, Li Y, Luo J, *et al.* The effect of surface charge on in vivo biodistribution of PEG-oligocholic acid based micellar nanoparticles. Biomaterials 2011; 32(13): 3435-46. [http://dx.doi.org/10.1016/j.biomaterials.2011.01.021] [PMID: 21295849]

[71] Albanese A, Tang PS, Chan WCW. The effect of nanoparticle size, shape, and surface chemistry on biological systems. Annu Rev Biomed Eng 2012; 14(1): 1-16. [http://dx.doi.org/10.1146/annurev-bioeng-071811-150124] [PMID: 22524388]

[72] Blanco E, Shen H, Ferrari M. Principles of nanoparticle design for overcoming biological barriers to drug delivery. Nat Biotechnol 2015; 33(9): 941-51. [http://dx.doi.org/10.1038/nbt.3330] [PMID: 26348965]

[73] Souris JS, Lee CH, Cheng SH, *et al.* Surface charge-mediated rapid hepatobiliary excretion of mesoporous silica nanoparticles. Biomaterials 2010; 31(21): 5564-74. [http://dx.doi.org/10.1016/j.biomaterials.2010.03.048] [PMID: 20417962]

[74] Yang B, Jiang J, Jiang L, *et al.* Chitosan mediated solid lipid nanoparticles for enhanced liver delivery of zedoary turmeric oil in vivo. Int J Biol Macromol 2020; 149: 108-15. [http://dx.doi.org/10.1016/j.ijbiomac.2020.01.222] [PMID: 31987952]

[75] Hirn S, Semmler-Behnke M, Schleh C, *et al.* Particle size-dependent and surface charge-dependent biodistribution of gold nanoparticles after intravenous administration. Eur J Pharm Biopharm 2011; 77(3): 407-16. [http://dx.doi.org/10.1016/j.ejpb.2010.12.029] [PMID: 21195759]

[76] Wang H, Thorling CA, Liang X, *et al.* Diagnostic imaging and therapeutic application of nanoparticles targeting the liver. J Mater Chem B Mater Biol Med 2015; 3(6): 939-58. [http://dx.doi.org/10.1039/C4TB01611D] [PMID: 32261972]

[77] Pafili K, Roden M. Nonalcoholic fatty liver disease (NAFLD) from pathogenesis to treatment concepts in humans. Mol Metab 2021; 50: 101122.
[http://dx.doi.org/10.1016/j.molmet.2020.101122] [PMID: 33220492]

[78] Mishra N, Yadav NP, Rai VK, *et al.* Efficient hepatic delivery of drugs: novel strategies and their significance. BioMed Res Int 2013; 2013: 1-20.
[http://dx.doi.org/10.1155/2013/382184] [PMID: 24286077]

[79] Tripathi D, Pandey P, Sharma S, Rai AK, Prabhu B H M. Advances in nanomaterials for precision drug delivery: Insights into pharmacokinetics and toxicity. Bioimpacts 2024; 15: 30573.
[http://dx.doi.org/10.34172/bi.30573] [PMID: 40256227]

CHAPTER 4

Liver Targeting Strategies with Nanocarriers

Afreen Usmani[1], **Mohd Aftab Siddiqui**[2,*], **Mohd Nazam Ansari**[3] and **Rania I.M. Almoselhy**[4]

[1] *Department of Pharmacology, MESCO Institute of Pharmacy, Amroha, Uttar Pradesh, India*

[2] *Faculty of Pharmacy, Integral University, Lucknow, Uttar Pradesh, India*

[3] *Department of Pharmacology and Toxicology, College of Pharmacy, Prince Sattam Bin Abdulaziz University, Alkharj, Saudi Arabia*

[4] *Oils and Fats Research Department, Food Technology Research Institute, Agricultural Research Center, Giza, Egypt*

Abstract: Fatty liver diseases, including nonalcoholic fatty liver disease (NAFLD) and alcoholic fatty liver disease (AFLD), have emerged as some of the most prevalent causes of chronic liver disorders worldwide. Treatment options remain limited due to poor drug bioavailability and nonspecific targeting, resulting in suboptimal therapeutic outcomes. In this context, nanocarriers have shown significant promise by improving drug delivery, enabling precise targeting, and thereby enhancing therapeutic efficacy in the management of fatty liver diseases. This chapter offers a comprehensive review of liver-targeting strategies using nanocarriers, with particular attention to the complexity of fatty liver disease. It examines various nanocarrier systems, such as liposomes, polymeric nanoparticles, dendrimers, and lipid-based carriers, focusing on their structural features and potential for targeted drug delivery. Emerging strategies, including receptor-mediated and stimulus-responsive delivery systems, are critically analyzed. Furthermore, this chapter explores the integration of nanocarriers with cutting-edge technologies, such as RNA-based therapeutics and CRISPR-Cas9 gene editing. Issues related to scalability, safety, and regulatory challenges are also discussed, alongside the latest advancements in preclinical and clinical research. Overall, this chapter serves as a valuable resource, outlining current knowledge and future directions for researchers, clinicians, and pharmaceutical developers working to advance liver-targeted therapies for fatty liver diseases.

Keywords: Fatty liver disease, Liver-targeted drug delivery, Liposomes and nanoparticles, Nanocarriers, RNA-based and gene-editing therapeutics, Stimuli-responsive systems.

[*] **Corresponding author Mohd Aftab Siddiqui:** Faculty of Pharmacy, Integral University, Lucknow, Uttar Pradesh, India; E-mail: aftab.uzaiz@gmail.com

Anjali Sharma, Devkant Sharma, Ajmer Singh Grewal, Geeta Deswal & Ganga Reddy Velma (Eds.)

INTRODUCTION

Fatty Liver Disease

Fatty liver disease refers to a condition characterized by excessive fat accumulation in liver cells not attributable to significant alcohol intake. It is broadly classified into two types: alcoholic fatty liver disease (AFLD) and nonalcoholic fatty liver disease (NAFLD). Of these, NAFLD, recently redefined as metabolic dysfunction-associated fatty liver disease (MAFLD), has gained prominence as a global health challenge owing to its increasing prevalence and close association with metabolic syndrome [1]. The reclassification of NAFLD to MAFLD in 2020 marks a paradigm shift, moving from exclusion-based diagnostic criteria to inclusion-based ones that center on metabolic dysfunction, including obesity, type 2 diabetes, and related risk factors [2, 3].

MAFLD is now the most common chronic liver condition worldwide. In Western countries, its prevalence ranges from 20–30%, while in China, it affects approximately 23.3% of the population, underscoring its global reach [4]. Its rising incidence parallels lifestyle transitions marked by increased caloric and fructose consumption, reduced physical activity, and the growing burden of obesity and metabolic syndrome. Notably, MAFLD is no longer restricted to adults; the escalating rates of childhood obesity have led to a concerning increase in pediatric cases, which could predispose affected individuals to lifelong complications. The condition is more common in men and postmenopausal women, suggesting a possible protective role of female sex hormones [5].

The burden of MAFLD extends far beyond liver-specific complications, such as cirrhosis, liver failure, and hepatocellular carcinoma. It is closely linked with systemic diseases like cardiovascular disease and type 2 diabetes, significantly contributing to increased morbidity and mortality [4, 5]. MAFLD arises from a complex interplay of genetic, environmental, and metabolic factors, with insulin resistance playing a central role in hepatic fat accumulation by enhancing lipogenesis and impairing lipid oxidation. Other key contributors include chronic inflammation, mitochondrial dysfunction, dyslipidemia, and oxidative stress. Central obesity, characterized by visceral fat accumulation, is a major driver of these metabolic disturbances [6].

High-fructose diets, sedentary behavior, and genetic mutations, particularly in the PNPLA3 gene, further exacerbate susceptibility. Disease progression spans a broad spectrum, beginning with simple steatosis and potentially advancing to nonalcoholic steatohepatitis (NASH), fibrosis, cirrhosis, and ultimately liver failure. Fibrosis, in particular, is associated with a markedly increased risk of liver-related mortality [7].

Early detection is essential to prevent disease progression. Non-invasive diagnostic tools, such as ultrasound and elastography, are widely used to assess hepatic steatosis and fibrosis, offering safer alternatives to liver biopsy [8]. Biomarkers and scoring systems, including the Fibrosis-4 (FIB-4) index, are gaining attention for their utility in disease staging and risk stratification. Management primarily revolves around correcting metabolic dysfunction, with lifestyle changes, especially weight loss through diet and exercise, as the cornerstone of treatment. While pharmacological therapies targeting insulin resistance, lipid metabolism, and inflammation are under development, their clinical effectiveness remains limited, reflecting the need for novel therapeutic approaches [9].

In this context, nanotechnology has emerged as a promising strategy, enabling the development of targeted drug-delivery systems that enhance therapeutic efficacy while minimizing off-target effects. Nanocarriers, such as liposomes, polymeric nanoparticles, and lipid-based nanoparticles, offer new avenues for delivering therapeutic agents directly to hepatocytes, thereby addressing the underlying mechanisms of MAFLD with greater precision.

Limitations of Conventional Therapies

Despite numerous advances, current treatments for fatty liver disease (NAFLD) face significant challenges due to the complexity of its pathophysiology. Pharmacological intervention remains limited by the lack of drugs that specifically target the disease or its advanced stage, NASH. Most therapies address associated metabolic conditions, such as obesity, type 2 diabetes, and dyslipidemia [10, 11], but not the underlying mechanisms, such as hepatic inflammation, lipid accumulation, and fibrosis. This creates a gap in treatment options, depriving patients of therapies capable of halting disease progression or reversing damage.

Diagnostic challenges further compound this gap. Accurate diagnosis is essential for timely treatment, but faces barriers. While liver biopsy is the gold standard for diagnosing and staging NAFLD, it is invasive, costly, and carries risks, such as bleeding and infection. Non-invasive imaging methods like ultrasound and transient elastography offer safer alternatives but often lack sensitivity, particularly in early or mild cases [12]. These limitations delay treatment initiation and complicate disease management. In addition to diagnostic and therapeutic challenges, implementing lifestyle interventions is also difficult. Changes in diet and physical activity are poorly adhered to due to a lack of motivation, time, and support [13, 14]. Few structured programs exist, and long-term adherence remains a challenge, especially in patients with advanced disease or comorbidities, often leading to suboptimal outcomes. These challenges highlight the need for innovative, personalized treatment strategies that address metabolic dysfunction, inflammation, and fibrosis. Interventions must also consider compliance, accessibility, and sustainability to improve outcomes for patients with NAFLD [10, 13].

In this context, nanotechnology-based approaches offer promising solutions. These therapies enable targeted delivery to liver tissues, reduce systemic side effects, and improve adherence through less frequent dosing. With further development, such strategies could address existing treatment gaps and redefine the therapeutic landscape for liver diseases. This chapter explores liver-targeting strategies using nanocarriers, examining their mechanisms, advantages, and barriers to clinical application. These strategies have the potential to improve the safety and effectiveness of NAFLD management.

NANOCARRIERS IN DRUG DELIVERY FOR LIVER DISEASES

Unique anatomical and physiological features of the liver, such as its high blood flow and specialized receptors on hepatocyte surfaces, make it an attractive target for nanomedicine [15]. In the literature, many nanocarriers have been designed for targeted delivery to the liver, each exhibiting specific advantages over others (Table **1**). Examples of such nanocarriers include the following:

Table 1. Nanocarriers for liver-targeted drug delivery.

Nanocarrier Types	Advantages	Challenges	References
Liposomes	Biocompatible, encapsulates both hydrophilic and lipophilic drugs, modifiable for active targeting (*e.g.*, galactose-ASGPR targeting)	Potential immunogenicity, stability, size, and surface charge optimization required	[15 - 19]
Polymeric Nanoparticles (PLGA, PEG, etc.)	Versatile, biodegradable, personalized for controlled release, can incorporate targeting ligands (*e.g.*, galactose, antibodies)	Possible toxicity, variable degradation rates, and efficient drug loading need optimization	[20, 21]
Solid Lipid Nanoparticles (SLNs)	High drug-loading capacity, improved stability, controlled release	Polymorphism, drug expulsion during storage, and limited drug loading capacity	[22, 23]
Inorganic Nanoparticles (SiNPs, CeO2 NPs)	SiNPs modulate hepatic lipid metabolism; CeO2 NPs provide antioxidant effects, and targeted resveratrol delivery	Potential toxicity and safety concerns limit clinical translation	[24]

(Table 1) cont.....

Nanocarrier Types	Advantages	Challenges	References
Albumin Nanoparticles	Biocompatible, biodegradable, improved drug circulation time, reduced immunogenicity	Limited drug loading capacity, stability concerns	[25 - 27]
Extracellular Vesicles (EVs)	Natural biocompatibility, engineered for specific liver targeting	Standardization, scalable production, and consistent cargo loading remain challenges	[28]
Low-density lipoprotein (LDL) Nanoparticles	Exploit natural LDL uptake for targeted hepatocyte delivery	Complex structure, potential off-target effects	[29]
Chitosan Nanoparticles (CSNPs)	Biodegradable, enhances hepatic uptake via ASGPRs, used for liver fibrosis and HCC therapy	Rapid clearance by RES, poor *in vivo* stability	[30 - 34]
Gold Nanoparticles (AuNPs)	Functionalizable for liver targeting, used in imaging and photothermal therapy	Long-term biocompatibility, cytotoxicity, and biodistribution concerns	[35 - 37]
Carbon-Based Nanocarriers (Fullerenes, CNTs, Graphene Derivatives)	Large surface area, high mechanical strength, electrical conductivity, functionalizable for liver targeting	Cytotoxicity, biodegradation issues, and clearance challenges	[38 - 40]
Dendrimers	Highly branched, controlled drug release, conjugation with hepatic-targeting ligands	Cytotoxicity, high production cost, and potential immunogenicity	[41 - 44]
Micelles	Solubilize hydrophobic drugs and provide controlled release	Instability, premature drug leakage, and rapid clearance	[45]
Metal-Organic Frameworks (MOFs)	High porosity, substantial drug loading, controlled hepatic drug release	Biocompatibility concerns, stability in physiological conditions, and scalability	[46]
Nanostructured Lipid Carriers (NLCs)	Superior to SLNs: higher drug loading, reduced drug expulsion, more flexible release kinetics for hepatic steatosis and inflammation control	Requires optimization of solid/liquid lipid ratios; long-term stability data needed	[47]
Carbon Quantum Dots (CQDs)	Excellent aqueous solubility, biocompatibility, intrinsic fluorescence for imaging, easy surface functionalization (*e.g.*, with galactose) for targeting	Potential long-term toxicity and biodistribution profiles require further investigation; scalable synthesis challenges	[48]
Nanosuspensions	Carrier-free; significantly enhances dissolution and bioavailability of poorly water-soluble drugs; enables passive liver targeting	Physical stability (*e.g.*, Ostwald ripening) requires stabilizers; potential for variable dosing in suspension form	[49]

(Table 1) cont.....

Nanocarrier Types	Advantages	Challenges	References
Nanogels	High water solubility, biocompatibility, can entrap diverse therapeutics (small molecules to proteins/nucleic acids); can be stimuli-responsive (pH, enzymes), and surface-functionalized for active targeting	Can have limited drug loading for some compounds; may exhibit swelling/deswelling behavior affecting release kinetics	[50]

Liposomes

Liposomes are probably one of the most widely studied drug nanocarriers; they are small, spherical vesicles composed of phospholipid bilayers [16]. Their biocompatibility, ability to encapsulate both hydrophilic and lipophilic drugs, and relative ease of modification make them attractive candidates for liver targeting [15]. Passive targeting, based on the enhanced permeability and retention (EPR) effect, can be exploited; however, this strategy is confronted by active targeting strategies using ligands, such as galactose, which bind to asialoglycoprotein receptors on hepatocytes, thereby significantly improving targeting efficiency [17]. Guo et al. demonstrated aptamer-functionalized ultrasound nanobubbles that target the delivery of resveratrol and copper-based nanoparticles to the liver in a NAFLD model [18]. Further modifications to liposome composition and surface chemistry could improve their stability, circulation time, and cell uptake. There are more challenges, though: for example, potential immunogenicity and optimization of size and surface charge for maximal liver accumulation [19].

Polymeric Nanoparticles

Polymeric nanoparticles allow for versatility in the choice of materials, size, shape, and surface modification to adjust drug delivery profiles. Polymers like PLGA (poly(lactic-co-glycolic acid)) and PEG (polyethylene glycol) are widely used due to their biodegradability and stealth properties, respectively. Targeting ligands, such as galactose or specific antibodies, can be incorporated to achieve liver-specific delivery [20]. For instance, glycogen-based nanoparticles for targeted delivery of resveratrol have been investigated [21], which demonstrated improved stability and activity as compared to free resveratrol. However, issues like possible toxicity, the rate of biodegradation, and efficient drug loading are the most critical parameters that need optimization [20].

Solid Lipid Nanoparticles

Solid Lipid Nanoparticles (SLNs), which are solid lipids dispersed in an aqueous phase, offer several advantages, including high drug-loading capacity, improved drug stability, and controlled drug release [22]. Their biocompatibility and ease of production make them attractive alternatives to liposomes and polymeric nanoparticles [23]. As with liposomes and polymeric nanoparticles, surface modification strategies can be used to enhance liver targeting. However, issues regarding polymorphism, drug expulsion during storage, and drug loading capacity need to be further explored [22].

Inorganic Nanoparticles

Inorganic nanoparticles, such as silica nanoparticles (SiNPs) and cerium oxide nanoparticles (CeO2 NPs), have also been tested for targeting the liver [20]. SiNPs, which hold great promise as drug carriers, have also been reported to influence hepatic lipid metabolism, potentially leading to lipid metabolic disorders [24]. CeO2 NPs, well known for their antioxidant activity, were incorporated into hollow mesoporous nanocarriers to deliver resveratrol effectively in NASH models [17]. However, the potential toxicity of some inorganic NPs warrants careful safety profiling before they can be used in clinical practice [20].

Albumin Nanoparticles

Albumin is a naturally occurring protein that is biocompatible and biodegradable and is often used in the formulation of nanocarriers [25]. Albumin nanoparticles can encapsulate drugs, improve their pharmacokinetics, and enhance their delivery to the liver [26]. The use of albumin as a nanocarrier also offers the advantages of increased circulation time and reduced immunogenicity. However, certain drawbacks concerning drug loading capacity and stability require further exploration [27].

Extracellular Vesicles

Extracellular Vesicles (EVs) secreted by cells are biologically engineered nanosized vesicles that have come into the limelight of science as drug delivery vehicles owing to their biocompatibility and low immunogenicity. EVs can be native or engineered to target the liver; one modification is to enhance their surface to improve the delivery of therapeutic cargo to hepatocytes. However, standardization of EV production, consistent cargo loading, and scalable production remain significant challenges for the clinical translation of those EVs [28].

Low-density Lipoprotein

Low-density lipoprotein (LDL) nanoparticles take advantage of the natural uptake of LDL by LDL receptors (LDLR) in the liver to achieve hepatocyte targeting. This receptor-mediated endocytosis enables targeted drug delivery to hepatocytes. Naturally and synthetically made LDL-based nanocarriers have been studied for their potential applications in targeted therapy and imaging. However, the complexity of the LDL structure and potential off-target effects are subjects under further investigation [29].

Chitosan Nanoparticles

Chitosan nanoparticles are promising for targeted drug delivery to the liver, leveraging their biodegradability and biocompatibility to enhance the therapeutic efficacy in diseases, such as liver fibrosis and hepatocellular carcinoma (HCC) [30, 31]. Modification with saccharides enhances the affinity of ASGPRs, which further facilitates hepatic uptake [30]. Recent studies have focused on the potential of CSNPs in the delivery of a variety of therapeutic agents, including cannabidiol for acute liver injury and curcumin for nonalcoholic fatty liver disease, due to their ability to enhance bioavailability while reducing off-target effects [32, 33]. However, the rapid clearance by the reticuloendothelial system (RES) and poor *in vivo* stability demand further optimization of these nanoparticles to enhance their clinical applicability [31, 34].

Gold Nanoparticles

Gold nanoparticles (AuNPs) are increasingly being considered for liver-targeted imaging and therapeutic applications due to their plasmonic properties, ease of functionalization with various molecules or groups, and stability. Due to their strong localized surface plasmon resonance (LSPR), they enhance detection and photothermal therapeutics, making the gold nanoparticles suitable for targeted delivery in liver cancer [35]. Functionalization with ligands, such as glycyrrhizin and lactobionic acid, was found to increase liver specificity, enabling selective accumulation in hepatic tissues [36]. Long-term biocompatibility, biodistribution, and cytotoxicity are, however, critical areas under research since the safety profile of AuNPs needs to be clearly understood for their effective application in clinical settings [37]. Taken together, while AuNPs provide promising avenues for theranostic applications in liver cancer, further investigations in this direction are necessary to overcome these safety concerns.

Carbon-based Nanocarriers

Carbon-based nanocarriers, such as fullerene, carbon nanotubes (CNTs), and graphene derivatives, possess superior physicochemical properties, including a large surface area, mechanical strength, and electrical conductivity. All these characteristics make them promising candidates for drug delivery systems, especially in the therapy of cancer [38]. The ability to functionalize, thereby increasing their targeting ability and improving the delivery to hepatocytes and tumor sites, is a key characteristic that must be met to have an effective liver cancer therapy [39, 40]. Despite their advantages, key challenges persist, such as possible cytotoxicity, problems related to biodegradation, and body clearance that impede their clinical application. Advanced functionalization techniques and improvement in biocompatibility are urgently needed to answer these concerns so that these nanocarriers can successfully translate into the clinical setting [40].

Dendrimers

Dendrimers, with the advantages of being nanosized and highly branched, show great promise in the treatment of liver diseases by offering precise control over size, functionality, and surface modification that enables targeted drug delivery and controlled release mechanisms [41]. Their tunable surface chemistry allows conjugation with specific ligands to enhance drug encapsulation efficiency and release, targeting the hepatic stellate cells (HSCs) in liver fibrosis [42]. Even though there are advantages to using dendrimers, critical barriers remain, including cytotoxicity, high production costs, and possible immunogenicity, to their clinical application [43]. Further research on considerable measure is needed to develop good, scalable synthesis methods and to elucidate further the safety profiles of the dendrimer-based systems, which may revolutionize drug delivery strategies in liver diseases [44].

Micelles

Micelles are self-assembling amphiphilic molecules that have been extensively utilized for hepatic drug delivery due to their ability to solubilize hydrophobic drugs and provide controlled drug release. Polymeric micelles functionalized with hepatotropic ligands, such as glycyrrhetinic acid, exhibit enhanced liver targeting.

However, challenges, including instability, premature drug leakage, and rapid systemic clearance, hinder their widespread application [45].

Metal-organic Frameworks

Metal-organic frameworks (MOFs) are hybrid nanostructures composed of metal ions and organic linkers characterized by high porosity and substantial drug-loading capacity. They have demonstrated significant potential in hepatic drug delivery due to their ability to provide sustained release and specificity toward liver cells. Nonetheless, issues such as long-term biocompatibility, structural stability under physiological conditions, and scalability present significant challenges to clinical adoption [46].

Nanostructured Lipid Carriers (NLCs)

Nano lipid carriers (NLCs) are nanostructures generated by the dissolution of lipids in aqueous glycerol and phospholipid solutions. A superior type of lipid nanoparticles is the Nanostructured Lipid Carriers (NLCs), which adopt a combination of solid and liquid lipids to form a less crystalline, perfect matrix. The structure is beneficial as it bypasses the essential drawbacks of SLNs in terms of drug loading capacity and reduction of possible drug expulsion during storage, as well as the ability to make the release kinetics more flexible to enhance the control of hepatic steatosis and inflammation [47].

Carbon Quantum Dots (CQDs)

Carbon Quantum Dots (CQDs) are a recent type of quasi-spherical carbon nanomaterials (<10 nm). They are very promising in liver theranostics because of their excellent solubility in aqueous solvents, biocompatibility, and easy surface functionalization to targeting ligands, such as galactose. Their intrinsic fluorescence can be imaged and tracked, and the therapeutics can be loaded onto their functionalized surfaces [48].

Nanosuspensions

Nanosuspensions are biphasic, colloidal suspensions containing pure drug particles developed through surfactant and having a nanometric size. It is their carrier-free method that is especially applicable to increase the dissolution speed and saturation solubility of drugs that are poorly water-soluble (BCS Class II and IV) and, in doing so, increase their oral bioavailability and passive liver targeting without having a traditional lipid or polymer matrix [49].

Nanogels

Nanogels are nanoparticles that are crosslinked and three-dimensional hydrogels made of polymers that are hydrophilic in nature. They are highly water-soluble and biocompatible and have an outstanding ability to entrap a broad diversity of therapeutic molecules, such as small hydrophilic molecules and larger biomacromolecules such as proteins and nucleic acids. Their surface may be functionalized to be actively targeted to the liver, and they may be stimuli-responsive (*e.g.*, to pH or enzymes) so that the release of the drug at the hepatic site of action can be controlled [50]. Nanocarriers for liver disease are shown in Fig. (**1**).

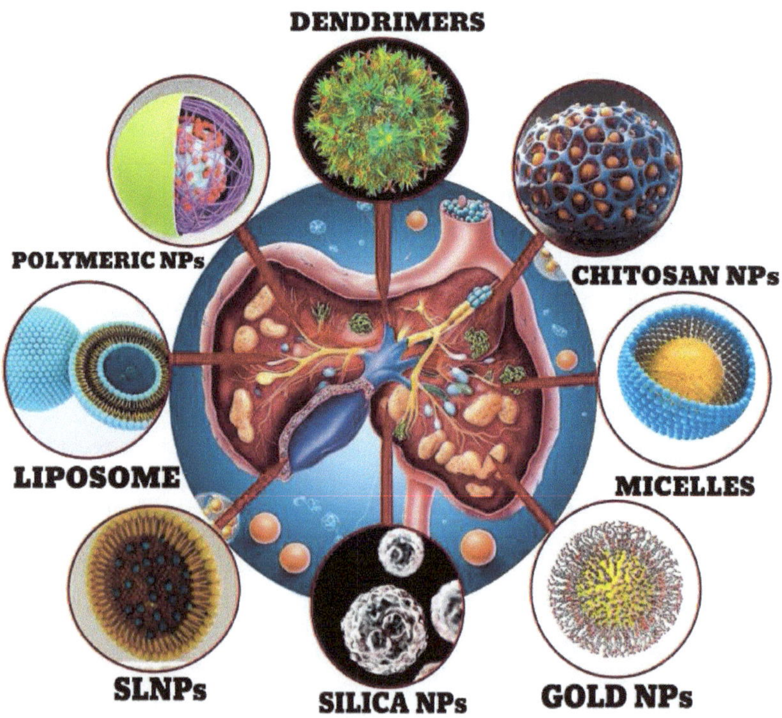

Fig. (1). Nanocarriers in drug delivery for liver diseases.

LIVER-TARGETING STRATEGIES

Advances in nanotechnology have opened new possibilities for targeted therapies in managing fatty liver disease and related disorders. Nanocarrier-based drug delivery systems are favored for enhancing efficacy and minimizing off-target effects [15 - 46]. These systems aim to improve treatment outcomes by delivering drugs directly to hepatic tissues, reducing systemic toxicity. Liver-targeting strategies, broadly classified into active and passive approaches, are central to this goal.

Active Targeting

Active targeting involves modifying nanocarriers with ligands or molecules that selectively bind to liver cell receptors, improving cellular uptake and therapeutic precision. For example, chitosan nanoparticles modified with saccharides target asialoglycoprotein receptors (ASGPR) on hepatocytes, enhancing drug delivery. Ligands like galactose and lactobionic acid further increase liver specificity by binding ASGPR, thus boosting drug accumulation. Antigen-based targeting, using monoclonal antibodies on nanocarriers, has shown promise in targeting hepatic stellate cells in liver fibrosis, reducing disease progression. This approach improves therapeutic precision while minimizing side effects [51].

Passive Targeting

Passive targeting makes use of the enhanced permeability and retention (EPR) effect, in which the nanoparticles are captured in diseased tissues of the liver with permeable vasculature, like tumours or fibrotic regions. This effect can be used in hepatocellular carcinoma to target drugs at tumor locations. An example of this mechanism used to enhance efficacy is liposomal doxorubicin. The size of nanoparticles, such as 10200 nm, and PEGylation are some of the factors that increase the circulation time and retention in pathological areas of the liver [52].

Synergistic Potential

Combining active and passive targeting offers a promising strategy for liver-specific drug delivery. Multifunctional nanocarriers designed for both ligand interaction and EPR optimization may overcome the limitations of conventional treatments. This dual strategy enhances specificity, reduces systemic toxicity, and marks a major step toward precision medicine in liver disease management, especially for conditions like NAFLD and liver fibrosis [15, 42].

Receptor-mediated Targeting Strategies

Receptor-mediated targeting strategies exploit hepatocyte-specific receptors to enhance drug specificity, thereby improving therapeutic outcomes and minimizing systemic toxicity. The asialoglycoprotein receptor (ASGPR), highly expressed on hepatocytes, is the most widely used, with ligands such as galactose and N-acetylgalactosamine enabling efficient receptor-mediated endocytosis. Emerging approaches include liver-targeting chimeras (LIVTACs), which bind ASGPR and intracellular proteins to achieve superior pharmacokinetics and sustained efficacy in liver cancer models. Additionally, lactobionic acid-functionalized gold nanoparticles demonstrate strong ASGPR affinity, significantly enhancing hepatocyte-specific gene delivery and transgene expression, highlighting their potential for liver-directed gene therapy [53].

Polysaccharide-based nanoparticles, particularly chitosan modified with galactose or mannose, have improved interaction with ASGPR. These functionalized carriers demonstrate enhanced cellular uptake, intracellular trafficking, and therapeutic outcomes in liver disease models, such as fibrosis and metabolic disorders [54].

Altogether, receptor-mediated targeting strategies mark a significant advance in hepatotropic drug delivery, enhancing specificity and reducing systemic toxicity. Continued research on ligand-receptor dynamics, nanocarrier design, and pharmacokinetics is essential for their clinical translation.

Stimuli-responsive Nanocarriers

Stimuli-responsive nanocarriers have transformed liver-targeted drug delivery, especially in hepatocellular carcinoma and chronic liver diseases. These systems release drugs in response to internal cues like pH, redox potential, or enzymes or external triggers, such as light or magnetic fields, ensuring site-specific accumulation and reduced systemic toxicity [28, 31].

Liposomal formulations are widely studied for their ability to encapsulate drugs within lipid bilayers, improving solubility, stability, and biodistribution. They exploit both passive (EPR effect) and active (ligand-mediated) targeting. pH- and enzyme-sensitive liposomes enhance controlled release and minimize off-target effects [15].

Polymeric nanoparticles (*e.g.*, PLGA, PEG) offer controlled release, extended circulation, and better hepatic accumulation when conjugated with targeting ligands. Redox- or pH-responsive polymeric micelles show added efficacy in tumor environments [55]. Inorganic platforms, like MSNs, gold, and magnetic nanoparticles, enable controlled release via stimuli-responsive gates. For example, glutathione-responsive gold nanoparticles enhance liver-specific delivery and bioavailability [56].

INTEGRATION WITH ADVANCED THERAPEUTICS

Nanocarriers significantly improve the delivery of novel therapeutics for fatty liver diseases such as MAFLD, NAFLD, and NASH by enhancing liver specificity and overcoming bioavailability issues.

RNA-based and siRNA Delivery

RNA interference (RNAi), especially siRNA, offers a targeted approach to silencing genes involved in NAFLD. Nanocarriers protect siRNA from degradation and facilitate liver-specific delivery [57 - 60]. Lipid nanoparticles (LNPs), especially those modified with PEG and GalNAc, target ASGPRs on hepatocytes for enhanced uptake and reduced off-target effects [58, 59]. siRNA-loaded SSLNPs show promise in liver fibrosis models [59]. Other platforms include polymeric nanoparticles, EVs, and vitamin E-coupled systems, which demonstrate effective delivery with minimal immune activation [28, 60 - 63].

CRISPR-Cas9 Delivery

CRISPR-Cas9 offers gene-level precision in treating MAFLD, but safe delivery remains a challenge. Nanocarriers such as lipoMSNs, peptide-based particles, and biomimetic mineralized nanoparticles have enabled effective in vivo editing and lipid reduction [61, 64 - 67]. LNPs co-delivering Cas9 mRNA and guide RNA target genes like *Angptl3* involved in lipid metabolism. However, concerns about off-target effects and safety persist.

Natural Compounds in Nanocarriers

Integrating natural compounds with nanocarriers enhances their bioactivity and delivery.

- *Curcumin* exhibits antioxidant and anti-inflammatory effects beneficial in MAFLD but suffers from low bioavailability. Lipid-based encapsulation improves its solubility and efficacy [22].
- *Berberine* has shown hepatoprotective effects and improved outcomes in MAFLD when delivered via chitosan nanoparticles [68].

These formulations enhance therapeutic potential by improving solubility, targeting, and sustained release, offering new avenues in managing NAFLD and NASH through natural, bioactive agents.

Targeting NAFLD and NASH with combination therapies

With the multifactorial nature of NAFLD and NASH, combination therapy targeting multiple pathways simultaneously is a must. Nanocarriers allow the co-delivery of bioactive compounds or drugs, enhancing therapeutic outcomes. A few of their examples are as follows:

Resveratrol and Astaxanthin

These compounds possess anti-inflammatory, antioxidative, and lipid-lowering properties. Encapsulation in nanocarriers enhances their bioavailability and synergistic effects on hepatic lipid metabolism [18, 69].

Fibrosis and Inflammation

Nanocarriers have been used to deliver anti-fibrotic agents, such as TSG-6, in combination with conventional drugs, including silybin or doxorubicin, to reduce liver fibrosis, inflammation, and steatosis [21, 68].

These new technologies show the revolutionary possibility of nanocarrier-based therapeutics for the treatment of NAFLD and NASH. Further research is imperative to optimize safety and efficacy in clinical practice [70, 71].

RECENT ADVANCES IN PRECLINICAL AND CLINICAL STUDIES

Success Stories and Ongoing Trials

Recent drug delivery advancements for fatty liver diseases, particularly for NAFLD and MASLD, bring to light new ways through which treatment outcomes could be optimized. Nanoemulsion technology has come up as a promising approach, offering enhanced drug-loading capabilities and targeted delivery to hepatic tissues, which are of utmost importance in the face of the global prevalence of the disease affecting approximately 32% of the world's population [10, 72]. These nanoemulsions increase the solubility and bioavailability of lipophilic drugs, hence making them an efficient platform for therapeutic intervention.

Cell membrane-derived nanoparticles (CMNs) have been successfully used to encapsulate rosuvastatin and have been shown to remarkably reduce lipid accumulation in hepatocytes. Such biomimetic nanocarriers offer several unique advantages, including immune evasion, extended circulation time, and highly efficient liver-targeted delivery, placing them as a potential candidate for future clinical applications [72].

Emerging Innovations in Nanomedicine for Liver Diseases

The whole class of nanocarrier-based therapies is revolutionizing the treatment of MASLD and NAFLD. Recent developments involving liposomes, lipid nanoparticles (LNPs), and polymeric nanocarriers have shown great promise in enhancing bioavailability, improving targeted drug delivery, and reducing systemic toxicity [15, 68, 73].

Lipid Nanoparticles (LNPs)

Lipid Nanoparticles are widely explored for encapsulating nucleic acid therapeutics (*e.g.*, mRNA and siRNA) to modulate gene expression and inflammatory pathways in hepatic disorders [73].

Cell Membrane-coated Nanoparticles (CMNPs)

These nanocarriers mimic the properties of natural cell membranes, allowing for immune evasion and improved liver-targeting efficiency [72].

Hybrid Nanocarrier Systems

Combining lipid, polymer, and inorganic nanomaterials might afford the hybrid carriers with higher stability, controlled drug release, and improved biocompatibility [74].

CRISPR and Gene Therapy Delivery Platforms

Researchers are actively developing nano-formulated CRISPR systems capable of precisely editing genes associated with lipid metabolism and fibrosis progression. These systems have the potential to cure MASLD and NAFLD [75].

Emerging Nanotechnology-based Pharmacological Agents in Clinical Trials for Liver Targeting

Nanotechnology is radically revolutionizing drug delivery, most specifically in liver-targeted therapies. Several nanoparticle-based pharmacological agents are under clinical investigation for the treatment of various liver diseases, including fibrosis, metabolic disorders, and liver cancer. In this, the main emerging agents under trial are as follows:

BMS-986263

BMS-986263 is an investigational therapy consisting of retinoid-conjugated lipid nanoparticles that encapsulate small interfering RNA (siRNA) against heat shock protein 47 (HSP47). HSP47 is a collagen-specific chaperone protein crucial in the development of fibrosis. BMS-986263 is an antisense oligonucleotide intended to knock down HSP47 expression in an effort to reduce the progression of fibrosis and promote improvement in liver function. An ongoing investigation involves a randomized, double-blind, placebo-controlled clinical trial in patients with advanced hepatic fibrosis following a virologic cure of hepatitis C, with NCT identifier NCT03420768 [76].

ARCT-810

Developed by Arcturus Therapeutics, ARCT-810 is an mRNA therapy in development using the LUNAR® lipid nanoparticle delivery system to deliver OTC-encoding mRNA directly into liver cells in order to treat ornithine transcarbamylase (OTC) deficiency. This urea cycle disorder prevents the body from getting rid of ammonia. It restores enzyme activity in hepatocytes by delivering functional OTC mRNA and, hence, halts hyperammonemia. A Phase 2a open-label study is currently underway to investigate its safety, tolerability, and pharmacokinetics in patients aged 12 years and older with OTC deficiency (NCT06488313) [76]. These emerging nanotechnology-based therapies demonstrate the potential of nanoparticles to improve drug targeting, reduce systemic toxicity, and improve treatment outcomes for liver diseases. The ongoing clinical trials will further establish their efficacy and pave the way for liver-targeted therapy in the near future.

SAFETY AND REGULATORY CONSIDERATIONS

Safety Considerations

While nanocarrier-based drug delivery shows great promise for treating fatty liver diseases like NAFLD and MASLD, safety and biocompatibility remain key concerns. Despite benefits such as targeted delivery and improved bioavailability with systems like liposomes, polymeric nanoparticles, and dendrimers, their potential toxicity and immune responses must be carefully considered for clinical use. The most pressing issue is nanocarrier-induced toxicity, including immune activation, inflammation, oxidative stress, and liver damage, especially since the liver plays a central role in metabolism and immune regulation [77]. Poorly designed nanoparticles may accumulate in liver tissue, causing off-target effects. Lipid nanoparticles, while promising, have been associated with liver toxicity, warranting cautious formulation [78]. Additionally, drug release profiles and particle size can influence toxicity; smaller nanoparticles, though better at targeting, may cross into non-target tissues and cause adverse effects [79]. Even lipid-based carriers, generally biocompatible, can degrade into toxic byproducts over time, raising long-term safety concerns [80].

Biocompatibility of Nanocarriers

Biocompatibility ensures that nanocarriers do not provoke immune or cellular toxicity. PEGylation, coating nanoparticles with PEG, helps prolong circulation and evade immune clearance. However, repeated administration may still trigger immune sensitization [81], highlighting the need for ongoing innovation. Polymeric nanoparticles, especially PLGA-based, offer low toxicity and biodegradability, with the added benefit of controlled drug release [82]. However, optimizing surface properties remains crucial to avoid rapid clearance or immune activation via the reticuloendothelial system (RES) [22].

Size, shape, and surface charge also govern interactions with liver cells and other tissues. Smaller nanoparticles can stay longer in circulation and enhance liver targeting via the EPR effect. However, they may also bind nonspecifically and accumulate in off-target organs [79]. A balanced design is essential to ensure safety and minimize toxicity.

Regulatory Challenges in Nanomedicine

The other regulatory challenge arises because complex nanoparticle-based drug formulations demand extensive safety assessment and long-term studies to establish an appropriate efficacy and safety profile. Stringent guidelines from regulatory agencies worldwide, including the U.S. Food and Drug Administration and the European Medicines Agency, ensure that nanomedicines are manufactured and have met quality and safety standards [73, 78]. The main regulatory hurdles include:

Standardization of Characterization Protocols

Detailed physicochemical characterization of nanomedicines, including particle size, charge, surface chemistry, and drug-loading efficiency, is required.

However, standardized testing protocols are still poorly established, complicating regulatory approval [73].

Long-term Safety Data

The majority of nanomedicine research is in the preclinical and early clinical stages, with only a few providing chronic exposure, biodistribution, and potential off-target toxicity data. In general, the absence of intense, long-term safety studies tends to delay regulatory approval in most cases [73].

Batch-to-batch Consistency and Scalability

Unlike small-molecule drugs, nanoparticle formulations may exhibit variability in their synthesis and stability during large-scale production. The regulatory agencies demand rigorous batch-to-batch reproducibility to ensure quality control and therapeutic consistency [78].

Risk-benefit Assessment

Because nanomedicine is new, regulatory bodies have to weigh the benefits of enhanced drug delivery against potential risks of nanoparticle accumulation and toxicity. This becomes of utmost importance for MASLD treatments due to the long-term administration that may be required for disease management [77].

CHALLENGES IN CLINICAL TRANSLATION

Despite encouraging preclinical studies' results, numerous challenges remain to translate nanocarrier-based therapies into clinical practice. While nanomedicine holds tremendous promise in improving treatment outcomes in MASLD, NAFLD, and NASH, several key barriers must be overcome for its widespread clinical adaptation.

Optimization of Drug Loading and Release Profiles

Achieving efficient drug loading and controlled release remains a major hurdle. Lipid-based and polymeric nanocarriers often suffer from low drug encapsulation, limiting their efficacy and requiring higher doses, which increase toxicity risks [20]. Strategies to address this include surface modifications for better drug affinity and stability, stimuli-responsive carriers that react to liver-specific cues, and hybrid systems like lipid-polymer combinations to improve solubility and bioavailability [74].

Immunogenicity and Biocompatibility Issues

Immunogenicity continues to be a major limitation. Nanocarriers must avoid rapid clearance by the mononuclear phagocyte system (MPS) while ensuring effective hepatocyte targeting. Even with PEGylation, immune reactions can occur, including hypersensitivity, cytokine storms, and anti-PEG antibody formation, reducing nanoparticle efficacy over time [75, 81]. Current strategies include developing biomimetic nanocarriers with immune-evasive membranes, non-immunogenic coatings using zwitterionic or carbohydrate-based polymers, and conducting long-term toxicity studies to assess chronic immune responses.

Manufacturing and Scalability Challenges

Another challenge is the large-scale production of consistent, stable, and effective nanocarriers. Unlike small-molecule drugs, nanocarriers require precise manufacturing to maintain uniformity, as variations in particle size and distribution affect their therapeutic performance. Major obstacles include scaling up production without quality loss and meeting GMP standards. Emerging solutions involve microfluidic synthesis for precise formulation, automated large-scale production for improved reproducibility, and regulatory collaboration to standardize nanoparticle manufacturing protocols [68, 75].

FUTURE PERSPECTIVES IN NANOCARRIER-BASED THERAPIES

The convergence of artificial intelligence (AI) with emerging nanotechnologies is poised to bring transformative progress in nanocarrier-based therapies for fatty liver diseases, particularly in the context of metabolic dysfunction-associated steatotic liver disease (MASLD). AI holds significant promise in optimizing nanocarrier design by predicting effective formulations based on physicochemical parameters such as particle size, surface charge, and drug-release kinetics, thereby reducing the reliance on time-consuming and costly experimental trials [83]. Furthermore, AI-driven approaches pave the way for personalized nanomedicine by enabling the customization of nanocarriers according to patient-specific genetic profiles and biomarkers, improving therapeutic efficacy while minimizing adverse effects [84]. Machine learning algorithms also assist in the interpretation of complex clinical data, facilitating the identification of patterns associated with drug toxicity and interindividual variability in response. This supports regulatory compliance and accelerates the translation of nanocarrier-based therapies from laboratory research to clinical application [68, 84]. Thus, the synergy between AI and nanotechnology not only enhances therapeutic precision but also catalyzes the development of innovative, patient-centered treatment strategies for MASLD [68].

Among emerging nanotechnological interventions, cell membrane-coated nanoparticles have demonstrated substantial promise in improving drug bioavailability and cellular uptake while mitigating lipid accumulation in hepatocytes, as exemplified in studies involving rosuvastatin delivery [72]. Advances in lipid nanoparticles for the co-delivery of small interfering RNA (siRNA) and small molecules are also gaining momentum. These systems target overexpressed receptors specific to MASLD, enabling more precise therapeutic delivery [73, 85]. Additionally, targeting hepatic stellate cells (HSCs) using nanosystems has shifted therapeutic strategies from systemic to localized treatment, enhancing specificity while reducing systemic toxicity [42]. Although polymeric and multifunctional nanoparticles continue to face challenges related to toxicity and long-term stability, their capacity to refine targeted drug delivery in liver diseases remains immense [75].

CONCLUSION

Nanocarrier-based drug delivery systems represent a pivotal advancement in the therapeutic management of fatty liver diseases, particularly NAFLD and MASLD. These platforms offer solutions to many limitations inherent in conventional treatments, including poor drug bioavailability, nonspecific distribution, and systemic side effects. The integration of various nanocarrier systems, such as liposomes, polymeric nanoparticles, dendrimers, lipid-based carriers, and extracellular vesicles, has enabled controlled drug release and hepatocyte-specific targeting, thereby enhancing therapeutic efficacy.

Moreover, the coupling of nanocarriers with novel therapeutic strategies, including RNA-based therapeutics and CRISPR-Cas9 gene-editing tools, presents promising opportunities for addressing the molecular underpinnings of fatty liver diseases. AI-driven approaches and personalized medicine frameworks further optimize treatment, allowing therapeutic interventions to be customized according to individual patient profiles.

Nevertheless, significant translational hurdles remain. Issues related to nanocarrier toxicity, large-scale manufacturing, long-term biocompatibility, and regulatory approval continue to impede clinical adoption. Addressing these challenges will require standardized fabrication protocols, robust long-term safety data, and cost-effective production methodologies. Moving forward, interdisciplinary collaboration, spanning nanotechnology, artificial intelligence, clinical hepatology, and regulatory sciences, will be crucial in closing the gap between preclinical innovation and clinical implementation. With sustained progress, nanocarrier-based therapies are well-positioned to revolutionize the treatment landscape of fatty liver diseases, offering safer, more effective, and highly individualized therapeutic options that can significantly improve long-term patient outcomes.

LIST OF ABBREVIATIONS

NAFLD	Nonalcoholic Fatty Liver Disease
AFLD	Alcoholic Fatty Liver Disease
MAFLD	Metabolic Dysfunction-Associated Fatty Liver Disease
NASH	Nonalcoholic Steatohepatitis
HCC	Hepatocellular Carcinoma
LDL	Low-Density Lipoprotein
PEG	Polyethylene Glycol
PLGA	Poly(lactic-co-glycolic acid)
SLNs	Solid Lipid Nanoparticles
EVs	Extracellular Vesicles
CSNPs	Chitosan Nanoparticles
AuNPs	Gold Nanoparticles
MOFs	Metal-Organic Frameworks
SiNPs	Silica Nanoparticles
CMNPs	Cell Membrane-Coated Nanoparticles
CeO2	Cerium Oxide Nanoparticles

REFERENCES

[1] Tang R, Li R, Li H, *et al.* Design of hepatic targeted drug delivery systems for natural products: insights into nomenclature revision of nonalcoholic fatty liver disease. ACS Nano 2021; 15(11): 17016-46.
[http://dx.doi.org/10.1021/acsnano.1c02158] [PMID: 34705426]

[2] Sharma S, Sharma A, Gupta P, *et al.* The green path to liver health: Herbal solutions for non-alcoholic steatohepatitis. Cardiovasc Hematol Disord Drug Targets 2025; 25(3): 168-92.
[http://dx.doi.org/10.2174/011871529X360903250211101856] [PMID: 40108906]

[3] Alsayegh AS, Alduaybi MA, Alanizi HG, *et al.* Fatty liver disease: An updated overview of risk factors. Int J Health Sci 2023; 7(S1): 3698-710.
[http://dx.doi.org/10.53730/ijhs.v7nS1.15308]

[4] Wu TL, Huang CW, Yen HH. Prevalence of fatty liver disease: A Taiwanese ultrasound cohort-based study. Ultrasound Med Biol 2024; 50: S51-2.
[http://dx.doi.org/10.1016/j.ultrasmedbio.2024.01.064]

[5] Darii F, Tagadiuc O. The burden of steatotic liver disease. Akademos. 2024;73(2):91–8. [http://dx.doi.org/10.52673/18570461.24.2-73.09]

[6] Abou Assi R, Abdulbaqi IM, Siok Yee C. The evaluation of drug delivery nanocarrier development and pharmacological briefing for metabolic-associated fatty liver disease (MAFLD): an update. Pharmaceuticals (Basel) 2021; 14(3): 215. [http://dx.doi.org/10.3390/ph14030215] [PMID: 33806527]

[7] Butcko AJ, Putman AK, Mottillo EP. The intersection of genetic factors, aberrant nutrient metabolism, and oxidative stress in the progression of cardiometabolic disease. Antioxidants 2024; 13(1): 87. [http://dx.doi.org/10.3390/antiox13010087] [PMID: 38247511]

[8] Dawod S, Brown K. Non-invasive testing in metabolic dysfunction-associated steatotic liver disease. Front Med (Lausanne) 2024; 11: 1499013. [http://dx.doi.org/10.3389/fmed.2024.1499013] [PMID: 39606621]

[9] Abdelhameed F, Kite C, Lagojda L, *et al.* Non-invasive scores and serum biomarkers for fatty liver in the era of metabolic dysfunction-associated Steatotic Liver Disease (MASLD): a Comprehensive Review from NAFLD to MAFLD and MASLD. Curr Obes Rep 2024; 13(3): 510-31. [http://dx.doi.org/10.1007/s13679-024-00574-z] [PMID: 38809396]

[10] Sarthi S, Bhardwaj H, Jangde RK. Recent progress in nanoemulsion technology for the management of hepatic diseases. Curr Nanomed 2024; 15: 25. [http://dx.doi.org/10.2174/0124681873323497240922153222]

[11] Portincasa P, Grattagliano I, Palmieri V, Palasciano G. Current pharmacological treatment of nonalcoholic fatty liver. Curr Med Chem 2005; 12(10): 1147-61. [PMID: 17073635]

[12] Sumida Y, Nakajima A, Itoh Y. Limitations of liver biopsy and non-invasive diagnostic tests for the diagnosis of nonalcoholic fatty liver disease/nonalcoholic steatohepatitis. World J Gastroenterol 2014; 20(2): 475-85. [http://dx.doi.org/10.3748/wjg.v20.i2.475] [PMID: 24574716]

[13] Bołdys A, Bułdak Ł, Maligłówka M, Surma S, Okopień B. Potential therapeutic strategies in the treatment of metabolic-associated fatty liver disease. Medicina (Kaunas) 2023; 59(10): 1789. [http://dx.doi.org/10.3390/medicina59101789] [PMID: 37893507]

[14] Armandi A, Schattenberg JM. Beyond the paradigm of weight loss in non-alcoholic fatty liver disease: From pathophysiology to novel dietary approaches. Nutrients 2021; 13(6): 1977. [http://dx.doi.org/10.3390/nu13061977] [PMID: 34201382]

[15] AbouSamra MM. Liposomal nano-carriers mediated targeting of liver disorders: mechanisms and applications. J Liposome Res 2024; 34(4): 728-43. [http://dx.doi.org/10.1080/08982104.2024.2377085] [PMID: 38988127]

[16] Bozzuto G, Molinari A. Liposomes as nanomedical devices. Int J Nanomedicine 2015; 10: 975-99. [http://dx.doi.org/10.2147/IJN.S68861] [PMID: 25678787]

[17] Tong Y, Yu X, Huang Y, Zhang Z, Mi L, Bao Z. Hepatic-targeted Nano-enzyme with resveratrol loading for precise relief of nonalcoholic Steatohepatitis. ChemMedChem 2023; 18(5): e202200468. [http://dx.doi.org/10.1002/cmdc.202200468] [PMID: 36380399]

[18] Guo X, Huang Z, Chen J, *et al.* Synergistic delivery of resveratrol and ultrasmall copper-based nanoparticles by aptamer-functionalized ultrasound nanobubbles for the treatment of nonalcoholic fatty liver disease. Front Physiol 2022; 13: 950141. [http://dx.doi.org/10.3389/fphys.2022.950141] [PMID: 36160874]

[19] Danaei M, Dehghankhold M, Ataei S, *et al.* Impact of particle size and polydispersity index on the clinical applications of lipidic nanocarrier systems. Pharmaceutics 2018; 10(2): 57. [http://dx.doi.org/10.3390/pharmaceutics10020057] [PMID: 29783687]

[20] Mitragotri S, Lahann J. Materials for drug delivery: innovative solutions to address complex biological hurdles. Adv Mater 2012; 24(28): 3717-23. [http://dx.doi.org/10.1002/adma.201202080] [PMID: 22807037]

[21] Li X, Chen XX, Xu Y, *et al.* Construction of glycogen-based nanoparticles loaded with resveratrol for the alleviation of high-fat diet-induced nonalcoholic fatty liver disease. Biomacromolecules 2022; 23(1): 409-23. [http://dx.doi.org/10.1021/acs.biomac.1c01360] [PMID: 34964604]

[22] Mishra V, Bansal KK, Verma A, *et al.* Solid lipid nanoparticles: Emerging colloidal nano drug delivery systems. Pharmaceutics 2018; 10(4): 191. [http://dx.doi.org/10.3390/pharmaceutics10040191] [PMID: 30340327]

[23] Montoto SS, Muraca G, Ruiz ME. Solid lipid nanoparticles for drug delivery: pharmacological and biopharmaceutical aspects. Front. Mol. Biosci. 2020 Oct 30; 7(1-24): 587997.

[24] Duan J, Liang S, Feng L, Yu Y, Sun Z. Silica nanoparticles trigger hepatic lipid-metabolism disorder in vivo and in vitro. Int J Nanomedicine 2018; 13: 7303-18. [http://dx.doi.org/10.2147/IJN.S185348] [PMID: 30519016]

[25] Karimi M, Bahrami S, Ravari SB, *et al.* Albumin nanostructures as advanced drug delivery systems. Expert Opin Drug Deliv 2016; 13(11): 1609-23. [http://dx.doi.org/10.1080/17425247.2016.1193149] [PMID: 27216915]

[26] Wang M, Zhang M, Fu L, *et al.* Liver-targeted delivery of TSG-6 by calcium phosphate nanoparticles for the management of liver fibrosis. Theranostics 2020; 10(1): 36-49. [http://dx.doi.org/10.7150/thno.37301] [PMID: 31903104]

[27] An FF, Zhang XH. Strategies for preparing albumin-based nanoparticles for multifunctional bioimaging and drug delivery. Theranostics 2017; 7(15): 3667-89. [http://dx.doi.org/10.7150/thno.19365] [PMID: 29109768]

[28] Jiang S, Tian S, Wang P, *et al.* Native and engineered extracellular vesicles: novel tools for treating liver disease. J Mater Chem B Mater Biol Med 2024; 12(16): 3840-56. [http://dx.doi.org/10.1039/D3TB01921G] [PMID: 38532706]

[29] Di L, Maiseyeu A. Low-density lipoprotein nanomedicines: mechanisms of targeting, biology, and theranostic potential. Drug Deliv 2021; 28(1): 408-21. [http://dx.doi.org/10.1080/10717544.2021.1886199] [PMID: 33594923]

[30] Herdiana Y, Febrina E, Nurhasanah S, Gozali D, Elamin KM, Wathoni N. Drug loading in chitosan-based nanoparticles. Pharmaceutics 2024; 16(8): 1043. [http://dx.doi.org/10.3390/pharmaceutics16081043] [PMID: 39204388]

[31] Liu J, Liu J, Mu W, *et al.* Delivery strategy to enhance the therapeutic efficacy of Liver Fibrosis *via* Nanoparticle Drug Delivery systems. ACS Nano 2024; 18(32): 20861-85. [http://dx.doi.org/10.1021/acsnano.4c02380] [PMID: 39082637]

[32] Yu Y, Wang Q, Huang X, Li Z. GA receptor targeted chitosan oligosaccharide polymer nanoparticles improve non-alcoholic fatty liver disease by inhibiting ferroptosis. Int J Biol Macromol 2024; 278(Pt 2): 134779. [http://dx.doi.org/10.1016/j.ijbiomac.2024.134779] [PMID: 39151850]

[33] Zhang X, Yi X, Gao X, Li Y, Shen X. Liver-targeted nanoparticles loaded with cannabidiol based on redox response for effective alleviation of acute liver injury. Foods 2024; 13(15): 2464. [http://dx.doi.org/10.3390/foods13152464] [PMID: 39123655]

[34] Hefnawy A, Abdelhamid AS, Abdelaziz MM, Elzoghby AO, Khalil IA. Recent advances in nano-based drug delivery systems for treatment of liver cancer. J Pharm Sci 2024; 113(11): 3145-72. [http://dx.doi.org/10.1016/j.xphs.2024.08.012] [PMID: 39151795]

[35] Duman H, Akdaşçi E, Eker F, Bechelany M, Karav S. Gold nanoparticles: Multifunctional properties,

synthesis, and future prospects. Nanomaterials (Basel) 2024; 14(22): 1805. [http://dx.doi.org/10.3390/nano14221805] [PMID: 39591046]

[36] Georgeous J, AlSawaftah N, Abuwatfa WH, Husseini GA. Review of gold nanoparticles: synthesis, properties, shapes, cellular uptake, targeting, release mechanisms and applications in drug delivery and therapy. Pharmaceutics 2024; 16(10): 1332. [http://dx.doi.org/10.3390/pharmaceutics16101332] [PMID: 39458661]

[37] Satapathy T, Diwakar MK. Molecular targets and nano-technological approaches in the treatment of hepatic carcinoma. Curr Cancer Drug Targets 2024; 24(1): 25. [http://dx.doi.org/10.2174/0113894501271207231127063431] [PMID: 39482912]

[38] Kataria T, Bose S, Kalia S, *et al.* Functionalized carbon nanotubes: An advanced tool with enhanced biomedical attributes. Curr Nanomed 2024; 15: 15. [http://dx.doi.org/10.2174/0124681873331266241003104137]

[39] Zaman M, Hameed H, Shazly GA, *et al.* Carbon nanotube marvels: unveiling synthetic methods and pharmaceutical frontiers in targeted delivery. In: Nanocomposites -Properties, Preparations and Applications. IntechOpen; 2024.

[40] Mendhe R, Dalal A. Carbon Nanotubes an Excellent Targeted Drug Delivery System. Res J Pharmacol Pharmacodyn 2024; 16: pp. 213-20.

[41] Vardhan H, Jain A, Singhai A. Potential of Dendrimers in Drug Delivery: An Updated Review. Asian J Pharm Res 2024; 14: 242-54.

[42] Yuan K, Lai K, Miao G, *et al.* Cholinized-polymer functionalized lipid-based drug carriers facilitate liver fibrosis therapy via ultrafast liver-targeting delivery. Biomacromolecules 2024; 25(10): 6526-38. [http://dx.doi.org/10.1021/acs.biomac.4c00691] [PMID: 39213520]

[43] N M, Ch S, B M, T RR. Dendrimers: An innovative tool of drug delivery system. International Journal of Zoological Investigations 2024; 10(2): 515-21. [http://dx.doi.org/10.33745/ijzi.2024.v10i02.048]

[44] Sztandera K, Rodríguez-García JL, Ceña V. *In Vivo* applications of dendrimers: A step toward the future of nanoparticle-mediated therapeutics. Pharmaceutics 2024.

[45] Huang W, Wang W, Wang P, *et al.* Glycyrrhetinic acid-functionalized degradable micelles as liver-targeted drug carrier. J Mater Sci Mater Med 2011; 22(4): 853-63. [http://dx.doi.org/10.1007/s10856-011-4262-2] [PMID: 21373811]

[46] Khafaga DSR, El-Morsy MT, Faried H, *et al.* Metal–organic frameworks in drug delivery: engineering versatile platforms for therapeutic applications. RSC Advances 2024; 14(41): 30201-29. [http://dx.doi.org/10.1039/D4RA04441J] [PMID: 39315019]

[47] Mukherjee S, Ray S, Thakur RS. Solid lipid nanoparticles: A modern formulation approach in drug delivery system. Indian J Pharm Sci 2009; 71(4): 349-58. [http://dx.doi.org/10.4103/0250-474X.57282] [PMID: 20502539]

[48] Baker SN, Baker GA. Luminescent carbon nanodots: emergent nanolights. Angew Chem Int Ed 2010; 49(38): 6726-44. [http://dx.doi.org/10.1002/anie.200906623] [PMID: 20687055]

[49] Müller RH, Keck CM. Twenty years of drug nanocrystals: Where are we, and where do we go? Eur J Pharm Biopharm 2012; 80(1): 1-3. [http://dx.doi.org/10.1016/j.ejpb.2011.09.012] [PMID: 21971369]

[50] Ma X, Li SJ, Liu Y, *et al.* Bioengineered nanogels for cancer immunotherapy. Chem Soc Rev 2022; 51(12): 5136-74. [http://dx.doi.org/10.1039/D2CS00247G] [PMID: 35666131]

[51] Wahi A, Bishnoi M, Raina N, *et al.* Recent updates on nano-phyto-formulations based therapeutic intervention for cancer treatment. Oncol Res 2024; 32(1): 19-47.

[http://dx.doi.org/10.32604/or.2023.042228] [PMID: 38188681]

[52] Maeda H, Wu J, Sawa T, Matsumura Y, Hori K. Tumor vascular permeability and the EPR effect in macromolecular therapeutics: a review. J Control Release 2000; 65(1-2): 271-84. [http://dx.doi.org/10.1016/S0168-3659(99)00248-5] [PMID: 10699287]

[53] Zenze M, Singh M. Receptor targeting using copolymer-modified gold nanoparticles for pCMV-Luc gene delivery to liver cancer cells *in vitro*. Int J Mol Sci 2024; 25(9): 5016. [http://dx.doi.org/10.3390/ijms25095016] [PMID: 38732235]

[54] Prabaharan M. Chitosan-based nanoparticles for tumor-targeted drug delivery. Int J Biol Macromol 2015; 72: 1313-22. [http://dx.doi.org/10.1016/j.ijbiomac.2014.10.052] [PMID: 25450550]

[55] Yang Y, Jun L, Cuili K, Shaoguo R, Xiaona Z. Research progress on non-alcoholic fatty liver disease induced by environmental pollutant. Asian J Ecotoxicol 2024; 19(3)

[56] Parra-Nieto J, de Carcer IA, García del Cid MA, Jiménez-Falcao S, Gónzalez-Larre J, Baeza A. Stimuli-responsive nanocarriers as active enhancers of antitumoral immunotherapy. Adv Mater Interfaces 2024; 11(30): 2400343. [http://dx.doi.org/10.1002/admi.202400343]

[57] Kalita T, Dezfouli SA, Pandey LM, Uludag H. siRNA functionalized lipid nanoparticles (LNPs) in management of diseases. Pharmaceutics 2022; 14(11): 2520. [http://dx.doi.org/10.3390/pharmaceutics14112520] [PMID: 36432711]

[58] Khaja F, Jayawardena D, Kuzmis A, Önyüksel H. Targeted sterically stabilized phospholipid siRNA nanomedicine for hepatic and renal fibrosis. Nanomaterials (Basel) 2016; 6(1): 8. [http://dx.doi.org/10.3390/nano6010008] [PMID: 28344266]

[59] Lorenzer C, Dirin M, Winkler AM, Baumann V, Winkler J. Going beyond the liver: Progress and challenges of targeted delivery of siRNA therapeutics. J Control Release 2015; 203: 1-15. [http://dx.doi.org/10.1016/j.jconrel.2015.02.003] [PMID: 25660205]

[60] Duan L, Yan Y, Liu J, *et al.* Target delivery of small interfering RNAs with vitamin E-coupled nanoparticles for treating hepatitis C. Sci Rep 2016; 6(1): 24867. [http://dx.doi.org/10.1038/srep24867] [PMID: 27113197]

[61] Xiao Y, Shi K, Qu Y, Chu B, Qian Z. Engineering nanoparticles for targeted delivery of nucleic acid therapeutics in tumor. Mol Ther Methods Clin Dev 2019; 12: 1-18. [http://dx.doi.org/10.1016/j.omtm.2018.09.002] [PMID: 30364598]

[62] Neumayer C, Ng D, Requena D, *et al.* GalNAc-conjugated siRNA targeting the DNAJB1-PRKACA fusion junction in fibrolamellar hepatocellular carcinoma. Mol Ther 2024; 32(1): 140-51. [http://dx.doi.org/10.1016/j.ymthe.2023.11.012] [PMID: 37980543]

[63] Holm A, Løvendorf MB, Kauppinen S. Development of siRNA therapeutics for the treatment of liver diseases. Design and delivery of SiRNA therapeutics. 2021: 57-75. [http://dx.doi.org/10.1007/978-1-0716-1298-9_5]

[64] Keeler AM, ElMallah MK, Flotte TR. Gene therapy 2017: progress and future directions. Clin Transl Sci 2017; 10(4): 242-8. [http://dx.doi.org/10.1111/cts.12466] [PMID: 28383804]

[65] Gong J, Wang HX, Lao YH, *et al.* A versatile nonviral delivery system for multiplex gene□Editing in the liver. Adv Mater 2020; 32(46): 2003537. [http://dx.doi.org/10.1002/adma.202003537] [PMID: 33053221]

[66] Guzman Gonzalez V, Grunenberger A, Nicoud O, *et al.* Enhanced CRISPR-Cas9 RNA system delivery using cell penetrating peptides-based nanoparticles for efficient in vitro and in vivo applications. J Control Release 2024; 376: 1160-75. [http://dx.doi.org/10.1016/j.jconrel.2024.11.008] [PMID: 39521064]

[67] Qiu M, Glass Z, Chen J, *et al.* Lipid nanoparticle-mediated codelivery of Cas9 mRNA and single-guide RNA achieves liver-specific in vivo genome editing of *Angptl3*. Proc Natl Acad Sci USA 2021; 118(10): e2020401118.
[http://dx.doi.org/10.1073/pnas.2020401118] [PMID: 33649229]

[68] Yang Y, Wang X. Nano-drug delivery systems (NDDS) in metabolic dysfunction-associated steatotic liver disease (MASLD): current status, prospects and challenges. Front Pharmacol 2024; 15: 1419384.
[http://dx.doi.org/10.3389/fphar.2024.1419384] [PMID: 39166109]

[69] Che T, Song Y, Su W, Xing S, Wang H, Tan M. Hepatic parenchymal cell and mitochondrial-targeted astaxanthin nanocarriers for relief of high fat diet-induced nonalcoholic fatty liver disease. Food Funct 2023; 14(6): 2908-20.
[http://dx.doi.org/10.1039/D2FO04036K] [PMID: 36883333]

[70] Fu J, Dong H, Wu J, Jin Y. Emerging progress of RNA-Based Antitumor therapeutics. Int J Biol Sci 2023; 19(10): 3159-83.
[http://dx.doi.org/10.7150/ijbs.83732] [PMID: 37416764]

[71] Torchilin VP. Multifunctional nanocarriers. Adv Drug Deliv Rev 2012; 64(Suppl): 302-15.

[72] Allen TM, Cullis PR. Liposomal drug delivery systems: From concept to clinical applications. Adv Drug Deliv Rev 2013; 65(1): 36-48.

[73] Peer D, Karp JM, Hong S, Farokhzad OC, Margalit R, Langer R. Nanocarriers as an emerging platform for cancer therapy. Nat Nanotechnol 2007; 2(12): 751-60.

[74] Blanco E, Shen H, Ferrari M. Principles of nanoparticle design for overcoming biological barriers to drug delivery. Nat Biotechnol 2015; 33(9): 941-51.

[75] Farokhzad OC, Langer R. Impact of nanotechnology on drug delivery. ACS Nano 2009; 3(1): 16-20.

[76] Duncan R, Izzo L. Dendrimer biocompatibility and toxicity. Adv Drug Deliv Rev 2005; 57(15): 2215-37.

[77] Kesharwani P, Jain K, Jain NK. Dendrimer as nanocarrier for drug delivery. Prog Polym Sci 2014; 39(2): 268-307.

[78] Bobo D, Robinson KJ, Islam J, Thurecht KJ, Corrie SR. Nanoparticle-based medicines: A review of FDA-approved materials and clinical trials. Pharm Res 2016; 33(10): 2373-87.

[79] Zhang L, Gu FX, Chan JM, Wang AZ, Langer RS, Farokhzad OC. Nanoparticles in medicine: Therapeutic applications and developments. Clin Pharmacol Ther 2008; 83(5): 761-9.

[80] Wang AZ, Langer R, Farokhzad OC. Nanoparticle delivery of cancer drugs. Annu Rev Med 2012; 63: 185-98.

[81] Sercombe L, Veerati T, Moheimani F, Wu SY, Sood AK, Hua S. Advances and challenges of liposome assisted drug delivery. Front Pharmacol 2015; 6: 286.

[82] Panyam J, Labhasetwar V. Biodegradable nanoparticles for drug and gene delivery to cells and tissue. Adv Drug Deliv Rev 2003; 55(3): 329-47.

[83] Sahoo SK, Labhasetwar V. Nanotech approaches to delivery and imaging drug. Drug Discov Today 2003; 8(24): 1112-20.

[84] Owens DE, Peppas NA. Opsonization, biodistribution, and pharmacokinetics of polymeric nanoparticles. Int J Pharm 2006; 307(1): 93-102.

[85] Wilhelm S, Tavares AJ, Dai Q, *et al.* Analysis of nanoparticle delivery to tumours. Nat Rev Mater 2016; 1: 16014.

CHAPTER 5

Lipid-based Nanocarriers for Fatty Liver Disease

Monika Sharma[1,*], **Diksha Sharma**[2], **Sonia Gupta**[2] and **Jasmine Bhatia**[2]

[1] *Bharat Institute of Pharmacy, Kurukshetra, Haryana, India*

[2] *Swami Devi Dyal Institute of Pharmacy, Panchkula, Haryana, India*

Abstract: Lipid-based nanocarriers (LBCs) have emerged as a promising strategy for the targeted treatment of fatty liver diseases, including non-alcoholic fatty liver disease (NAFLD) and non-alcoholic steatohepatitis (NASH). These nanocarriers offer several advantages, including enhanced bioavailability, controlled release, and targeted delivery of therapeutic agents, all of which are crucial for improving treatment outcomes in hepatic disorders. Solid lipid nanoparticles (SLNs), liposomes, and nanostructured lipid carriers (NLCs) are lipid nanoparticles that have been extensively studied for their ability to encapsulate lipophilic drugs, antioxidants, and gene therapies, offering efficient liver-specific drug-delivery solutions. This chapter explains the different ways LBC can deliver drugs to the liver, the formulation techniques used, and how they may help reduce the pathophysiology of fatty liver diseases. Additionally, it examines the challenges, potential applications, and clinical implications of developing lipid-based nanocarrier systems for liver-targeted therapies.

Keywords: Lipid-based nanocarriers, Liposomes, Non-alcoholic fatty liver disease, Nanostructured lipid carriers.

INTRODUCTION TO FATTY LIVER DISEASES

Non-alcoholic fatty liver disease (NAFLD) is a common disorder characterized by an excessive buildup of fat in the liver in people, especially those who consume little to no alcohol. NAFLD, which includes a range from simple steatosis to non-alcoholic steatohepatitis (NASH), is characterized by liver inflammation, cell injury, and fibrosis, significantly raising the risk of cirrhosis, liver failure, and carcinomas, which are closely associated with obesity, type 2 diabetes, and high cholesterol. Up to 25% of people worldwide suffer from NAFLD, with a higher prevalence in Western nations as a result of the growing frequency of metabolic diseases. Even though it is less frequent, NASH is predicted to rise as more instances of NAFLD develop into this severe type. Imaging techniques, such as

* **Corresponding author Monika Sharma:** Bharat Institute of Pharmacy, Kurukshetra, Haryana, India; E-mail: 21dikshsharma@gmail.com

Anjali Sharma, Devkant Sharma, Ajmer Singh Grewal, Geeta Deswal & Ganga Reddy Velma (Eds.)

ultrasound or MRI, are usually used for diagnosis, with biopsy employed in more advanced stages [1, 2].

CURRENT THERAPEUTIC APPROACHES AND THEIR LIMITATIONS

For the treatment of NAFLD and NASH, current strategies primarily focus on reducing liver fat content and improving liver function tests. Other therapeutic interventions are as follows:

- Lifestyle Modifications
- Weight Loss
- Dietary Adjustments
- Physical Activity

However, they are not sufficient to reverse the more severe forms of liver damage seen in NASH, such as fibrosis and cirrhosis [3]. For targeting the underlying pathophysiological mechanisms of NAFLD and NASH, pharmacological therapies have been explored, but are associated with side effects. For example

- Thiazolidinediones improve insulin sensitivity and have shown promise, but weight gain and edema side effects limit their use [4].
- Statins and lipid-lowering medications possess the potential to reduce liver inflammation and fibrosis, but their effectiveness specifically for NASH remains uncertain [5].

Moreover, the antioxidant vitamin E has demonstrated some benefit in reducing liver inflammation in non-diabetic individuals with NASH; however, its long-term safety and efficacy are still awaited [6].

ROLE OF NANOTECHNOLOGY IN THE TREATMENT OF LIVER DISEASE

Liver diseases like NAFLD and NASH could be managed using nanotechnology due to its site-specific drug delivery and lower systemic toxicity. API can be delivered directly to the liver using nanoparticle engineering. Enhanced bioavailability and improved treatment with reduced side effects are the primary objectives of nanotechnology. It allows for precise delivery at the cellular or molecular level. Furthermore, nanoparticles can be used as sophisticated imaging agents that enable non-invasive monitoring and detection of liver fibrosis and inflammation using techniques, such as CT and MRI [7 - 10].

Role of Nanocarriers in the Management of NASH and NAFLD

Nanocarriers are compact particles in the size range of 1-1000 nanometers that are used to deliver drugs, genes, or other agents to specific hepatic sites. Due to their small size, nanocarriers can easily navigate biological barriers, such as cell membranes, making them highly effective for targeted drug delivery to hepatic cells.

Lipid-based Nano Carriers (LBCs) in the Management of NASH and NAFLD

LBCs are an emerging class of drug delivery systems that use lipids as the primary material for encapsulating therapeutic agents for liver delivery. The various types of LBCs, along with their properties, are shown in Table **1**. These nanocarriers are designed to enhance the solubility, stability, and bioavailability of hydrophobic drugs. Additionally, their biocompatibility, biodegradability, and enhanced targeting capabilities have made them attractive platforms for pharmaceutical and biomedical applications. The most common LBCs include:

Table 1. Types of LBCs with their properties.

Feature	SLNs	NLCs	Liposomes
Structure	Solid lipid core with surfactant shell	Blend of solid and liquid lipids forming a hybrid matrix	One or more phospholipid bilayers forming spherical vesicles
Size Range	50–1000 nm	50–300 nm	Variable 50–500 nm
Drug Encapsulation	Mainly lipophilic drugs	Enhanced loading for hydrophobic drugs	Both hydrophilic (core) and hydrophobic (bilayer) drugs
Targeting Ability	Passive targeting, potential for nucleic acid delivery	Passive targeting, improved cellular uptake	Naturally targets liver (RES uptake); can be surface-modified
Stability	Good thermal stability (up to 37 °C)	Long-Term stability due to lipid matrix flexibility	Structurally similar to cell membranes but prone to physical instability
Formulation Methods	- High-pressure homogenization - Solvent evaporation -Microemulsion method	- Hot/cold homogenization -Ultrasonication - Solvent diffusion	- Thin film hydration - Reverse-phase evaporation
Applications	-Vaccine delivery (Hepatitis B) -siRNA & DNA delivery	-Delivery of hydrophobic drugs -Controlled release systems	-Gene therapy - Liver-targeted drug delivery - Antioxidant delivery
References	[11 - 15]	[16 - 18]	[19, 20]

- Solid-lipid nanoparticles (SLNs)
- Nano-structured lipid carriers (NLCs)
- Liposomes

LIVER-TARGETED DRUG DELIVERY SYSTEMS

Liver-targeted drug delivery systems are designed to selectively deliver API to hepatic tissue, thereby maximizing efficacy and minimizing systemic side effects. There are different mechanisms through which a therapeutic agent could reach a specific site [21 - 23].

Liver Targeting Mechanisms

Passive Targeting

Passive targeting relies on the natural physiology of the liver. Kupffer cells and the reticuloendothelial system (RES) play a major role by phagocytosing circulating nanoparticles and foreign particles. The fenestrated structure of liver sinusoids, along with its dual blood supply from the portal vein and hepatic artery, allows easier accumulation of therapeutic agents. Moreover, the enhanced permeability and retention (EPR) effect and the interaction of particles with sinusoidal endothelial cells contribute to nanoparticle trapping and retention within the liver. The curcumin-loaded solid lipid nanoparticle formulation showed significantly enhanced liver uptake, improved bioavailability, and sustained release compared to the free drug. The system successfully reduced hepatic lipid accumulation, improved liver enzyme profiles, and exhibited protective effects in an animal/cellular model of NAFLD [24, 25].

Active Targeting

Active targeting involves receptor-mediated uptake of therapeutic agents using specific ligands or antibodies. The Asialoglycoprotein receptor (ASGPR), abundantly expressed on hepatocytes, recognizes desialylated glycoproteins and is widely used for hepatocyte-specific drug delivery. [47]. Doxorubicin-loaded nanoparticles functionalised with pullulan/arabinogalactan ligands achieved a remarkable hepatocyte-to–non-parenchymal cell uptake ratio of approximately 85:15 [26].

Reticuloendothelial System (RES):

The body's **RES** is made up of macrophages and dendritic cells in the liver, spleen, and bone marrow that play a major role in how nanocarriers behave once injected. In the liver, macrophages clear nanoparticles from the bloodstream by recognizing them as "foreign," ingesting and degrading them. **By opsonization**, nanocarriers are coated with proteins like immunoglobulins, complement proteins, or apolipoproteins, which makes them more visible to Kupffer cells (macrophages) and speeds their uptake. For example, Cai R et al. demonstrated that nanoparticles that acquire a corona enriched in opsonin proteins, such as complement C3 and immunoglobulins, show markedly higher uptake by macrophages [27].

Effect of Surface Modifications for Enhanced Liver Targeting

In drug delivery systems, surface alterations for improved liver targeting are a crucial research topic, especially for the treatment of liver-related conditions, such as cirrhosis, hepatitis, and liver cancer. The capacity of ligands to selectively target liver cells, including asialoorosomucoid, galactose, and mannose, has been thoroughly investigated. For example, galactose-modified nanocarriers (Gal-OSL/Res) were used to deliver resveratrol (RSV), a compound known for its anti-inflammatory and antioxidant effects. Gal-OSL/Res significantly enhanced cellular uptake of RSV in steatotic HepG2 cells and effectively reduced triglyceride accumulation [28, 29].

Folic Acid Conjugation for Targeting

As liver cancer cells exhibit large numbers of folate receptors, folic acid is a well-known ligand for targeting liver cells, especially hepatocellular carcinoma. Folic acid conjugation to nanoparticle surfaces enhances liver-specific targeting. One of the primary factors influencing a nanoparticle's ability to target the liver is its size. For hepatic uptake, nanoparticles in the 20–200 nm size range are optimal. Folate receptor–mediated endocytosis increases the cellular uptake of curcumin, thereby enhancing its therapeutic efficacy against NASH progression [30 - 32] (Table **2**).

Table 2. Various examples of LBCs in the management of NASH and NAFLD.

Examples of LBCs	Model System Used	Result	Reference
Dual-ligand nanostructured lipid carriers (NLCs) (Dehydrocavidine, **Glycyrrhetinic acid, Galactose-PEG2000-NH$_2$)**	***In vitro***: aHSC-T6 (rat hepatic stellate cell line) -***In vivo***: Rat model of liver fibrosis	- Enhanced liver targeting and apoptosis of aHSCs (via increased Bax expression). - Reduced extracellular matrix deposition. - Greater anti-fibrotic effects than GA- or GalNH$_2$-only NLCs.	[33]
Semaglutide-loaded lipid nanocapsules	MASLD (dietary mouse model)	Oral nanocapsule delivery of the glucagon-like peptide-1 (GLP-1) analog semaglutide improved glucose homeostasis and markers of inflammation better than oral suspension, and prevented progression towards more severe disease.	[34]
Lipid nanocapsules (LNCs) loaded with GLP-1	NAFLD/NASH (genetic and dietary models of mouse)	Oral LNCs increased glucagon-like peptide 1 levels, improved glucose homeostasis and insulin resistance better than subcutaneous analogs, and mitigated the progression of disease.	[35]
Nanostructured lipid carriers cantaining Astragaloside IV	TGF-β1-activated HSCs	Significantly higher uptake for PDGFR-β-targeting/ Astragaloside IV NLCs compared to non-targeted NLCs.	[36]
Liposome-allicin-aptamer (LAA)	Genetic and dietary models of the mouse	LAA showed superior performance in improving NAFLD compared with free allicin. *In vitro* results showed that allicin loaded in liposome reduced oleic acid-induced intracellular lipid droplet accumulation and triglyceride synthesis in HepG2 cells and *in vivo*. It significantly reduced lipid accumulation and improved liver injury than free allicin.	[37]

(Table 2) cont.....

Examples of LBCs	Model System Used	Result	Reference
Galactose-Functionalized Nanoemulsion Co-Loaded with Resveratrol and β-Carotene	High-fat diet (HFD)-induced NASH in rodents	Treatment with galactose-functionalized nanoemulsion loaded with resveratrol and β-carotene showed significant improvement in liver pathology and biochemical markers compared to controls.	[38]

OPTIMIZATION AND SCALE-UP STRATEGIES FOR LBC

LBC offers a biocompatible, versatile drug-delivery platform across multiple administration routes. However, successful clinical translation requires meticulous formulation optimization and robust scale-up strategies to ensure consistency and minimize variations.

Scale-up Challenges

Transitioning LBC from laboratory-scale research to industrial-scale production for NASH and NAFLD therapy requires strategic optimization of both formulation and process parameters. Particle size (ideally 100–200 nm), zeta potential, and drug encapsulation efficiency must be controlled to ensure effective hepatic targeting with maximum systemic performance.

Moreover, lipid selection plays a critical role. Biocompatible solid lipids, such as glyceryl monostearate and stearic acid, and liquid lipids, such as oleic acid and medium-chain triglycerides, are often preferred for their stability and ability to encapsulate lipophilic drugs. The surfactant class and concentration, typically 1–5% w/w (*e.g.*, Tween 80 or Poloxamer 188), must be optimized to stabilize the nanocarriers and prevent aggregation without compromising cellular compatibility or scalability.

Furthermore, ligand modifications, such as folic acid, galactose, and glycyrrhizin conjugation, enable active targeting via receptor-mediated hepatocyte uptake (*e.g.*, ASGPR), thereby enhancing drug accumulation in diseased liver tissues.

Microfluidization or high-pressure homogenization (HPH) ensures uniform nanocarrier distribution and improves liver uptake by controlling particle size.

For industrial-scale manufacturing, scalable techniques, such as ultrasonication systems, high-shear homogenizers, high-pressure homogenizers (*e.g.*, Microfluidizer®), and tangential flow filtration for purification, are essential.

To reduce production costs and enhance commercial viability, robust quality control systems, continuous manufacturing technologies, and automated emulsification processes should be integrated. Ultimately, by fine-tuning surfactant concentration, selecting optimal lipid types, and adopting industrial-scale equipment, LBC for NASH and NAFLD can be efficiently scaled up while maintaining therapeutic performance and regulatory compliance [39, 40].

CLINICAL IMPLICATIONS AND CHALLENGES

LBCs hold considerable clinical promise, yet concerns regarding their toxicity, biocompatibility, and stability remain significant. The lipid, surfactant, and stabilizer composition can impact cytotoxicity, immunogenicity, and systemic tolerance, necessitating thorough *in vitro* and *in vivo* evaluations. Stability and storage are critical for clinical application; factors, such as temperature sensitivity, oxidation, and aggregation, can compromise long-term viability. Optimizing lipid composition and maintaining careful storage conditions are essential. Regulatory challenges, including stringent safety, efficacy, and GMP compliance requirements, further complicate their translation into clinical use. Overcoming these obstacles is quite crucial for realizing the full therapeutic potential of lipid-based nanocarriers [41, 42].

FUTURE DIRECTIONS IN LIPID NANOCARRIER RESEARCH

Advancements in lipid nanocarriers are revolutionizing targeted drug delivery, improving therapeutic efficacy while minimizing systemic toxicity. Innovations, such as stimuli-responsive, multifunctional lipid-based systems enable precise, site-specific drug release. Personalized medicine is also gaining momentum, particularly for conditions like fatty liver disease, where patient-specific biomarkers optimize treatment outcomes.

Emerging Trends

- Integration with Gene and Immunotherapy: Combining LBCs with gene therapy, immunotherapy, and targeted small-molecule drugs enhances treatment strategies for complex diseases.
- Smart Lipid Systems: High drug-loading nanoformulations and nano-pruning techniques enable biologically responsive drug release.
- Intelligent Lipid Monolayers: Designed to dynamically respond to physiological conditions, facilitating precise drug and nutrient delivery.
- Nano-Micro Hybrid Carriers: Combining nanoscale and microscale systems expands therapeutic applications.

Challenges and Regulatory Considerations

Regulatory approval remains a major hurdle, requiring 5–10 years of preclinical studies to establish safety and efficacy. Large-scale viability and compliance with stringent regulations are crucial for clinical translation. Despite these challenges, continued advancements promise safer, more effective treatments across various diseases [43 - 45].

CONCLUSION

The role of lipid-based nanocarriers in targeting the liver, especially for NAFLD and NASH, has been found indispensable, with multiple merits, including biocompatibility, enhanced solubility, reduced toxicity, and controlled release. By developing multiple preparation methods, such as HSH, solvent evaporation, emulsification-dispersion, and microemulsion techniques, their manufacturing costs are reduced, and their availability is increased. The detailed applications of SLNs, NLCs, and liposomes revealed that lipid-based nanocarriers occupy a vast section of the pharmaceutical market.

LIST OF ABBREVIATIONS

API	Active Pharmaceutical Ingredient
ASGPR	Asialoglycoprotein Receptor
EPR	Enhanced Permeability and Retention
GLP-1	Glucagon-Like Peptide-1
HSH	High Shear Homogenization
LBCs	Lipid-Based Nanocarriers
LNPs	Lipid Nanoparticles
MRI	Magnetic Resonance Imaging
NAFLD	Non-Alcoholic Fatty Liver Disease
NASH	Non-Alcoholic Steatohepatitis
NLCs	Nanostructured Lipid Carriers
RES	Reticuloendothelial System
RNA	Ribonucleic Acid
SLNs	Solid Lipid Nanoparticles
MASLD	Metabolic dysfunction-associated steatotic liver disease
aHSCs	Activated hepatic stellate cells

REFERENCES

[1] Younossi ZM, Koenig AB, Abdelatif D, Fazel Y, Henry L, Wymer M. Global epidemiology of nonalcoholic fatty liver disease—Meta-analytic assessment of prevalence, incidence, and outcomes.

Hepatology 2016; 64(1): 73-84.
[http://dx.doi.org/10.1002/hep.28431] [PMID: 26707365]

[2] Chalasani N, Younossi Z, Lavine JE, *et al.* The diagnosis and management of nonalcoholic fatty liver disease: Practice guidance from the american association for the study of liver Diseases. Hepatology 2018; 67(1): 328-57.
[http://dx.doi.org/10.1002/hep.29367] [PMID: 28714183]

[3] Vilar-Gomez E, Martinez-Perez Y, Calzadilla-Bertot L, Torres-Gonzalez A, Gra-Oramas B, Gonzalez-Fabian L, *et al.* Weight loss through lifestyle modification significantly reduces features of nonalcoholic steatohepatitis. Gastroenterology 2015; 149(2): 367-78.e5.
[http://dx.doi.org/10.1053/j.gastro.2015.04.005] [PMID: 25865049]

[4] He L, Liu X, Wang L, Yang Z, *et al.* Thiazolidinediones for nonalcoholic steatohepatitis: a meta-analysis of randomized clinical trials. Medicine (Baltimore) 2016; 95(42): e4947.
[http://dx.doi.org/10.1097/MD.0000000000004947] [PMID: 27759627]

[5] Doumas M, Imprialos K, Dimakopoulou A, Stavropoulos K, Binas A, Athyros VG. The role of statins in the management of nonalcoholic fatty liver disease. Curr Pharm Des 2019; 24(38): 4587-92.
[http://dx.doi.org/10.2174/1381612825666190117114305] [PMID: 30652643]

[6] Shah RA, Kowdley KV, *et al.* Obeticholic acid for the treatment of nonalcoholic steatohepatitis. Expert Rev Gastroenterol Hepatol 2018; 14(5): 311-21.
[http://dx.doi.org/10.1080/17474124.2020.1748498] [PMID: 32241197]

[7] Wang S, Wu Y, Yuan M, *et al.* Nanotechnology-Enabled Diagnosis and Treatment of Hepatocellular Carcinoma: Theranostics, Combination Regimens, and Translation. International Journal of Nanomedicine 2026 Dec 31; 581911.

[8] Müller RH, Radtke M, Wissing SA. Solid lipid nanoparticles (SLN) and nanostructured lipid carriers (NLC) in cosmetic and dermatological preparations. Adv Drug Deliv Rev 2002; 54 (Suppl. 1): S131-55.
[http://dx.doi.org/10.1016/S0169-409X(02)00118-7] [PMID: 12460720]

[9] Müller RH, Mäder K, Gohla S. Solid lipid nanoparticles (SLN) for controlled drug delivery: a review of the state of the art. Eur J Pharm Biopharm 2000; 50(1): 161-77.

[10] Kim MW, Jeong HY, Kang SJ, *et al.* Cancer-targeted nucleic acid delivery and quantum dot imaging using EGF receptor aptamer-conjugated lipid nanoparticles. Sci Rep 2017; 7: 9474.
[http://dx.doi.org/10.1038/s41598-017-09555-w] [PMID: 28842588]

[11] Bukke SPN, Venkatesh C, Bandenahalli Rajanna S, *et al.* Solid lipid nanocarriers for drug delivery: design innovations and characterization strategies—a comprehensive review. Discover Applied Sciences 2024; 6: 279.
[http://dx.doi.org/10.1007/s42452-024-05897-z]

[12] Amoabediny G, Haghiralsadat F, Naderinezhad S, *et al.* Overview of preparation methods of polymeric and lipid-based (niosome, solid lipid, liposome) nanoparticles: A comprehensive review. Int J Polym Mater 2018; 67(6): 383-400.
[http://dx.doi.org/10.1080/00914037.2017.1332623]

[13] Harde H, Das M, Jain S. Solid lipid nanoparticles: an oral bioavailability enhancer vehicle. Expert Opin Drug Deliv 2011; 8(11): 1407-24.
[http://dx.doi.org/10.1517/17425247.2011.604311] [PMID: 21831007]

[14] Geszke-Moritz M, Moritz M. Solid lipid nanoparticles as attractive drug vehicles: Composition, properties and therapeutic strategies. Mater Sci Eng C 2016; 68: 982-94.
[http://dx.doi.org/10.1016/j.msec.2016.05.119] [PMID: 27524099]

[15] Hao J, Wang F, Wang X, *et al.* Development and optimization of baicalin-loaded solid lipid nanoparticles prepared by coacervation method using central composite design. Eur J Pharm Sci 2012; 47(2): 497-505.

[http://dx.doi.org/10.1016/j.ejps.2012.07.006] [PMID: 22820033]

[16] Andrade LN, Oliveira DML, Chaud MV, *et al.* Praziquantel-solid lipid nanoparticles produced by supercritical carbon dioxide extraction: physicochemical characterization, release profile, and cytotoxicity. Molecules 2019; 24(21): 3881.
[http://dx.doi.org/10.3390/molecules24213881] [PMID: 31661906]

[17] Shahgaldian P, Da Silva E, Coleman AW, Rather B, Zaworotko MJ. Para-acyl-calix-arene based solid lipid nanoparticles (SLNs): a detailed study of preparation and stability parameters. Int J Pharm 2003; 253(1-2): 23-38.
[http://dx.doi.org/10.1016/S0378-5173(02)00639-7] [PMID: 12593934]

[18] Qushawy M, Nasr A. Solid lipid nanoparticles (SLNs) as nano drug delivery carriers: preparation, characterization and application. Int J Appl Pharm 2020; 12(1): 1-9.
[http://dx.doi.org/10.22159/ijap.2020v12i1.35312]

[19] Mohammadi-Samani S, Ghasemiyeh P. Solid lipid nanoparticles and nanostructured lipid carriers as novel drug delivery systems: applications, advantages and disadvantages. Res Pharm Sci 2018; 13(4): 288-303.
[http://dx.doi.org/10.4103/1735-5362.235156] [PMID: 30065762]

[20] Mukherjee S, Ray S, Thakur RS. Solid lipid nanoparticles: A modern formulation approach in drug delivery system. Indian J Pharm Sci 2009; 71(4): 349-58.
[http://dx.doi.org/10.4103/0250-474X.57282] [PMID: 20502539]

[21] Bon C, Hofer T, Bousquet-Mélou A, Davies MR, Krippendorff BF. Capacity limits of asialoglycoprotein receptor-mediated liver targeting. MAbs 2017; 9(8): 1360-9.
[http://dx.doi.org/10.1080/19420862.2017.1373924] [PMID: 28876162]

[22] Ise H, Nikaido T, Negishi N, *et al.* Effective hepatocyte transplantation using rat hepatocytes with low asialoglycoprotein receptor expression. Am J Pathol 2004; 165(2): 501-10.
[http://dx.doi.org/10.1016/S0002-9440(10)63315-9] [PMID: 15277224]

[23] Ellipilli S, Wang H, Binzel DW, Shu D, Guo P. Ligand-displaying-exosomes using RNA nanotechnology for targeted delivery of multi-specific drugs for liver cancer regression. Nanomedicine 2023; 50: 102667.
[http://dx.doi.org/10.1016/j.nano.2023.102667] [PMID: 36948369]

[24] Verma NK, Roshan A, Singh VK, *et al.* Liver specific targeted drug delivery system: a review. Asian J Phytomed Clin Res 2019; 7(1): 49-66.

[25] Meng X, Zhu G, Yang YG, Sun T. Targeted delivery strategies: The interactions and applications of nanoparticles in liver diseases. Biomed Pharmacother 2024; 175: 116702.
[http://dx.doi.org/10.1016/j.biopha.2024.116702] [PMID: 38729052]

[26] Landschulz KT, Pathak RK, Rigotti A, Krieger M, Hobbs HH. Regulation of scavenger receptor, class B, type I, a high density lipoprotein receptor, in liver and steroidogenic tissues of the rat. J Clin Invest 1996; 98(4): 984-95.
[http://dx.doi.org/10.1172/JCI118883] [PMID: 8770871]

[27] Nel A, Xia T, Mädler L, Li N, Hoek EM, Somasundaran P, *et al.* Toxic potential of materials at the nanolevel. Science 2006; 311(5761): 622-7.
[http://dx.doi.org/10.1126/science.1114397] [PMID: 16456071]

[28] Wang Q, Zhang L, Hu W, *et al.* Norcantharidin-associated galactosylated chitosan nanoparticles for hepatocyte-targeted delivery. Nanomedicine 2010; 6(2): 371-81.
[http://dx.doi.org/10.1016/j.nano.2009.07.006] [PMID: 19699319]

[29] Yang KW, Li XR, Yang ZL, Li PZ, Wang F, Liu Y. Novel polyion complex micelles for liver-targeted delivery of diammonium glycyrrhizinate: *In vitro* and *in vivo* characterization. J Biomed Mater Res A 2009; 88A(1): 140-8.
[http://dx.doi.org/10.1002/jbm.a.31866] [PMID: 18260143]

[30] Kim SI, Shin D, Choi TH, *et al.* Systemic and specific delivery of small interfering RNAs to the liver mediated by apolipoprotein A-I. Mol Ther 2007; 15(6): 1145-52.
[http://dx.doi.org/10.1038/sj.mt.6300168] [PMID: 17440441]

[31] Longmuir KJ, Haynes SM, Baratta JL, Kasabwalla N, Robertson RT. Liposomal delivery of doxorubicin to hepatocytes *in vivo* by targeting heparan sulfate. Int J Pharm 2009; 382(1-2): 222-33.
[http://dx.doi.org/10.1016/j.ijpharm.2009.07.030] [PMID: 19664697]

[32] Zhang Q, Li X, Zhang X, *et al.* Folic acid-conjugated curcumin nanoparticles for targeted treatment of non-alcoholic steatohepatitis. Int J Nanomedicine 2021; 16: 2309-22.

[33] Su X, Zhong H, Zeng Y, *et al.* Dual-ligand-functionalized nanostructured lipid carriers as a novel dehydrocavidine delivery system for liver fibrosis therapy. Colloids Surf B Biointerfaces 2025; 246: 114376.
[http://dx.doi.org/10.1016/j.colsurfb.2024.114376] [PMID: 39551037]

[34] Domingues I, Yagoubi H, Zhang W, *et al.* Effects of semaglutide-loaded lipid nanocapsules on metabolic dysfunction-associated steatotic liver disease. Drug Deliv Transl Res 2024; 14(10): 2917-29.
[http://dx.doi.org/10.1007/s13346-024-01576-z] [PMID: 38615156]

[35] Domingues I, Michalowski CB, Marotti V, *et al.* Exploiting the biological effect exerted by lipid nanocapsules in non-alcoholic fatty liver disease. J Control Release 2023; 356: 542-53.
[http://dx.doi.org/10.1016/j.jconrel.2023.03.012] [PMID: 36907563]

[36] Zhang S, Zhang X, Wang M, Guo L, Tan S. Corrigendum to "pPB peptide-modified nanostructured lipid carriers loaded with astragaloside IV as a potential strategy for enhanced antifibrosis therapy" [Int. J. Biol. Macromol. 319 (2025) 145221]. Int J Biol Macromol 2025; 319(Pt 2): 146243.
[http://dx.doi.org/10.1016/j.ijbiomac.2025.146243] [PMID: 40713255]

[37] Li J, Huang K, Song Y, Wang Y, Li J, He X, *et al.* Synergistic effect on nonalcoholic fatty liver disease by aptamer-functionalized liposome loading allicin. J Funct Foods 2024; 114: 104003.
[http://dx.doi.org/10.1016/j.jfutfo.2024.04.003]

[38] Fan Y, Bai H, Liu T, Wang R, Wang Z. The role of galactose and chitosan in novel targeted nanoemulsion delivery carriers: Synthesis, in vitro stability, and anti-Hepa 1–6 cell activity. Carbohydr Polym 2025; 358: 123515.
[http://dx.doi.org/10.1016/j.carbpol.2025.123515] [PMID: 40383575]

[39] Khairnar SV, Pagare P, Thakre A, *et al.* Review on the scale-up methods for the preparation of solid lipid nanoparticles. Pharmaceutics 2022; 14(9): 1886.
[http://dx.doi.org/10.3390/pharmaceutics14091886] [PMID: 36145632]

[40] Upadhyay P, Aslam R, Tiwari V, Upadhyay S. Lipid-based nanocarrier drug delivery approach for biomedical application. Curr Nanomater 2024; 9(2): 92-108.
[http://dx.doi.org/10.2174/2405461508666230508140508]

[41] Patel J, Roy H, Khobragade DS, *et al.* Natural lipid-based nanoformulations for enhancing hepatoprotective activity: mechanisms, efficacy, and clinical translation. Health Nanotechnology 2025; 1(1): 11.
[http://dx.doi.org/10.1186/s44301-025-00010-8]

[42] Hassan AAA, Ramadan E, Kristó K, Regdon G Jr, Sovány T. Lipid-polymer hybrid nanoparticles as a smart drug delivery system for peptide/protein delivery. Pharmaceutics 2025; 17(6): 797.
[http://dx.doi.org/10.3390/pharmaceutics17060797] [PMID: 40574109]

[43] Cheng Z, Fobian SF, Gurrieri E, *et al.* Lipid-based nanosystems: the next generation of cancer immune therapy. J Hematol Oncol 2024; 17(1): 53.
[http://dx.doi.org/10.1186/s13045-024-01574-1] [PMID: 39030582]

[44] Huang T, Peng L, Han Y, *et al.* Lipid nanoparticle-based mRNA vaccines in cancers: Current advances and future prospects. Front Immunol 2022; 13: 922301.

[http://dx.doi.org/10.3389/fimmu.2022.922301] [PMID: 36090974]

[45] Cheng Z, Li M, Dey R, Chen Y. Nanomaterials for cancer therapy: current progress and perspectives. J Hematol Oncol 2021; 14(1): 85.
[http://dx.doi.org/10.1186/s13045-021-01096-0] [PMID: 34059100]

CHAPTER 6

Polymeric Nanocarriers for Fatty Liver Disease

Kshama Srivastava[1], **Deepika Rani**[2], **Vinit K Sharma**[3] and **Ranjit Singh**[4,*]

[1] *Department of Pharmaceutics, School of Pharmaceutical Sciences, Maharishi University of Information Technology, Noida, Uttar Pradesh, India*

[2] *Department of Pharmaceutics, School of Pharmacy and Emerging Sciences, Baddi University of Emerging Sciences and Technology, Baddi, Himachal Pradesh, India*

[3] *Department of Pharmacology, Adarsh Vijendra Institute of Pharmaceutical Sciences, Shobhit University, Gangoh, Uttar Pradesh, India*

[4] *Department of Pharmaceutics, Adarsh Vijendra Institute of Pharmaceutical Sciences, Shobhit University, Gangoh, Uttar Pradesh, India*

Abstract: An essential organ in our body, the liver performs a wide range of functions, including detoxification, metabolism, digestion, immune responses, and the storage of minerals and vitamins. As a result, liver function abnormalities caused by a variety of hepatic conditions, including transplant rejection, non-alcoholic steatohepatitis, hepatitis B virus infection, hepatic fibrosis, and hepatocellular cancer, represent a serious threat to human health worldwide. Compared with traditional therapeutic agents, polymer-based nanomedicines, which are readily customisable and possess ideal physicochemical properties and functions, offer significant advantages in the treatment of liver diseases, including improved therapeutic outcomes and reduced side effects. This chapter discusses the structure and function of the liver, treatment approaches for hepatic diseases, liver-targeting strategies, and the intrahepatic effects of polymeric nanomedicines, while also highlighting the challenges and opportunities associated with their use in managing hepatic disorders.

Keywords: Nanotechnology, polymeric nanoparticles, liver disease, drug delivery, liver fibrosis.

INTRODUCTION

Overview of Fatty Liver Disease (NAFLD and NASH)

Fatty liver disease, or hepatic steatosis, refers to the accumulation of excess fat in liver cells, affecting about one in three adults in many Western countries. It can

* **Corresponding author Ranjit Singh:** Department of Pharmaceutics, Adarsh Vijendra Institute of Pharmaceutical Sciences, Shobhit University, Gangoh, Uttar Pradesh, India; E-mail: ranjitsps@gmail.com

Anjali Sharma, Devkant Sharma, Ajmer Singh Grewal, Geeta Deswal & Ganga Reddy Velma (Eds.)

result from heavy alcohol use (alcoholic fatty liver disease) or metabolic factors, such as obesity and diabetes (nonalcoholic hepatic steatosis (NASH), nonalcoholic fatty liver disease (NAFLD), or metabolic-associated fatty liver disease, MAFLD). In most cases, fatty liver is asymptomatic but may occasionally cause fatigue or discomfort in the upper right abdomen. Over time, persistent fat accumulation can lead to inflammation and scarring, escalating to steatohepatitis and progressing to fibrosis and cirrhosis, potentially resulting in irreversible liver damage or even liver cancer. Diagnosis often depends on medical history, laboratory tests, and imaging studies, and management includes addressing risk factors like alcohol intake, diet, and body weight, with early intervention offering a favorable prognosis [1].

Fatty liver disease can result from a range of factors, predominantly obesity, type 2 diabetes, metabolic syndrome, and high triglycerides, with alcohol abuse being the primary cause of alcoholic fatty liver. Less common causes include certain medications (such as methotrexate and tamoxifen), rapid weight loss, malnutrition, viral hepatitis, and genetic conditions affecting fat metabolism. The initial stage, simple steatosis, may remain stable for years. However, with additional triggers like infection or hormonal imbalance, it can progress to inflammation (steatohepatitis), fibrosis, and eventually cirrhosis or liver cancer. Diagnosis typically relies on blood tests for liver enzymes and metabolic markers, viral hepatitis screening, and imaging studies, such as abdominal ultrasound, CT, or MRI, to detect and quantify liver fat. Definitive staging of steatohepatitis and fibrosis may require a liver biopsy. Management centers on lifestyle interventions, weight loss via healthy diet and exercise, controlling diabetes and lipid levels, and abstinence from alcohol, while drugs affecting the liver should be discontinued, and patients at risk should be monitored for complications and comorbidities [2].

Current Therapeutic Challenges

Current therapeutic challenges in the treatment of fatty liver disease include a lack of approved pharmacological therapies, the heterogeneous pathogenesis of the disease, and difficulties in identifying patients who will benefit most from specific interventions. Lifestyle modification, including dietary changes and increased physical activity, remains the cornerstone of management, but many patients struggle with adherence and sustainable weight loss, limiting overall effectiveness. Pharmacologic agents like pioglitazone and GLP-1 receptor agonists show benefit in nonalcoholic steatohepatitis (NASH). Yet, concerns about side effects, limited efficacy in reversing fibrosis, and a lack of long-term data limit widespread use. Furthermore, the biological complexity of fatty liver disease, encompassing metabolic, inflammatory, and fibrotic pathways, hampers therapeutic development, with most novel drugs still in clinical trials, underscoring an urgent need for personalized, combination, or multi-targeted strategies [3].

Furthermore, therapeutic management is complicated by the need for coordinated care across specialties, insufficient awareness and education for both patients and healthcare providers, and socioeconomic barriers, such as healthcare access and medication availability. Effective management requires the creation of multidisciplinary strategies, digital health monitoring, and policy-level interventions to address the underlying metabolic risk factors and promote early detection, sustained weight management, and patient empowerment. As novel therapies are developed, long-term studies and better personalized approaches, including combination and multi-targeted regimens, will be crucial to overcome the current limitations and achieve successful outcomes in fatty liver disease [4].

Role of Nanotechnology in Liver-targeted Therapy

The liver, one of the most vital organs in the human body, performs a wide array of essential functions, including protein synthesis, nutrient metabolism, immune regulation, hormonal balance, and detoxification. Consequently, any impairment of liver function, whether caused by viral hepatitis, fatty liver disease, fibrosis, cirrhosis, or hepatocellular carcinoma (HCC), poses a serious threat to human health, contributing to nearly two million deaths worldwide each year [5]. A variety of therapeutic approaches have been employed in the clinical management of liver diseases, including interventional procedures, surgical resection, immunotherapy, antiviral therapy, chemotherapy, radiotherapy, and liver transplantation [6, 7]. Despite notable progress, several challenges continue to limit the effectiveness of these treatments. For instance, incomplete tumor removal often results in recurrence, while conventional drug therapies may lead to drug resistance, systemic toxicity, and reduced efficacy due to their lack of specificity. Furthermore, following liver transplantation (LT), patients must take lifelong immunosuppressants to prevent graft rejection, which can cause severe adverse effects and compromise quality of life [8, 9]. Complex conditions, such as non-alcoholic steatohepatitis (NASH) and hepatic fibrosis, still lack standardized therapies, despite some agents showing promise in clinical trials [10, 11]. Recent advances in nanomedicine (NMs) offer new opportunities to address these limitations. By facilitating targeted drug delivery to the liver, nanomedicines can improve therapeutic efficacy while minimizing systemic side effects. This approach has been applied to a wide range of therapeutics, including natural extracts, chemotherapeutic agents, and nucleic acid–based therapies, demonstrating considerable potential in overcoming the shortcomings of conventional treatments.

Over the past five decades, nanomedicine has witnessed remarkable progress in both diagnostics and therapy [12, 13]. Since the introduction of the first liposomes by Gregoriadis and colleagues in 1974 [14], a wide variety of nanodrug delivery systems have been developed. These systems typically consist of biomacromolecules (proteins), polymers, viral capsids, inorganic materials, or lipids, and they exhibit unique physicochemical properties that provide substantial therapeutic advantages. Such properties include enhanced pharmacokinetics, the ability to penetrate biological barriers, improved accumulation at disease sites through active or passive targeting, controlled drug release, the ability to overcome multidrug resistance, high-contrast imaging capabilities, and reduced systemic toxicity [15].

The clinical translation of nanomedicines has already led to the commercialization of several formulations, such as Rezdiffra, an FDA-approved medicine for the treatment of steatohepatitis [16, 17]. Additionally, nanomedicines designed specifically for liver diseases have been developed [18]. Among these, polymer- and lipid-based nanomedicines are the most widely utilized, owing to their biocompatibility, biodegradability, and well-established methods of synthesis and characterization. However, lipid-based nanomedicines face certain limitations, including low structural stability (*e.g.*, fragile liposomal bilayers) and challenges in functionalization [19]. In contrast, polymeric nanomedicines offer greater flexibility, as their physicochemical properties can be tailored to optimize stability, responsiveness to biological stimuli, and targeted delivery. This has led to their extensive development for the treatment of a broad spectrum of liver disorders, including NASH, hepatitis B virus (HBV) infection, liver fibrosis, HCC, and host-versus-graft disease (HVGD).

Despite these successes, further research and innovation are required to advance the development of polymer-derived nanomedicines for the effective treatment of liver diseases.

ANATOMY OF THE LIVER

The liver, the largest smooth-surfaced organ in the human body, accounts for approximately 2–3% of total body weight. On average, it weighs about 1,800 grams in males and 1,400 grams in females. It is located in the upper right abdomen beneath the right hemidiaphragm and is protected by the surrounding ribs. Except for the area adjacent to the diaphragm, the liver is entirely enclosed by the Glisson's capsule [20 - 24]. The falciform ligament attaches the liver to the anterior abdominal wall and externally divides it into the right and left lobes. The ligamentum teres, found at the base of the liver, represents the remnant of the umbilical vein. The liver has two main surfaces: the diaphragmatic surface and the visceral surface, which encompasses the anterior, lateral, superior, and posterior regions [23]. Blood supply to the liver is primarily from the portal vein, which accounts for about 75% of total blood flow, while the hepatic artery supplies the remaining 25% and delivers nearly 75% of the oxygen requirement. Structurally, the liver is composed of parenchymal and non-parenchymal cells (NPCs). Hepatocytes, the dominant parenchymal cells, constitute 70–80% of the total liver cell population [24]. The NPCs include hepatic stellate cells (HSCs), Kupffer cells (KCs), and liver sinusoidal endothelial cells (LSECs) [25]. LSECs, which form the inner lining of hepatic sinusoids, contain fenestrae with pore diameters ranging from 100 to 200 nm [26, 27]. The hepatic lobule, the liver's fundamental anatomical and functional unit, measures approximately 2.0 × 0.7 mm. It consists of hepatocyte plates arranged in a hexagonal pattern around a central vein, with an intricate sinusoidal network that distributes mixed portal and arterial blood to the hepatocytes. At each corner of the lobule lies the portal triad, composed of a branch of the hepatic artery, a branch of the portal vein, and a bile duct [28 - 32]. Hepatic sinusoids, with diameters of about 5–10 μm, facilitate efficient exchange of substances between the blood and the perisinusoidal space.

Bile is a vital physiological fluid that aids in the elimination of toxins that cannot be excreted by the kidneys. It plays a crucial role in fat digestion and absorption by releasing bile acids and salts. Bile is a complex mixture of water, electrolytes, bile acids, bile pigments, bilirubin, cholesterol, phospholipids, and other components, all produced by hepatocytes. The bile secreted by hepatocytes enters the bile ducts and flows through a network of channels, eventually reaching the duodenum or being stored in the gallbladder for later use. Components of bile that are not excreted are recycled; intestinal bacteria convert them into bile acids, which are absorbed by the ileum and transported back to the liver [31]. In addition, the liver is essential for the storage and processing of fat-soluble vitamins. For example, α- and γ-tocopherol (forms of vitamin E) are transported to the liver, whereas vitamin K, required by the hepatic enzyme γ-glutamyl carboxylase, is not stored or metabolized in the liver. The liver also plays a central role in metabolic detoxification, converting endogenous and exogenous substances, including drugs and hormones, into less active or less harmful metabolites, which are subsequently excreted via the kidneys or intestines. Furthermore, the liver detoxifies harmful substances, such as alcohol, amphetamines, steroids, hormones, and barbiturates, thereby preventing their accumulation and reducing potential toxic effects.

PATHOPHYSIOLOGY OF FATTY LIVER DISEASE

Fatty liver disease develops through a complex interplay of metabolic and cellular processes, resulting in excessive lipid accumulation within liver cells. Central pathogenic mechanisms include increased hepatic uptake of circulating free fatty acids (FFAs), primarily driven by insulin resistance and enhanced adipose tissue lipolysis, alongside upregulated de novo lipogenesis in hepatocytes, where glucose and other substrates are converted to fatty acids via key enzymes such as acetyl-CoA carboxylase and fatty acid synthase. Fatty acids within the liver undergo conditional partitioning: they are either oxidized for energy, stored as triglycerides, exported as very-low-density lipoproteins (VLDL), or accumulate as hepatocellular lipid droplets. Collectively, fatty liver disease exemplifies a disease of lipid overload and metabolic derangement, evolving from simple steatosis toward steatohepatitis and fibrosis under the influence of insulin resistance, oxidative stress, and dysregulated hepatic lipid handling [32, 33].

STRATEGIES FOR HEPATIC-TARGETED DRUG DELIVERY

Liver-targeted drug delivery systems have been extensively developed to address a wide range of hepatic disorders. Nanomedicines (NMs) can exploit both passive and active targeting strategies to reach diseased liver tissues. In passive targeting, the accumulation of NPs within the liver depends on several factors, including the physicochemical properties of the NPs, the architecture of hepatic lobules, the pathophysiological changes associated with liver diseases, and the specific drug delivery route employed. This process enhances the local concentration of therapeutic agents in diseased regions while minimizing their distribution to healthy tissues, thereby improving cellular uptake and therapeutic efficacy.

In contrast, active targeting relies on the functionalization of NPs with cell-specific ligands that selectively bind to receptors expressed on target cells. This approach not only facilitates precise drug delivery but also reduces off-target toxicity to healthy hepatocytes and non-parenchymal liver cells. In practice, passive and active targeting mechanisms often work synergistically. Typically, NPs first accumulate passively in the liver and are subsequently internalized by target cells through receptor-mediated endocytosis, ensuring improved specificity and therapeutic outcomes.

Passive Targeting

NP properties, including surface charge, size, and shape, play critical roles in their biodistribution and hepatic uptake. Highly charged NPs, particularly those with strong surface charges, tend to adsorb proteins rapidly after intravenous injection. This protein corona triggers immunological responses that promote its clearance by Kupffer cells (KCs) in hepatic sinusoids [34, 35]. Studies have shown that hepatocytes preferentially internalize positively charged NPs, whereas negatively charged NPs are more efficiently eliminated by the liver's reticuloendothelial system (RES) [36]. Similarly, hydrophobic NPs are cleared more rapidly by the

RES compared to hydrophilic NPs. To overcome these limitations, surface functionalization with polyethylene glycol (PEG) is frequently employed. PEGylation reduces protein adsorption, prolongs circulation time, and minimizes RES-mediated uptake. The size of NPs is equally important for the effective targeting of liver diseases. NPs with diameters below 200 nm generally evade uptake by KCs and are able to traverse the fenestrations of liver sinusoidal endothelial cells into the space of Disse. This enables their diffusion and uptake by hepatocytes [37]. Interestingly, even larger nanocarriers, up to ~400 nm, have been reported to penetrate the Disse space by a forced extrusion mechanism through sinusoidal fenestrations [38]. NP shape also influences biodistribution; compared with spherical particles, rod- and worm-like NPs with high aspect ratios exhibit reduced clearance by KCs, thereby enhancing their availability for therapeutic action [39]. Passive accumulation of nanomedicines (NMs) is particularly advantageous in solid tumors, such as hepatocellular carcinoma (HCC), due to the enhanced permeability and retention (EPR) effect. This phenomenon arises from the aberrant tumor vasculature and deficient lymphatic drainage [40 - 43]. In human tumors, vascular fenestrations typically range in diameter from 400 to 600 nm [44]. Consequently, NPs are widely employed for passive targeting in HCC therapy by exploiting the EPR effect [45 - 47]. Studies suggest that an NP diameter of 70–200 nm is optimal for effective tumor penetration and therapeutic efficacy [48].

Beyond NP physicochemical properties, the biodistribution and uptake of NMs are strongly influenced by the pathophysiological characteristics of HCC, the architecture of hepatic lobules, and the delivery method. To improve diagnostic accuracy and therapeutic outcomes, several administration routes have been explored, including hydrodynamic injection, intra-arterial infusion, intratumoral delivery, and intrabiliary infusion.

Active Targeting

To improve the selective uptake of NM by target cells, active targeting, also known as ligand–receptor-mediated targeting, makes use of certain molecules affixed to the surface of NPs [49]. Antibodies, proteins, peptides, aptamers, carbohydrates, and vitamins (including retinol and folate) are examples of targeting ligands that can be made to attach to surface molecules or receptors that are overexpressed on sick cells [50]. As previously mentioned, liver cells express a variety of receptors that can be leveraged to develop nanomedicines (NM) targeted specifically to the liver. The concept of targeted NPs has been studied for over 40 years, but only a small number have advanced to clinical trials, and none have yet received approval for clinical use. The targeting efficiency of NPs is influenced by several factors, including:

- The route of administration, such as oral, intramuscular, intravenous, or intratumoral delivery.
- The physicochemical properties of NPs, which include the type and density of ligands, as well as particle size, material composition, shape, charge, and surface hydrophobicity.

Enhancing the active targeting capabilities of NM is crucial for their successful clinical translation.

OVERVIEW OF POLYMERIC NPS

Speiser and his colleagues were the first to suggest using polymeric NPs for medication delivery in 1969 [51]. To treat liver diseases, many polymeric NPs have been developed for the targeted delivery of vaccines, nucleic acids, natural bioactive substances, and small molecules. These developments center on polymeric NPs that provide benefits, such as hydrophilicity, bloodstream stability, nucleic acid protection, effective lysosomal escape, and an ideal surface charge to improve drug transfer.

Broadly, solid polymeric nanoparticles can be divided into nanospheres and nanocapsules, depending on how the drug or therapeutic payload is associated with the polymer matrix. This classification is based on structural differences that influence drug encapsulation, release mechanisms, and therapeutic outcomes [52, 53]. The various methods of preparing polymeric nanoparticles are mentioned in Table **1**.

Table 1. Various methods for the preparation of polymeric nanocarriers

Category	Emulsion Diffusion	Nanoprecipitation	Solvent Evaporation	Salting Out	Dialysis	Reference
Physicochemical Properties	Based on the reciprocal diffusion of solvent and non-solvent.	Determines stability and biological activity	Influenced by viscosity, volatility, diffusivity, material properties, surface tension, and vapor pressure.	Uses high-concentration salt to reduce solubility, inducing precipitation/crystallization, improving purity and stability	Hydrophobic drugs are dissolved in a water-miscible organic solvent, eliminating the need for surfactants.	[64]
Encapsulation of Drugs	Hydrophilic drugs	Hydrophilic and hydrophobic drugs	Hydrophilic and hydrophobic drugs	Lipophilic drugs	Hydrophobic drugs	[64, 65]

(Table 1) cont.....

Category	Emulsion Diffusion	Nanoprecipitation	Solvent Evaporation	Salting Out	Dialysis	Reference
Solvents Used	Ethyl acetate	Dimethyl sulfoxide, ethanol	Chloroform, dichloromethane, ethyl acetate	Tetrahydrofuran, acetone, acetonitrile, ethanol	Acetone, methanol	[64]
Drug Loading Capacity	100%	27.2 wt%	81%	66.5 wt%	35%	[65]
Types of Particles	Nanoparticles (NPs)	NPs	Nanospheres and NPs	Polymeric NPs (protein-based)	Hydrophilic NPs, quantum dots, polymeric NPs	[65]
Drug Delivery Function	Organic solvent diffuses out of the droplet into the external phase	Enables controlled and prolonged release, enhancing bioavailability	A versatile method allowing active incorporation of various polymers and drugs	Creates an extended lag time, masking immediate drug release and improving bioavailability	Nanocarrier system effectively encapsulates, protects drugs, and improves bioavailability.	[65]

Nanospheres

Nanospheres are defined as matrix-type polymeric nanoparticles in which the drug is uniformly dispersed throughout the polymeric network. In this configuration, the active pharmaceutical ingredient (API) can be molecularly dissolved, adsorbed, or physically entrapped within the polymeric structure. Unlike reservoir systems, nanospheres lack a distinct core–shell architecture; instead, they are homogenous, solid colloids in which both the surface and the bulk of the particle can serve as sites for drug localization [54, 55].

Structural Characteristics

Nanospheres are typically spherical, although irregular morphologies may be observed depending on the preparation technique. Their structure provides a large surface area-to-volume ratio, which can enhance drug interactions with the biological environment and facilitate the rapid release of surface-adsorbed molecules. The degree of drug entrapment and distribution within nanospheres is influenced by polymer type, hydrophobicity, molecular weight, and the synthesis method.

Drug Release Mechanisms

Drug release from nanospheres typically follows two mechanisms: Diffusion-controlled release of drug molecules from the polymer matrix, and polymer degradation-controlled release, where erosion or hydrolysis of the polymer facilitates sustained drug liberation. In practice, a combination of these mechanisms often occurs, allowing tunable release kinetics depending on polymer composition [56].

Applications

Nanospheres have been widely explored for the management of fatty liver disease, especially nonalcoholic fatty liver disease. Several studies have reported that these are used exclusively to improve drug bioavailability and drug delivery to the liver.

Nanocapsules

Nanocapsules are vesicular, reservoir-type polymeric nanoparticles in which the drug is confined to a central cavity surrounded by a thin polymeric shell or membrane. Unlike nanospheres, which are homogeneous solid matrices, nanocapsules possess a distinct core–shell structure. The inner core can be either oily (for hydrophobic drugs) or aqueous (for hydrophilic drugs), while the outer polymeric shell stabilizes the system and controls drug release [57].

Structural Characteristics

Nanocapsules typically consist of a liquid or semi-liquid core surrounded by a biodegradable polymeric wall. This architecture offers higher encapsulation efficiency for lipophilic drugs compared to nanospheres, as the oily core serves as a reservoir that solubilizes poorly water-soluble compounds. The polymeric membrane regulates drug diffusion and can be engineered for controlled release [58].

Drug Release Mechanisms

Drug release from nanocapsules occurs primarily through diffusion across the polymeric shell, polymer degradation or erosion, which gradually liberates the encapsulated drug, and core leakage, especially if the capsule wall is thin or unstable. This release can be engineered to respond to physiological conditions, such as pH, temperature, or enzymatic activity [59].

Applications

Nanocapsules are widely used for targeting fatty liver disease by safely delivering genetic drugs (siRNA) into liver cells, silencing the SPTLC2 gene, which is responsible for the production of ceramide, a driving factor in liver fat buildup [60 - 63].

PCL is a biodegradable polymer that has proven highly effective for sustained and controlled drug release due to its gradual degradation rate [66]. It can be used to encapsulate chemotherapeutic agents for liver cancer treatment [67]. Liver-targeted delivery was achieved by functionalizing PCL NPs with specific ligands, enhancing drug efficacy while minimizing toxicity to healthy tissues.

PREPARATION OF POLYMERIC NPS

Depending on their intended uses, a variety of techniques have been devised for the manufacture of NPs [68]. Based on how monomers are polymerized, these techniques can be roughly divided into two groups:

- **Two-step procedures**: This method involves emulsification preparation before NP synthesis.
- **One-step procedures**: This method does not require emulsification for NP synthesis.

Polymer-based NM for Liver Disease Treatment

Liver disorders are associated with harmful alterations in the assembly and function of liver cells, typically triggered by internal or external pathogenic elements [69 - 72]. Building on current understanding of the cellular pathophysiological mechanisms of liver diseases and knowledge of both macroscopic and microscopic liver anatomy, researchers have developed a range of drug delivery systems in recent years. The next section explores the advancements in the development of various polymer-based nanocarriers, highlighting their potential for targeted delivery of therapeutic agents for conditions, such as NASH, HBV infection, HCC, liver fibrosis, and HVGD post-LT.

Hepatitis

In addition to inflammation and the presence of inflammatory cells and substances, hepatitis is characterized by damage to the liver cells. Liver damage can result from long-term alcohol use, exposure to dangerous drugs, and bacterial or viral infections. There are currently no viable treatments for the two most prevalent chronic liver disorders, NASH and HBV infection. Many attempts have been made recently to increase the efficacy of hepatitis therapies.

HBV Infection

HBV is a liver-targeting DNA virus capable of causing chronic infection. Its replication within liver cells can result in fibrosis, cirrhosis, and HCC. While HBV surface-antigen vaccines effectively prevent infection, eradicating HBV from infected cells remains a major challenge. Various antiviral agents, including interferons, nucleic acids, and small molecules, have been used to manage HBV infections. However, these treatments often cause dose-limiting side effects and may contribute to drug resistance development [73]. To overcome these challenges, polymeric nanocarriers have been developed to deliver conventional antiviral agents, such as vaccines, nucleic acids, and small molecules, directly to hepatocytes, improving drug efficacy while reducing side effects.

The HBV vaccine is based on inactivated HBsAg, serving as the cornerstone for preventing HBV. Nonetheless, the inadequate absorbability, minimal immunogenicity, and low patient adherence to traditional vaccination hinder the advancement of vaccines. To address these challenges, alternative methods of administration have been developed. The nasal mucosa, with its dense network of capillaries, facilitates the rapid absorption of vaccines into the bloodstream. Thus, N, N, N-trimethyl chitosan (N-TMC) NPs were created by Subbiah *et al.* as a nanocarrier for HBsAg nasal administration. *In-vitro*, these NPs demonstrated prolonged antigen release and improved drug-loading capability. Additionally, immunological research showed that their adjuvant effect was more efficient and persistent *in-vivo* than traditional vaccines. Similarly, nasal immunization with CS-based nanovaccines containing PCL and HBsAg leveraged CS's mucoadhesive and immunostimulatory properties, as well as PCL's blood stability. The immunological response was greatly enhanced by the synergistic action of PCL and CS together [74].

To deliver HBsAg, Dewangan *et al.* created a variety of NPs using PLGA and refined the formulation using a central composite design. Their results demonstrated that intramuscular delivery of the nanovaccine markedly improved humoral and cellular immune responses [75, 76]. Similarly, Zhu *et al.* added HBsAg to mannose-modified PLGA NPs, which improved antigen presentation to lymphocytes and enabled progressive release of HBsAg, thereby extending immunity. Their research showed that RAW 264.7 cells and bone marrow-derived dendritic cells (BMDCs) significantly increased their uptake of NP. Additionally, in animal models, subcutaneous delivery of these NPs enhanced cellular immune responses and successfully preserved humoral immunity [77].

NASH and Nanomaterial-based Therapeutics

Alcohol consumption has a limited influence on non-alcoholic steatohepatitis (NASH), an inflammatory subtype of non-alcoholic fatty liver disease (NAFLD) [77 - 80]. The pathogenesis of NASH involves multiple molecular pathways, with heterogeneous pathogenic factors leading to variable disease progression and clinical manifestations [81]. A widely accepted explanation highlights the liver's impaired ability to metabolize excess carbohydrates and fatty acids, resulting in hepatocellular accumulation of toxic lipid species [82, 83]. These metabolic disturbances cause hepatocyte stress, injury, and apoptosis, which in turn promote fibrogenesis, genomic instability, and progression to cirrhosis and hepatocellular carcinoma (HCC). To improve therapeutic outcomes for NAFLD, innovative polymer-based nanomaterials (NMs) have been developed.

Natural extract delivery: Resveratrol (Res), a phytoalexin found in grapes and other foods, has demonstrated cholesterol-lowering, glucose-stabilizing, and anti-metabolic disease properties. However, its clinical translation is limited by poor stability and low bioavailability. To overcome these challenges, Res was encapsulated in a galactose (Gal)-modified polymeric carrier, which significantly improved its physicochemical stability and markedly inhibited NAFLD progression compared to free Res [84]. Similarly, silymarin, the principal bioactive constituent of milk thistle, and chitosan (CS), a naturally occurring cationic amino polysaccharide, are both known for their lipid-lowering potential. Liang *et al.* designed core–shell CS-modified, silymarin-encapsulated lipophilic nanoparticles (LPH NPs) with a polymeric core and phospholipid shell. This formulation enhanced silymarin's oral bioavailability and improved its lipid-lowering efficacy in the treatment of NAFLD [85].

Synthetic small-molecule delivery: De novo lipogenesis (DNL), regulated by sterol regulatory element-binding protein (SREBP)-1c, is markedly upregulated in NAFLD and represents an attractive therapeutic target. Zhao *et al.* developed mPEG-PLGA NP encapsulating rapamycin (RAPA), which effectively reduced hepatic lipid accumulation, alleviated steatosis, and promoted liver tissue repair in mice. Likewise, Cao *et al.* engineered biodegradable polyurethane NP loaded with the peroxisome proliferator-activated receptor α (PPARα) agonist fenofibrate (FNB). This system lowered triglyceride levels in vitro and in vivo, while simultaneously improving plasma FNB concentrations in mice. Nifedipine (NFD), another candidate for NAFLD therapy, restores cytosolic calcium balance, enhances autophagy, and promotes lysosomal degradation to prevent the accumulation of p62 and ubiquitinated protein aggregates induced by a high-fat diet. Recent work on PLGA-based NFD-loaded NP (NFD-NPs) demonstrated improved NFD bioavailability, enhanced lipid metabolism, facilitated autophagy-mediated hepatic clearance, and improved insulin sensitivity, thereby reducing glucose intolerance in NAFLD models.

Liver Fibrosis

Liver fibrosis represents the leading cause of mortality among individuals with chronic liver disease [86]. It commonly develops as a consequence of chronic hepatitis B or C infections, excessive alcohol intake, non-alcoholic fatty liver disease (NAFLD), autoimmune liver disorders, and certain genetic conditions [87].

The progression of fibrogenesis is a multifactorial process, primarily driven by:

- **Oxidative stress and inflammation:** Reactive oxygen species (ROS) and related oxidative stress factors initiate persistent inflammation, which in turn activates hepatic stellate cells (HSCs) [88, 89].
- **Extracellular vesicle signaling:** Vesicles released by injured or apoptotic hepatocytes modulate multiple cell types, thereby amplifying inflammation, fibrosis, and angiogenesis [90].
- **Excessive extracellular matrix (ECM) deposition:** An imbalance between collagen production and degradation, along with increased levels of tissue inhibitors of metalloproteinases (TIMPs), leads to the excessive accumulation of ECM proteins, particularly type I and III collagen, resulting in structural and functional liver impairment.

Currently, no antifibrotic drugs have been approved for clinical use. Given these therapeutic limitations, nanotechnology has emerged as a promising approach for antifibrotic drug development.

Natural Extract Delivery

Natural extracts are rich in bioactive compounds with antifibrotic, antioxidant, and hepatoprotective properties [91]. For instance, Li *et al.* developed silibinin-loaded hyaluronic acid (HA) micelles that selectively target CD44 receptors, highly expressed on activated hepatic stellate cells (aHSCs). These micelles exhibited enhanced delivery to fibrotic liver tissue, efficiently eliminating aHSCs and producing significant antifibrotic effects [92]. Similarly, Lin *et al.* designed a dual-sensitive micelle encapsulating polydatin (PD-MC) using a PEG-based block polymer responsive to ROS and acidic environments. This system not only suppressed oxidative stress and inflammation but also reduced hepatocyte apoptosis and the activation of both macrophages and HSCs [93]. Beyond plant-derived compounds, animal-based extracts have also shown promise. For example, astaxanthin, a keto-carotenoid from marine organisms with strong antioxidant and anti-inflammatory activity, was encapsulated in NP using a stearic acid–chitosan conjugate (SA-CS) and sodium caseinate. These NPs significantly enhanced bioactivity in LX-2 cells, lowering the expression of fibrogenic genes such as α-SMA and COL1A1 compared to free astaxanthin [94].

Hepatocellular Carcinoma

Hepatocellular carcinoma (HCC) is the most common form of liver cancer, representing around 90% of liver cancer cases [95]. Over 90% of HCC cases occur in individuals with chronic liver diseases, primarily due to liver inflammation [96]. In the early stages of HCC, treatment options include surgical resection, liver transplantation, or nonsurgical local ablation methods. For intermediate-stage HCC, trans arterial chemoembolization (TACE) has been the standard treatment for the past two decades [97]. In advanced stages, systemic treatments involving standard chemotherapeutics, immune checkpoint inhibitors (ICIs), tyrosine kinase inhibitors (TKIs), or monoclonal antibodies (mAbs) are typically used. Sorafenib and Lenvatinib are the most effective single-agent treatments among anticancer drugs.

However, the limited distribution of drugs within tumors and the multidrug resistance of cancer cells significantly reduce the efficacy of anticancer therapies. Utilizing appropriate drug carriers can enhance therapeutic outcomes and reduce side effects [98]. Several polymeric nanocarrier systems have shown promise in experimental studies for the treatment of HCC, including those designed for natural extracts, chemotherapy agents, and nucleic acids.

Natural extract administration: Natural compounds are increasingly being studied as potential anticancer agents due to their significant therapeutic benefits. To improve the efficacy of these compounds, various advanced drug delivery platforms have been developed. For example, a smart core-crosslinked camptothecin (CPT) prodrug micelle was created using a phenylboronic acid-modified PEG-polyglutamic acid polymer with disulfide-linked CPT. This micelle demonstrated enhanced cellular uptake, reduced sensitivity, and strong antitumor effects both *in vitro* and *in vivo* [99]. Ursolic acid, a pentacyclic triterpene acid found in many plants, offers various pharmacological advantages, including antioxidant, anti-inflammatory, antibacterial, anticancer, and antifungal properties. Shen *et al.* developed an amphiphilic self-assembled nanodrug using ursolic acid, lactobionic acid, and low-polyamidoamine dendrimers. This formulation enhanced cytotoxicity against liver cancer and reduced SMMC7721 cell migration and adhesion by inhibiting MMP-9 expression. Polyphenols, plant-derived compounds known for preventing chronic diseases, such as cardiovascular disorders, neurodegenerative diseases, and cancers, have also shown promise. For example, curcumin was encapsulated in poly-l-lysine (PLL)-derived NPs for pH-responsive release. These NPs enhanced curcumin uptake by Hep3B liver cancer cells through electrostatic endocytosis and extended the drug's circulation time in the bloodstream.

Chemotherapeutic drug delivery: Chemotherapy drugs face challenges, such as poor solubility and short half-lives, in the bloodstream. To address these issues, various polymeric nanocarriers have been developed. Naturally occurring polysaccharides, such as chitosan (CS)-based NPs, have been used for delivering doxorubicin (DOX) due to their biocompatibility, biodegradability, and low immunogenicity [100]. All-trans retinoic acid (ATRA), an effective Pinl inhibitor, has shown limited efficacy in solid tumors due to its short half-life in the bloodstream. To overcome this limitation, Yang *et al.* developed a novel ATRA formulation using poly-l-lactic acid for effective treatment of hepatocellular carcinoma (HCC). This formulation significantly enhanced ATRA's ability to inhibit HCC cell proliferation, increasing its half maximal inhibitory concentration (IC50) more than threefold compared to free ATRA [101]. Additionally, sorafenib-loaded polymeric NPs were prepared by self-assembly of TPGS-b-poly(caprolactone) (TPGS-b-PCL), Pluronic P123, and sorafenib, and were conjugated with an anti-GPC3 antibody for targeted liver cancer therapy. These antibody-conjugated NPs showed improved cellular uptake in HepG2 cells and greater cytotoxicity than untargeted NPs.

Host-versus-Graft Disease (HVGD)

Liver transplantation (LT) is the only viable treatment for advanced liver diseases, such as acute liver failure, a severe systemic complication of liver disease, as well as liver-related metabolic disorders or cirrhosis associated with conditions like HCC, variceal bleeding from portal hypertension, ascites, hepatorenal syndrome, and encephalopathy [102, 103]. Nonetheless, HVGD, the most prevalent form of immune rejection post-LT, may lead to irregular liver function and potentially graft dysfunction [104, 105]. Consequently, patients who undergo liver transplantation need to use immunosuppressants for life to prevent transplant rejection. Commonly used immunosuppressants include calcineurin inhibitors (cyclosporine and tacrolimus), glucocorticoids, cytotoxic agents (azathioprine), mycophenolate mofetil (MMF), and mTOR inhibitors (sirolimus and everolimus).

However, immunosuppressants pose several challenges, including a narrow therapeutic window, poor water solubility, low bioavailability, and significant interindividual variability in response. Additionally, these drugs can cause serious side effects, such as infections, nephrotoxicity, hepatotoxicity, increased risk of tumors, pneumonitis, and bone marrow suppression [106]. Nanocarriers provide a promising solution to enhance the physicochemical properties of immunosuppressants, enabling targeted delivery to liver tissues while minimizing adverse effects. This section explores recent advancements in polymer-based carriers designed for the efficient delivery of immunosuppressants.

Tacrolimus (Tac), an immunosuppressant that inhibits interleukin-2 (IL-2) synthesis to prevent T-cell activation and proliferation, faces challenges in clinical application due to its poor solubility and instability. To address these issues, Tac-loaded micelles have been developed using various biodegradable polymers, such as poly(ε-caprolactone)-PEG-poly(ε-caprolactone), PEG-poly(d,l-lactide), PEG-poly(ε-caprolactone), poly(methyl vinyl ether-co-maleic anhydride)-graf--hydroxypropyl-β-cyclodextrin, and ethyl cellulose (EC). These formulations are designed to enhance Tac's bioavailability, solubility, and circulation time [104 - 112].

The Fate of NPs in the Liver:

Understanding the fate of NPs in the liver remains crucial as NP-based technologies for diagnosing and treating liver diseases continue to evolve. As the largest organ in the reticuloendothelial system (RES), the liver can capture between 30- 99% of NPs introduced into the bloodstream. Research indicates that the following outcomes are commonly observed for these NPs [113]:

Uptake by kupffer cells: KCs, which serve as the liver's primary defence mechanism, play a key role in eliminating foreign substances through scavenger receptors. As a result, KCs are more likely to engulf NPs compared to other liver cells. After internalization, NPs may undergo endolysosomal and autophagic processing. These pathways aid in particle sequestration, nanomaterial breakdown, reduction of toxicity, and alleviation of cellular stress [114].

Hepatobiliary excretion: NPs that are not taken up or retained by Kupffer cells (KCs) but are smaller than the fenestrations of liver sinusoids (typically ranging from 100 to 200 nm) can pass through these fenestrations into the space of Disse. Once there, hepatocytes can engulf the particles, degrade them using various enzymatic systems, and eventually excrete them into the biliary tract. However, the distribution and metabolism of NPs may be affected in liver diseases due to alterations in liver anatomy and function.

FUTURE PROSPECTS

The state of the liver poses a serious risk to human health, and while polymer-based NM offers great promise in addressing these challenges, its clinical application remains limited due to several obstacles.

Although many promising treatments have shown success in animal models, their effectiveness in humans has often been limited. Several factors contribute to this discrepancy: (i) The precise types and amounts of receptors on liver cells remain unclear, and ligands that work in animal models may not bind effectively to human receptors. (ii) NPs, as foreign substances, can activate immune responses upon entering the bloodstream, making targeted drug delivery challenging. (iii) Animal models fail to accurately replicate the clinical progression of liver diseases, which in humans progress slowly over several years.

More accurate and representative animal models are therefore essential to better evaluate the therapeutic potential of NMs.

Secondly, polymeric micelles hold great promise in enhancing the bioavailability of unbound drugs but face challenges in physiological environments. Parameters, such as temperature, pH, ionic strength, and biological molecules, can destabilize micelle structures. Cross-linked polymer micelles, utilizing dynamic covalent or non-covalent interactions, are emerging as more stable and effective drug delivery systems. Future research must continue to optimize micelle architecture and preparation methods.

Third, a major challenge remains the effective targeting of liver cells. While the liver absorbs 30–99% of injected NPs, many are predominantly taken up by Kupffer cells (KCs). Understanding how NPs interact with the space of Disse and cross fenestrations without degradation is critical. PEGylation continues to be used for reducing RES uptake, and the development of multifunctional nanocarriers that combine imaging and therapy offers a promising direction aligned with personalized medicine. Radiolabeled NPs and immunohistochemical analysis could further enable precise monitoring of NP distribution and efficacy. Fourth, stimulus-responsive drug delivery systems are a growing area of interest. NMs that respond to endogenous (*e.g.*, redox potential, enzymes, pH) or external (*e.g.*, light, ultrasound, temperature) stimuli may significantly improve site-specific drug release, enhance therapeutic effects while minimizing side effects.

Lastly, comprehensive biosafety evaluations are essential. Immunogenicity, degradation product safety, hepatocyte functionality, and long-term pharmacokinetics must all be rigorously assessed, especially given the immunocompromised status of many liver disease patients. Sensitive serum markers for monitoring liver function during treatment must also be explored to support effective and adaptive therapeutic strategies [115].

CONCLUSION

Polymer-based NMs present significant potential for the targeted diagnosis and treatment of liver diseases, offering enhanced therapeutic efficacy and reduced systemic toxicity. Despite promising preclinical outcomes, numerous challenges, including immune response activation, poor targeting accuracy, micelle instability, and insufficient clinical model fidelity, have hindered their translation to clinical practice.

To bridge this gap, future efforts must prioritize the development of more representative disease models, stable and responsive nanocarrier systems, and thorough safety evaluations. Advancements in these areas will not only facilitate the clinical success of polymeric NMs but also support the broader goals of precision and personalized medicine in hepatology.

LIST OF ABBREVIATIONS

HCC	Hepatocellular Carcinoma
LT	Liver Transplantation
NM	Nanomedicine
NPs	Nanoparticles
NPCs	Non-Parenchymal Cells
HSCs	Hepatic Stellate Cells
KCs	Kupffer Cells
LSECs	Liver Sinusoidal Endothelial Cells
HVGD	Host-Versus-Graft Disease
PLGA	Poly (Lactic-co-Glycolic Acid)
RES	Reticuloendothelial System
PEG	Polyethylene Glycol
EPR	Enhanced Permeability and Retention
Ca^{2+}	Calcium Ions
α-SMA	Alpha-Smooth Muscle Actin
aHSCs	Activated Hepatic Stellate Cells
BMDCs	Bone Marrow-Derived Dendritic Cells
CD44	Cluster of Differentiation 44 (cell surface receptor)
COL1A1	Collagen Type I Alpha 1 Chain

DNL	De Novo Lipogenesis
ECM	Extracellular Matrix
FDA	Food and Drug Administration
HA	Hyaluronic Acid
HBV	Hepatitis B Virus
HBsAg	Hepatitis B Surface Antigen
HPMA	N-(2-Hydroxypropyl)methacrylamide
LP-NPs / LPH NPs	Lipophilic Nanoparticles
NAFLD	Non-Alcoholic Fatty Liver Disease
NASH	Non-Alcoholic Steatohepatitis
NFD	Nifedipine
N-TMC	N,N,N-Trimethyl Chitosan
PBCA	Polybutylcyanoacrylate
PCL	Polycaprolactone
PD-MC	Polydatin-Loaded Micelle
PEGylation	Covalent attachment of PEG chains to molecules
PMMA	Polymethyl Methacrylate
PNPs	Polymeric Nanoparticles
PPARα	Peroxisome Proliferator-Activated Receptor Alpha
Res	Resveratrol
RAPA	Rapamycin
ROS	Reactive Oxygen Species
SA-CS	Stearic Acid–Chitosan
SLB-HA	Silibinin-Loaded Hyaluronic Acid
SREBP-1c	Sterol Regulatory Element-Binding Protein 1c
TIMPs	Tissue Inhibitors of Metalloproteinases

REFERENCES

[1] Lazarus JV, Aithal GP, Lemoine M, Younossi Z, Marchesini G, Bugianesi E, *et al.* Advancing the global public health agenda for NAFLD: a consensus statement. Nat Rev Gastroenterol Hepatol 2022; 19(1): 60-78.
[http://dx.doi.org/10.1038/s41575-021-00523-4] [PMID: 34707258]

[2] Malnick SDH, Alin P, Somin M, Neuman MG. Fatty liver disease-alcoholic and non-alcoholic: similar but different. Int J Mol Sci 2022; 23(24): 16226.
[http://dx.doi.org/10.3390/ijms232416226] [PMID: 36555867]

[3] Iqbal U, Perumpail BJ, Akhtar D, Kim D, Ahmed A. The epidemiology, risk profiling and diagnostic challenges of nonalcoholic fatty liver disease. Medicines (Basel) 2019; 6(1): 41.
[http://dx.doi.org/10.3390/medicines6010041] [PMID: 30889791]

[4] Godoy-Matos AF, Silva Júnior WS, Valerio CM. NAFLD as a continuum: from obesity to metabolic syndrome and diabetes. Diabetol Metab Syndr 2020; 12(1): 60.
[http://dx.doi.org/10.1186/s13098-020-00570-y] [PMID: 32684985]

[5] Asrani SK, Devarbhavi H, Eaton J, Kamath PS. Burden of liver diseases in the world. J Hepatol 2019; 70(1): 151-71.
[http://dx.doi.org/10.1016/j.jhep.2018.09.014] [PMID: 30266282]

[6] Llovet JM, Kelley RK, Villanueva A, *et al.* Hepatocellular carcinoma. Nat Rev Dis Primers 2021; 7(1): 6.
[http://dx.doi.org/10.1038/s41572-020-00240-3] [PMID: 33479224]

[7] Singh L, Indermun S, Govender M, *et al.* Drug delivery strategies for antiviral against hepatitis B virus. Viruses 2018; 10(5): 267.
[http://dx.doi.org/10.3390/v10050267] [PMID: 29772748]

[8] Geissler EK, Schlitt HJ. Immunosuppression for liver transplantation. Gut 2009; 58(3): 452-63.
[http://dx.doi.org/10.1136/gut.2008.163527] [PMID: 19052024]

[9] Lohitesh K, Chowdhury R, Mukherjee S. Resistance a major hindrance to chemotherapy in hepatocellular carcinoma: an insight. Cancer Cell Int 2018; 18(1): 44.
[http://dx.doi.org/10.1186/s12935-018-0538-7] [PMID: 29568237]

[10] Sheka AC, Adeyi O, Thompson J, Hameed B, Crawford PA, Ikramuddin S. Nonalcoholic Steatohepatitis. JAMA 2020; 323(12): 1175-83.
[http://dx.doi.org/10.1001/jama.2020.2298] [PMID: 32207804]

[11] Bataller R, Brenner DA. Liver fibrosis. J Clin Invest 2005; 115(2): 209-18.
[http://dx.doi.org/10.1172/JCI24282] [PMID: 15690074]

[12] Reddy LH, Couvreur P. Nanotechnology for therapy and imaging of liver diseases. J Hepatol 2011; 55(6): 1461-6.
[http://dx.doi.org/10.1016/j.jhep.2011.05.039] [PMID: 21801699]

[13] Mitchell MJ, Billingsley MM, Haley RM, Wechsler ME, Peppas NA, Langer R. Engineering precision nanoparticles for drug delivery. Nat Rev Drug Discov 2021; 20(2): 101-24.
[http://dx.doi.org/10.1038/s41573-020-0090-8] [PMID: 33277608]

[14] Gregoriadis G, Swain CP, Wills EJ, Tavill AS. Drug-carrier potential of liposomes in cancer chemotherapy. Lancet 1974; 303(7870): 1313-6.
[http://dx.doi.org/10.1016/S0140-6736(74)90682-5] [PMID: 4134296]

[15] Li L, Wang H, Ong ZY, *et al.* Polymer- and lipid-based nanoparticle therapeutics for the treatment of liver diseases. Nano Today 2010; 5(4): 296-312.
[http://dx.doi.org/10.1016/j.nantod.2010.06.007]

[16] Moosavian SA, Sathyapalan T, Jamialahmadi T, Sahebkar A. The emerging role of nanomedicine in the management of nonalcoholic fatty liver disease: a state-of-the-art review. Bioinorg Chem Appl 2021; 2021: 4041415.
[http://dx.doi.org/10.1155/2021/4041415.] [PMID: 34659388]

[17] Li X, Wang J, Zhang L, Huang D, Li Y, Chen X. Nanomedicines in the treatment of liver fibrosis: Advances and perspectives. Int J Nanomedicine 2025; 20: 9641-65.
[http://dx.doi.org/10.2147/IJN.S524078] [PMID: 40785947]

[18] Ma Z, Zhang B, Fan Y, *et al.* Traditional Chinese medicine combined with hepatic targeted drug delivery systems: A new strategy for the treatment of liver diseases. Biomed Pharmacother 2019; 117: 109128.
[http://dx.doi.org/10.1016/j.biopha.2019.109128] [PMID: 31234023]

[19] Siepmann J, Faham A, Clas SD, *et al.* Lipids and polymers in pharmaceutical technology: Lifelong companions. Int J Pharm 2019; 558: 128-42.

[http://dx.doi.org/10.1016/j.ijpharm.2018.12.080] [PMID: 30639218]

[20] Abdel-Misih SRZ, Bloomston M. Liver Anatomy. Surg Clin North Am 2010; 90(4): 643-53. [http://dx.doi.org/10.1016/j.suc.2010.04.017] [PMID: 20637938]

[21] Juza RM, Pauli EM. Clinical and surgical anatomy of the liver: A review for clinicians. Clin Anat 2014; 27(5): 764-9. [http://dx.doi.org/10.1002/ca.22350] [PMID: 24453062]

[22] Llewellyn J, Fede C, Loneker AE, *et al.* Glisson's capsule matrix structure and function is altered in patients with cirrhosis irrespective of aetiology. JHEP Rep 2023; 5(9): 100760. [http://dx.doi.org/10.1016/j.jhepr.2023.100760] [PMID: 37534230]

[23] Mahadevan V. Anatomy of the gallbladder and bile ducts. Surgery 2020; 38(8): 432-6. [http://dx.doi.org/10.1016/j.mpsur.2014.10.003]

[24] Zhou Z, Xu MJ, Gao B. Hepatocytes: a key cell type for innate immunity. Cell Mol Immunol 2016; 13(3): 301-15. [http://dx.doi.org/10.1038/cmi.2015.97] [PMID: 26685902]

[25] Racanelli V, Rehermann B. The liver as an immunological organ. Hepatology 2006; 43(2) (Suppl. 1): S54-62. [http://dx.doi.org/10.1002/hep.21060] [PMID: 16447271]

[26] Sørensen KK, Simon-Santamaria J, McCuskey RS, Smedsrød B. Liver sinusoidal endothelial cells. Compr Physiol 2015; 5(4): 1751-74. [http://dx.doi.org/10.1002/j.2040-4603.2015.tb00660.x] [PMID: 26426467]

[27] Braet F, Wisse E. Structural and functional aspects of liver sinusoidal endothelial cell fenestrae: a review. Comp Hepatol 2002; 1(1): 1. [http://dx.doi.org/10.1186/1476-5926-1-1] [PMID: 12437787]

[28] Mccuskey RS. The hepatic microvascular system in health and its response to toxicants. Anat Rec (Hoboken) 2008; 291(6): 661-71. [http://dx.doi.org/10.1002/ar.20663] [PMID: 18484612]

[29] Trefts E, Gannon M, Wasserman DH. The liver. Curr Biol 2017; 27(21): R1147-51. [http://dx.doi.org/10.1016/j.cub.2017.09.019] [PMID: 29112863]

[30] Lachman N, Pawlina W. The liver and biliary apparatus: basic structural anatomy and variations. In: Talley NJ, Lindor KD, Vargas HE, Eds. Practical Gastroenterology and Hepatology: Liver and Biliary Disease. Oxford: Blackwell Publishing Ltd 2010; pp. 1-16. [http://dx.doi.org/10.1002/9781444325249.ch1]

[31] Kalra A, Yetiskul E, Wehrle CJ, Tuma F. Physiology, liver. In: StatPearls [Internet]. Treasure Island (FL): StatPearls Publishing; 2023. https://www.ncbi.nlm.nih.gov/books/NBK535438

[32] Smith GI, Shankaran M, Yoshino M, *et al.* Insulin resistance drives hepatic de novo lipogenesis in nonalcoholic fatty liver disease. J Clin Invest 2020; 130(3): 1453-60. [http://dx.doi.org/10.1172/JCI134165] [PMID: 31805015]

[33] Donnelly KL, Smith CI, Schwarzenberg SJ, Jessurun J, Boldt MD, Parks EJ. Sources of fatty acids stored in liver and secreted via lipoproteins in patients with nonalcoholic fatty liver disease. J Clin Invest 2005; 115(5): 1343-51. [http://dx.doi.org/10.1172/JCI23621] [PMID: 15864352]

[34] Walkey CD, Chan WCW. Understanding and controlling the interaction of nanomaterials with proteins in a physiological environment. Chem Soc Rev 2012; 41(7): 2780-99. [http://dx.doi.org/10.1039/C1CS15233E] [PMID: 22086677]

[35] Cheng SH, Li FC, Souris JS, *et al.* Visualizing dynamics of sub-hepatic distribution of nanoparticles using intravital multiphoton fluorescence microscopy. ACS Nano 2012; 6(5): 4122-31. [http://dx.doi.org/10.1021/nn300558p] [PMID: 22486639]

[36] Ogawara K, Yoshida M, Higaki K, *et al.* Hepatic uptake of polystyrene microspheres in rats: Effect of particle size on intrahepatic distribution. J Control Release 1999; 59(1): 15-22.
[http://dx.doi.org/10.1016/S0168-3659(99)00015-2] [PMID: 10210718]

[37] Romero EL, Morilla MJ, Regts J, Koning GA, Scherphof GL. On the mechanism of hepatic transendothelial passage of large liposomes. FEBS Lett 1999; 448(1): 193-6.
[http://dx.doi.org/10.1016/S0014-5793(99)00364-6] [PMID: 10217439]

[38] Champion JA, Mitragotri S. Shape induced inhibition of phagocytosis of polymer particles. Pharm Res 2009; 26(1): 244-9.
[http://dx.doi.org/10.1007/s11095-008-9626-z] [PMID: 18548338]

[39] Zhang YN, Poon W, Tavares AJ, McGilvray ID, Chan WCW. Nanoparticle–liver interactions: Cellular uptake and hepatobiliary elimination. J Control Release 2016; 240: 332-48.
[http://dx.doi.org/10.1016/j.jconrel.2016.01.020] [PMID: 26774224]

[40] Gu FX, Karnik R, Wang AZ, *et al.* Targeted nanoparticles for cancer therapy. Nano Today 2007; 2(3): 14-21.
[http://dx.doi.org/10.1016/S1748-0132(07)70083-X]

[41] Matsumura Y, Maeda H. A new concept for macromolecular therapeutics in cancer chemotherapy: mechanism of tumoritropic accumulation of proteins and the antitumor agent smancs. Cancer Res 1986; 46(12 Pt 1): 6387-92.
[PMID: 2946403]

[42] Maeda H, Wu J, Sawa T, Matsumura Y, Hori K. Tumor vascular permeability and the EPR effect in macromolecular therapeutics: a review. J Control Release 2000; 65(1-2): 271-84.
[http://dx.doi.org/10.1016/S0168-3659(99)00248-5] [PMID: 10699287]

[43] Bertrand N, Wu J, Xu X, Kamaly N, Farokhzad OC. Cancer nanotechnology: The impact of passive and active targeting in the era of modern cancer biology. Adv Drug Deliv Rev 2014; 66: 2-25.
[http://dx.doi.org/10.1016/j.addr.2013.11.009] [PMID: 24270007]

[44] Yuan F, Dellian M, Fukumura D, *et al.* Vascular permeability in a human tumor xenograft: molecular size dependence and cutoff size. Cancer Res 1995; 55(17): 3752-6.
[PMID: 7641188]

[45] Farra R, Musiani F, Perrone F, *et al.* Polymer-mediated delivery of siRNAs to hepatocellular carcinoma: variables affecting specificity and effectiveness. Molecules 2018; 23(4): 777.
[http://dx.doi.org/10.3390/molecules23040777] [PMID: 29597300]

[46] Wu H, Wang MD, Liang L, *et al.* Nanotechnology for hepatocellular carcinoma: from surveillance, diagnosis to management. Small 2021; 17(6)2005236
[http://dx.doi.org/10.1002/smll.202005236] [PMID: 33448111]

[47] Malla RR, Kumari S, Kgk D, Momin S, Nagaraju GP. Nanotheranostics: Their role in hepatocellular carcinoma. Crit Rev Oncol Hematol 2020; 151102968
[http://dx.doi.org/10.1016/j.critrevonc.2020.102968] [PMID: 32416345]

[48] Gaumet M, Vargas A, Gurny R, Delie F. Nanoparticles for drug delivery: The need for precision in reporting particle size parameters. Eur J Pharm Biopharm 2008; 69(1): 1-9.
[http://dx.doi.org/10.1016/j.ejpb.2007.08.001] [PMID: 17826969]

[49] Byrne JD, Betancourt T, Brannon-Peppas L. Active targeting schemes for nanoparticle systems in cancer therapeutics. Adv Drug Deliv Rev 2008; 60(15): 1615-26.
[http://dx.doi.org/10.1016/j.addr.2008.08.005] [PMID: 18840489]

[50] Danhier F, Feron O, Préat V. To exploit the tumor microenvironment: Passive and active tumor targeting of nanocarriers for anti-cancer drug delivery. J Control Release 2010; 148(2): 135-46.
[http://dx.doi.org/10.1016/j.jconrel.2010.08.027] [PMID: 20797419]

[51] Hassan S, Prakash G, Bal Ozturk A, *et al.* Evolution and clinical translation of drug delivery

nanomaterials. Nano Today 2017; 15: 91-106.
[http://dx.doi.org/10.1016/j.nantod.2017.06.008] [PMID: 29225665]

[52] Soppimath KS, Aminabhavi TM, Kulkarni AR, Rudzinski WE. Biodegradable polymeric nanoparticles as drug delivery devices. J Control Release 2001; 70(1-2): 1-20.
[http://dx.doi.org/10.1016/S0168-3659(00)00339-4] [PMID: 11166403]

[53] Crucho CIC, Barros MT. Polymeric nanoparticles: A study on the preparation variables and characterization methods. Mater Sci Eng C 2017; 80: 771-84.
[http://dx.doi.org/10.1016/j.msec.2017.06.004] [PMID: 28866227]

[54] Allemann E, Gurny R, Doelker E. Drug-loaded nanoparticles—Preparation methods and drug targeting issues. Eur J Pharm Biopharm 1993; 39(1): 173-91.

[55] Panyam J, Labhasetwar V. Biodegradable nanoparticles for drug and gene delivery to cells and tissue. Adv Drug Deliv Rev 2003; 55(3): 329-47.
[http://dx.doi.org/10.1016/S0169-409X(02)00228-4] [PMID: 12628320]

[56] Danhier F, Ansorena E, Silva JM, Coco R, Le Breton A, Préat V. PLGA-based nanoparticles: An overview of biomedical applications. J Control Release 2012; 161(2): 505-22.
[http://dx.doi.org/10.1016/j.jconrel.2012.01.043] [PMID: 22353619]

[57] Couvreur P, Dubernet C, Puisieux F. Controlled drug delivery with nanoparticles: Current possibilities and future trends. Eur J Pharm Biopharm 1995; 41(1): 2-13.

[58] Vauthier C. Bouchemal K. Methods for the preparation and manufacture of polymeric nanoparticles. Pharmaceutics 2009; 1(1): 1-28.

[59] Mora-Huertas CE, Fessi H, Elaissari A. Polymer-based nanocapsules for drug delivery. Int J Pharm 2010; 385(1-2): 113-42.
[http://dx.doi.org/10.1016/j.ijpharm.2009.10.018] [PMID: 19825408]

[60] Li Y, Chen X, Li W, Li J, Huang D, Lin Y, *et al.* RNA-based therapy targeting SPTLC2 inhibits ceramide synthesis and reverses metabolic disorders in mice with nonalcoholic fatty liver disease. Nat Commun 2025; 16(1): 1-16.
[PMID: 39746907]

[61] Domingues I, Michalowski CB, Marotti V, *et al.* Exploiting the biological effect exerted by lipid nanocapsules in non-alcoholic fatty liver disease. J Control Release 2023; 356: 542-53.
[http://dx.doi.org/10.1016/j.jconrel.2023.03.012] [PMID: 36907563]

[62] Benoit JP, Lagarce F. Exploiting the biological effect exerted by lipid nanocapsules in non-alcoholic fatty liver disease. J Control Release 2020; 327: 724-35.

[63] Zhang Y, Li X, Zhang L, Wang J. Lipid nanocapsules improve glucose tolerance and insulin resistance in mice with nonalcoholic fatty liver disease. Biomaterials 2022; 280: 121-32.

[64] Jung K, Corrigan N, Wong EHH, Boyer C. Bioactive synthetic polymers. Adv Mater 2022; 34(2)2105063
[http://dx.doi.org/10.1002/adma.202105063] [PMID: 34611948]

[65] D'souza AA, Shegokar R. Polyethylene glycol (PEG): a versatile polymer for pharmaceutical applications. Expert Opin Drug Deliv 2016; 13(9): 1257-75.
[http://dx.doi.org/10.1080/17425247.2016.1182485] [PMID: 27116988]

[66] Jevševar S, Kunstelj M, Porekar VG. PEGylation of therapeutic proteins. Biotechnol J 2010; 5(1): 113-28.
[http://dx.doi.org/10.1002/biot.200900218] [PMID: 20069580]

[67] Moreira LS, Chagas AC, Ames-Sibin AP, *et al.* Alpha-tocopherol-loaded polycaprolactone nanoparticles improve the inflammation and systemic oxidative stress of arthritic rats. J Tradit Complement Med 2022; 12(4): 414-25.
[http://dx.doi.org/10.1016/j.jtcme.2021.12.003] [PMID: 35747358]

[68] Bhardwaj H, Jangde RK. Current updated review on preparation of polymeric nanoparticles for drug delivery and biomedical applications. Next Nanotechnology 2023; 2: 100013. [http://dx.doi.org/10.1016/j.nxnano.2023.100013]

[69] Krenkel O, Tacke F. Liver macrophages in tissue homeostasis and disease. Nat Rev Immunol 2017; 17(5): 306-21. [http://dx.doi.org/10.1038/nri.2017.11] [PMID: 28317925]

[70] Hammoutene A, Rautou PE. Role of liver sinusoidal endothelial cells in non-alcoholic fatty liver disease. J Hepatol 2019; 70(6): 1278-91. [http://dx.doi.org/10.1016/j.jhep.2019.02.012] [PMID: 30797053]

[71] Yin C, Evason KJ, Asahina K, Stainier DYR. Hepatic stellate cells in liver development, regeneration, and cancer. J Clin Invest 2013; 123(5): 1902-10. [http://dx.doi.org/10.1172/JCI66369] [PMID: 23635788]

[72] Gissen P, Arias IM. Structural and functional hepatocyte polarity and liver disease. J Hepatol 2015; 63(4): 1023-37. [http://dx.doi.org/10.1016/j.jhep.2015.06.015] [PMID: 26116792]

[73] Asselah T, Loureiro D, Boyer N, Mansouri A. Targets and future direct-acting antiviral approaches to achieve hepatitis B virus cure. Lancet Gastroenterol Hepatol 2019; 4(11): 883-92. [http://dx.doi.org/10.1016/S2468-1253(19)30190-6] [PMID: 31609242]

[74] Jesus S, Soares E, Costa J, Borchard G, Borges O. Immune response elicited by an intranasally delivered HBsAg low-dose adsorbed to poly-ε-caprolactone based nanoparticles. Int J Pharm 2016; 504(1-2): 59-69. [http://dx.doi.org/10.1016/j.ijpharm.2016.03.013] [PMID: 26976502]

[75] Dewangan HK, Pandey T, Maurya L, Singh S. Rational design and evaluation of HBsAg polymeric nanoparticles as antigen delivery carriers. Int J Biol Macromol 2018; 111: 804-12. [http://dx.doi.org/10.1016/j.ijbiomac.2018.01.073] [PMID: 29343454]

[76] Dewangan HK, Pandey T, Singh S. Nanovaccine for immunotherapy and reduced hepatitis-B virus in humanized model. Artif Cells Nanomed Biotechnol 2018; 46(8): 2033-42. [PMID: 29179600]

[77] Zhu J, Qin F, Ji Z, *et al.* Mannose-modified PLGA nanoparticles for sustained and targeted delivery in hepatitis B virus immunoprophylaxis. AAPS PharmSciTech 2020; 21(1): 13. [http://dx.doi.org/10.1208/s12249-019-1526-5] [PMID: 31807947]

[78] Brunt EM, Wong VWS, Nobili V, *et al.* Nonalcoholic fatty liver disease. Nat Rev Dis Primers 2015; 1(1): 15080. [http://dx.doi.org/10.1038/nrdp.2015.80] [PMID: 27188459]

[79] Friedman SL, Neuschwander-Tetri BA, Rinella M, Sanyal AJ. Mechanisms of NAFLD development and therapeutic strategies. Nat Med 2018; 24(7): 908-22. [http://dx.doi.org/10.1038/s41591-018-0104-9] [PMID: 29967350]

[80] Wang XJ, Malhi H. Nonalcoholic fatty liver disease. Ann Intern Med 2018; 169(9): ITC65-80. [http://dx.doi.org/10.7326/AITC201811060] [PMID: 30398639]

[81] Alonso C, Fernández-Ramos D, Varela-Rey M, *et al.* Metabolomic identification subtypes nonalcoholic steatohepatitis. Gastroenterology 2017; 152(6): 1449-1461.e7. [http://dx.doi.org/10.1053/j.gastro.2017.01.015] [PMID: 28132890]

[82] Cusi K. Role of obesity and lipotoxicity in the development of nonalcoholic steatohepatitis: pathophysiology and clinical implications. Gastroenterology 2012; 142(4): 711-725.e6. [http://dx.doi.org/10.1053/j.gastro.2012.02.003] [PMID: 22326434]

[83] Neuschwander-Tetri BA. Hepatic lipotoxicity and the pathogenesis of nonalcoholic steatohepatitis. Hepatology 2010; 52(2): 774-88.

[http://dx.doi.org/10.1002/hep.23719] [PMID: 20683968]

[84] Zhao R, Zhu M, Zhou S, Feng W, Chen H. Rapamycin-loaded mPEG-PLGA nanoparticles ameliorate hepatic steatosis and liver injury in non-alcoholic fatty liver disease. Front Chem 2020; 8: 407. [http://dx.doi.org/10.3389/fchem.2020.00407] [PMID: 32548088]

[85] Cao Y, Baiyisaiti A, Wong CW, Hsu S, Qi R. Polyurethane nanoparticle-loaded fenofibrate exerts inhibitory effects on nonalcoholic fatty liver disease in mice. Mol Pharm 2018; 15(10): 4550-7. [http://dx.doi.org/10.1021/acs.molpharmaceut.8b00548] [PMID: 30188729]

[86] Marcellin P, Kutala BK. Liver diseases: A major, neglected global public health problem requiring urgent actions and large-scale screening. Liver Int 2018; 38 (Suppl. 1): 2-6. [http://dx.doi.org/10.1111/liv.13682] [PMID: 29427496]

[87] Lee YA, Wallace MC, Friedman SL. Pathobiology of liver fibrosis: a translational success story. Gut 2015; 64(5): 830-41. [http://dx.doi.org/10.1136/gutjnl-2014-306842] [PMID: 25681399]

[88] Novo E, Parola M. Redox mechanisms in hepatic chronic wound healing and fibrogenesis. Fibrogenesis Tissue Repair 2008; 1(1): 5. [http://dx.doi.org/10.1186/1755-1536-1-5] [PMID: 19014652]

[89] Novo E, Cannito S, Paternostro C, Bocca C, Miglietta A, Parola M. Cellular and molecular mechanisms in liver fibrogenesis. Arch Biochem Biophys 2014; 548: 20-37. [http://dx.doi.org/10.1016/j.abb.2014.02.015] [PMID: 24631571]

[90] Parola M, Pinzani M. Liver fibrosis: Pathophysiology, pathogenetic targets and clinical issues. Mol Aspects Med 2019; 65: 37-55. [http://dx.doi.org/10.1016/j.mam.2018.09.002] [PMID: 30213667]

[91] Latief U, Ahmad R. Herbal remedies for liver fibrosis: A review on the mode of action of fifty herbs. J Tradit Complement Med 2018; 8(3): 352-60. [http://dx.doi.org/10.1016/j.jtcme.2017.07.002] [PMID: 29992106]

[92] Li W, Zhou C, Fu Y, *et al.* Targeted delivery of hyaluronic acid nanomicelles to hepatic stellate cells in hepatic fibrosis rats. Acta Pharm Sin B 2020; 10(4): 693-710. [http://dx.doi.org/10.1016/j.apsb.2019.07.003] [PMID: 32322471]

[93] Lin L, Gong H, Li R, *et al.* Nanodrug with ROS and pH dual-sensitivity ameliorates liver fibrosis via multicellular regulation. Adv Sci (Weinh) 2020; 7(7): 1903138. [http://dx.doi.org/10.1002/advs.201903138] [PMID: 32274310]

[94] Hu Q, Hu S, Fleming E, Lee JY, Luo Y. Chitosan-caseinate-dextran ternary complex nanoparticles for potential oral delivery of astaxanthin with significantly improved bioactivity. Int J Biol Macromol 2020; 151: 747-56. [http://dx.doi.org/10.1016/j.ijbiomac.2020.02.170] [PMID: 32084488]

[95] Villanueva A. Hepatocellular Carcinoma. N Engl J Med 2019; 380(15): 1450-62. [http://dx.doi.org/10.1056/NEJMra1713263] [PMID: 30970190]

[96] Kanwal F, Kramer J, Asch SM, Chayanupatkul M, Cao Y, El-Serag HB. Risk of hepatocellular cancer in HCV patients treated with direct-acting antiviral agents. Gastroenterology 2017; 153(4): 996-1005.e1. [http://dx.doi.org/10.1053/j.gastro.2017.06.012] [PMID: 28642197]

[97] Llovet JM, Bruix J. Systematic review of randomized trials for unresectable hepatocellular carcinoma: Chemoembolization improves survival. Hepatology 2003; 37(2): 429-42. [http://dx.doi.org/10.1053/jhep.2003.50047] [PMID: 12540794]

[98] Elnaggar MH, Abushouk AI, Hassan AHE, *et al.* Nanomedicine as a putative approach for active targeting of hepatocellular carcinoma. Semin Cancer Biol 2021; 69: 91-9. [http://dx.doi.org/10.1016/j.semcancer.2019.08.016] [PMID: 31421265]

[99] Huang Y, Zhang W, Xu Y, *et al.* Dynamic core crosslinked camptothecin prodrug micelles with reduction sensitivity and boronic acid-mediated enhanced endocytosis: An intelligent tumor-targeted delivery nanoplatform. Int J Pharm 2020; 580: 119250.
[http://dx.doi.org/10.1016/j.ijpharm.2020.119250] [PMID: 32209369]

[100] Yang T, Du G, Cui Y, *et al.* pH-sensitive doxorubicin-loaded polymeric nanocomplex based on β-cyclodextrin for liver cancer-targeted therapy. Int J Nanomedicine 2019; 14: 1997-2010.
[http://dx.doi.org/10.2147/IJN.S193170] [PMID: 30962684]

[101] Yang D, Luo W, Wang J, *et al.* A novel controlled release formulation of the Pin1 inhibitor ATRA to improve liver cancer therapy by simultaneously blocking multiple cancer pathways. J Control Release 2018; 269: 405-22.
[http://dx.doi.org/10.1016/j.jconrel.2017.11.031] [PMID: 29170140]

[102] O'Leary JG, Lepe R, Davis GL. Indications for liver transplantation. Gastroenterology 2008; 134(6): 1764-76.
[http://dx.doi.org/10.1053/j.gastro.2008.02.028] [PMID: 18471553]

[103] EASL clinical practice guidelines: liver transplantation. J Hepatol 2016; 64(2): 433-85.
[http://dx.doi.org/10.1016/j.jhep.2015.10.006] [PMID: 26597456]

[104] Afzali B, Lechler RI, Hernandez-Fuentes MP. Allorecognition and the alloresponse: clinical implications. Tissue Antigens 2007; 69(6): 545-56.
[http://dx.doi.org/10.1111/j.1399-0039.2007.00834.x] [PMID: 17498264]

[105] Demetris AJ, Batts KP, Dhillon AP, *et al.* Banff schema for grading liver allograft rejection: an international consensus document. Hepatology 1997; 25(3): 658-63.
[http://dx.doi.org/10.1002/hep.510250328] [PMID: 9049215]

[106] Halloran PF, Kreepala C, Einecke G, Loupy A, Sellarés J. Therapeutic approaches to organ transplantation. In: Li XC, Jevnikar AM, Eds. Transplant immunology. Hoboken: Wiley 2015.
[http://dx.doi.org/10.1002/9781119072997.ch10]

[107] Wang Y, Wang C, Fu S, *et al.* Preparation of Tacrolimus loaded micelles based on poly(ε-caprolactone)–poly(ethylene glycol)–poly(ε-caprolactone). Int J Pharm 2011; 407(1-2): 184-9.
[http://dx.doi.org/10.1016/j.ijpharm.2011.01.018] [PMID: 21251958]

[108] Wang Y, Wang C, Wang Y, Luo F, Yan X, Qian Z. Micelles of methoxy poly(ethylene glycol)-poly(epsilon-caprolactone) as a novel drug delivery vehicle for tacrolimus. J Biomed Nanotechnol 2013; 9(2): 147-57.
[http://dx.doi.org/10.1166/jbn.2013.1489] [PMID: 23627041]

[109] Xu W, Ling P, Zhang T. Toward immunosuppressive effects on liver transplantation in rat model: Tacrolimus loaded poly(ethylene glycol)-poly(d,l-lactide) nanoparticle with longer survival time. Int J Pharm 2014; 460(1-2): 173-80.
[http://dx.doi.org/10.1016/j.ijpharm.2013.10.035] [PMID: 24172796]

[110] Zhang D, Pan X, Wang S, *et al.* Multifunctional poly(methyl vinyl ether- *co* -maleic anhydride)- *graft* -hydroxypropyl-β-cyclodextrin amphiphilic copolymer as an oral high-performance delivery carrier of tacrolimus. Mol Pharm 2015; 12(7): 2337-51.
[http://dx.doi.org/10.1021/acs.molpharmaceut.5b00010] [PMID: 26024817]

[111] Shin TH, Ho MJ, Kim SR, *et al.* Formulation and in vivo pharmacokinetic evaluation of ethyl cellulose-coated sustained release multiple-unit system of tacrolimus. Int J Biol Macromol 2018; 109: 544-50.
[http://dx.doi.org/10.1016/j.ijbiomac.2017.12.111] [PMID: 29277422]

[112] Wang M, Sun J, Zhai Y, *et al.* Enteric polymer based on pH-responsive aliphatic polycarbonate functionalized with vitamin E to facilitate oral delivery of tacrolimus. Biomacromolecules 2015; 16(4): 1179-90.
[http://dx.doi.org/10.1021/bm501847u] [PMID: 25714622]

[113] Hopf U, Ramadori G. [Physiology and pathophysiology of the reticuloendothelial system of the liver (author's transl)]. Leber Magen Darm 1980; 10(5): 277-83.
[PMID: 7464416]

[114] Hirn S, Semmler-Behnke M, Schleh C, *et al.* Particle size-dependent and surface charge-dependent biodistribution of gold nanoparticles after intravenous administration. Eur J Pharm Biopharm 2011; 77(3): 407-16.
[http://dx.doi.org/10.1016/j.ejpb.2010.12.029] [PMID: 21195759]

[115] Poon W, Zhang YN, Ouyang B, *et al.* Elimination pathways of nanoparticles. ACS Nano 2019; 13(5): 5785-98.
[http://dx.doi.org/10.1021/acsnano.9b01383] [PMID: 30990673]

CHAPTER 7

Dendrimers and Hybrid Nanocarriers for Fatty Liver Disease

Minky Mukhija[1], **Himanshu Sharma**[2], **Jyoti Monga**[1], **Ankush Sundriyal**[3] and **Jasmine Chaudhary**[4,*]

[1] *Department of Pharmacognosy, Ch. Devi Lal College of Pharmacy, Jagadhri, Haryana, India*

[2] *Chitkara College of Pharmacy, Chitkara University, Rajpura, Punjab, India*

[3] *Department of Pharmacognosy, School of Pharmaceutical Sciences, Sardar Bhagwan Singh Post Graduate Institute of Biomedical Sciences and Research, Dehradun, Uttarakhand, India*

[4] *Department of Pharmaceutical Chemistry, Maharishi Markandeshwar (Deemed to be University), Mullana, Haryana, India*

Abstract: Liver problems continue to be a major worldwide health concern despite advances in medical understanding, and pharmacological therapy is usually complicated by drug toxicity. Fatty liver disease, which comprises both alcoholic and non-alcoholic forms, is defined by an excessive buildup of hepatic fat. Nanotechnology may be employed to deliver drugs to the liver. Dendrimers and hybrid nanocarriers are two unique approaches for effective drug delivery. Dendrimers are artificial polymers. They have a central core, branches, and functional groups at their ends. The specific qualities of dendrimers, such as their high water solubility, well-defined structure, biocompatibility, and high encapsulation efficiency, make them excellent for a range of nanomedicine research. Conjugates of organic and inorganic materials produced by different techniques that combine the benefits of the materials in a synergistic manner are known as hybrid nanocarriers. In drug transport, hybrid nanocarriers combine the benefits of two or more nanocarrier systems, overcoming their flaws to build a new, perhaps safer, and more effective nanocarrier structure. This chapter discusses the chemistry and structure of dendrimers and hybrid nanocarriers, with a focus on their potential value in the treatment of fatty liver disease. It also covers the most recent advances in preliminary studies on these nanotechnologies for the treatment of fatty liver disease. This chapter also covers the challenges and opportunities for developing a framework for better fatty liver disease treatment.

Keywords: Dendrimers, Drug delivery, Fatty liver disease, Hybrid nanocarriers, Nanotechnology.

[*] **Corresponding author Jasmine Chaudhary:** Department of Pharmaceutical Chemistry, Maharishi Markandeshwar (Deemed to be University), Mullana, Haryana, India;
E-mail: jasmine.jain@mmumullana.org

Anjali Sharma, Devkant Sharma, Ajmer Singh Grewal, Geeta Deswal & Ganga Reddy Velma (Eds.)

INTRODUCTION

Triglyceride accumulation in hepatocytes, known as “fatty liver,” can lead to steatohepatitis [1]. Alcohol usage is the major cause of alcoholic fatty liver disease, whereas insulin resistance and metabolic syndrome are the main reasons for NAFLD [2]. Regardless of other traits of the metabolic syndrome, NAFLD is a risk factor in and of itself, and there is growing evidence associating it with an increased risk of atherosclerosis and cardiovascular disease [3]. Studies demonstrated that between 9% and 53% of Indians suffer from NAFLD, and that fatty liver is a major worldwide pandemic [4, 5]. The initial stage of NAFLD is marked by simple hepatic steatosis, which may develop into cirrhosis, fibrosis, hepatocellular cancer, or NASH [6]. Given India's enormous population, fatty liver disease can have a detrimental effect on the nation's limited resources and impose a significant strain on the healthcare system.

CONVENTIONAL THERAPEUTIC APPROACHES FOR FATTY LIVER DISEASE

Lifestyle Modifications

Lifestyle modification aimed at weight loss and increased physical activity is vital in managing all patients with NAFLD, irrespective of their underlying liver histology. An appropriate diet, such as the Mediterranean diet (whole grains, vegetables, fruits, lean protein, and healthy fats), is beneficial for reducing liver fat and inflammation [7]. Patients should be encouraged to avoid a sedentary lifestyle by increasing daily activities, undertaking regular exercise, and eating a healthy diet. Overall, lifestyle interventions, including behavioral, dietary, and exercise changes, can be very effective in reducing body weight.

Pharmacological Interventions

- ***Insulin Sensitizers***

Insulin resistance is a hallmark of NAFLD; therefore, targeting this pathway has been a significant focus of many studies. Insulin sensitizers, such as metformin and TZDs, have been relatively well studied. Newer agents in this class include GLP-1 agonists and DPP-4 inhibitors (*i.e.*, incretins) [8].

• ***Metformin***

Metformin has been evaluated in several small studies on nondiabetic NAFLD patients. It has been shown to improve transaminase levels and hepatic steatosis [9]. However, its effect on inflammation was less robust, and improvement in fibrosis was demonstrated in only one study. Most of these were small, short-duration trials, and, unfortunately, histological follow-up was incomplete. The results of the most extensive study on metformin, the treatment of NAFLD in children (TONIC) trial, which evaluated metformin, vitamin E, and placebo in a pediatric population, were recently published [10].

LIMITATIONS OF CONVENTIONAL TREATMENTS

Conventional treatment for FLD, in particular, faces many limitations. Firstly, managing NAFLD involves lifestyle changes, such as weight loss through regular exercise, which can improve liver health by reducing inflammation and fat accumulation [11]. However, these changes are often challenging to maintain over a long time, and there are no standard pharmacological treatments explicitly approved for NAFLD. In improving insulin resistance, liver fat-reducing pharmacological interventions have shown some benefit, for example, metformin and TZDs. However, their effects are dependent on weight loss and may not persist after discontinuation of the medicine. Additionally, TZDs are associated with their side effects, i.e., weight gain and edema, which can limit their use. The anti-diabetic drugs, including GLP-1 receptor agonists, such as liraglutide, show promising results in reducing liver fat and enhancing insulin sensitivity, but they can cause side effects in the GIT [12].

For morbidly obese patients with NAFLD, bariatric surgery is another way to improve the metabolic syndrome and liver histology. However, bariatric surgery is not suitable for all patients, particularly those who have cirrhosis and fibrosis, because of the increased surgical risks [13]. Moreover, the direct liver benefit is not demonstrated in anti-obesity drugs, and some have been withdrawn from the market due to safety issues. In summary, the cornerstone of NAFLD management is lifestyle changes. They require sustained effort and may not be sufficient for all patients. Current pharmacological options have limitations in safety and efficacy, and they need more targeted management and more effective [14]. Continued research into novel therapies, such as lipase inhibitors and FGF21 analogues, offers hope for future advances in the management of fatty liver disease [15].

NANOTECHNOLOGY IN THE TREATMENT OF FATTY LIVER DISEASE

Advantages of Nanocarriers in Liver Targeting

In targeting liver diseases, the nanocarrier has emerged as a tool, including FLD, because of its ability to deliver the drug specifically to the liver while minimizing its side effects on healthy tissues [16]. Targeted drug delivery capability is one of the primary advantages of nanocarriers, which can achieve both active and passive targeting. Active targeting involves modifying the nanocarrier surface with specific ligands, while passive targeting relies on the improved retention and permeability that bind to receptors overexpressed in liver tissues or cells [17]. The prolonged circulation in the bloodstream is crucial, and without causing any harm to autogenous tissues, the nanocarrier offers biodegradability and biocompatibility. A diverse array of pharmaceuticals may be conjugated and encapsulated by their production from lipids, other materials, and inorganic compounds [18]. The development of multifunctional nanoparticles is not only for delivering drugs but also serves as a diagnostic tool and provides real-time imaging of liver tissue. In the context of FLD, the nanocarrier is designed to target specific cells involved in disease progression, such as macrophages and HSCs [19]. The key components of FLD progression can be addressed by delivering drugs directly to these cells, and the nanocarrier can help suppress inflammation and fibrosis. The nanocarrier safeguards medications against prolonged circulation and premature metabolism, enhancing their pharmacological attributes and yielding superior outcomes.

Despite these benefits, challenges remain, including instability of nanomaterials and potential toxicity, necessitating further research to optimize their functionality and design. Nonetheless, ongoing research on nanocarrier development holds significant promise for improving the treatment of FLD by enabling efficient, targeted drug delivery and safer therapeutic options [20].

Types of Nanocarriers Used for FLD Therapy

To enhance the safety and efficacy of treatment for fatty liver disease, nanotechnologies have emerged as a promising approach by utilizing various nanocarrier types [21]. FLD, including NAFLD, the MASLD, and its more severe form, poses significant challenges in management due to limitations in current treatments and its complex pathogenesis.

- ***Liposomes:*** Liposomes are vesicular structures composed of lipids. Liposomes are particularly effective for drug delivery because they can be taken up by sinusoidal endothelial cells [22]. Both lipophilic and hydrophilic drugs are encapsulated in liposomes, but they differ in FLD treatment.
- ***Micelles:*** Micelle structures are self-assembled from amphiphilic molecules and are also helpful in the delivery of hydrophobic drugs [23]. Micelles improve drug solubility and the pharmacokinetic profile.
- ***Polymeric nanoparticles:*** These include nanoparticles made from materials such as polylactic-co-glycolic acid and polylactic acid. They can be engineered to release drugs in a controlled manner and are biocompatible [24]. For instance, polylactic-co-glycolic acid nanoparticles are used to encapsulate siRNA targeting inflammatory receptors and are also effective at reducing markers of liver disease in animal models.
- ***Nano-emulsions:*** Nano-emulsions enhance the lipophilic drug solubility and facilitate their delivery to liver tissues due to their stable mixtures of oil, surfactants, and water [25].
- ***Cell membrane-delivered nanoparticles:*** These nanoparticles are engineered for drug delivery and are derived from cell membranes, *e.g.*, reducing lipid accumulation and increasing rosuvastatin uptake by hepatocytes [26].

DENDRIMERS IN LIVER DISEASE

Structure and Properties of Dendrimers

Dendrimers are three-dimensional, highly structured, and hyper-branched macromolecules. In the field of pharmaceutical therapy, they have attracted significant attention due to their distinct properties and functionalities [27]. Dendrimers consist of a central core surrounded by layers of branching units that terminate in terminal groups. Dendrimers are monodispersed, meaning they have a uniform weight distribution, which improves functionality and reliability in many applications. Dendrimers are globular in shape, a result of their adaptable surfaces, which enable them to interact effectively with other molecules and encapsulate guest molecules within their internal cavities.

Dendrimer's properties are largely influenced by the functional group on its surface, which is designed to facilitate specific biological interactions. Dendrimers are suitable for drug delivery applications if they are made water-soluble by functionalizing their outer shell with hydrophilic groups [28]. Higher-generation dendrimers have more surface groups for modification, allowing precise control over their physicochemical properties. The concept of dendrimer therapy offers various benefits. The unique properties and structure of dendrimers make them an exciting area of research in pharmaceutical therapy, particularly in drug delivery systems.

Mechanisms of Hepatic Targeting Using Dendrimers

Due to their molecular flexibility and plasticity, dendrimers are promising carriers for targeted delivery to the liver. The use of specific ligands to modify dendrimers that bind receptors expressed by hepatocytes is known as liver targeting [29]. The hepatocyte-specific ASGPR, for instance, binds galactose-conjugated dendrimers and is especially responsive to galactose, lactose, and glucose. By avoiding the reticuloendothelial processes that usually limit drug transport to hepatocytes, these multivalent binding traits allow dendrimer internalisation and efficient targeting within these cells. Another method is to release dendrimers modified with lactobionic acid, which binds to ASGPR to target cells.

Furthermore, these lactobionic acid-modified dendrimers might boost specific efficiency and cytocompatibility, especially in liver cancer cells. The PEG spacer enhances the stability of the dendrimer-drug complex and reduces non-specific interactions, allowing for more effective delivery of the therapeutic agents to liver cancer cells. The design of dendrimers for targeting hepatic cells often involves surface and size modifications to ensure they can navigate through liver sinusoidal endothelial cells and reach hepatocytes without being cleared prematurely. This targeted delivery not only increases therapeutic efficacy but also reduces systemic side effects by minimizing their exposure to nontarget tissues. Overall, dendrimers offer a unique platform for developing targeted therapies for liver disease, including acute liver injuries and liver cancer, by leveraging specific receptor-mediated uptake mechanisms [30].

Dendrimer-based drug delivery systems for FLD

For FLD, there is currently very little research, particularly in dendrimer-based drug delivery. Some diseases, such as nervous system disorders and cancer, for which dendrimers show remarkable potential for targeted drug delivery due to their biocompatibility and functionality [31]. Dendrimer-based drug delivery systems have shown promise in reducing lipid aggregation, effectively targeting liver cells, and mitigating oxidative stress in hepatocytes. For FLD treatment, the dendrimer-based drug delivery system can be adapted by leveraging its ability to encapsulate drugs and deliver them to specific target tissues. For example, it enhances delivery to liver cells by surface-modifying dendrimers with targeting moieties. In addition, for improving drug bioavailability and drug solubility, the dendrimer's ability can help deliver therapeutic agents to the liver [32]. Fig. (**1**) shows a dendrimer as a nanocarrier for drug delivery and targeting therapeutics. The principles of dendrimer-based drug delivery are not specifically applied to FLD; however, they could be applied to develop new management strategies for this condition by using dendrimer modification to target liver tissue and enhance the delivery of therapeutic compounds.

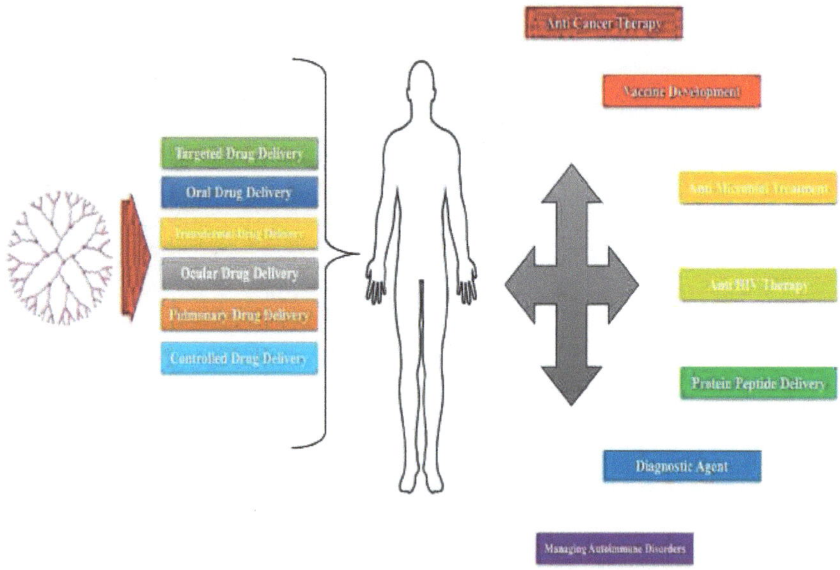

Fig. (1). Dendrimer as a nanocarrier for drug delivery and targeting therapeutics.

RECENT ADVANCEMENTS IN DENDRIMER-BASED THERAPIES

Recent advancements in dendrimer-based therapies have created promising avenues for addressing liver diseases, including FLD and related conditions. Dendrimers are spherical molecules that carry therapeutic drugs, which improve drug efficacy and delivery [33]. For delivering medication that targets liver conditions, the ability of dendrimers is beneficial, as they enhance drug bioavailability and solubility. In liver disease, nanotechnology has been explored for delivering medication to specific liver cells, i.e., HSCs, which play a vital role in liver fibrosis, an advanced complication of NAFLD. HSC activation pathways are shown in Fig. (**2**) for further research on the use of dendrimers in the treatment of NAFLD. Pharmacological treatments, including glucagon-like peptide agonists, as well as dietary and lifestyle modifications, are crucial components of NAFLD treatment. Further exploring the potential of dendrimers to enhance drug delivery in NAFLD could be beneficial for future studies.

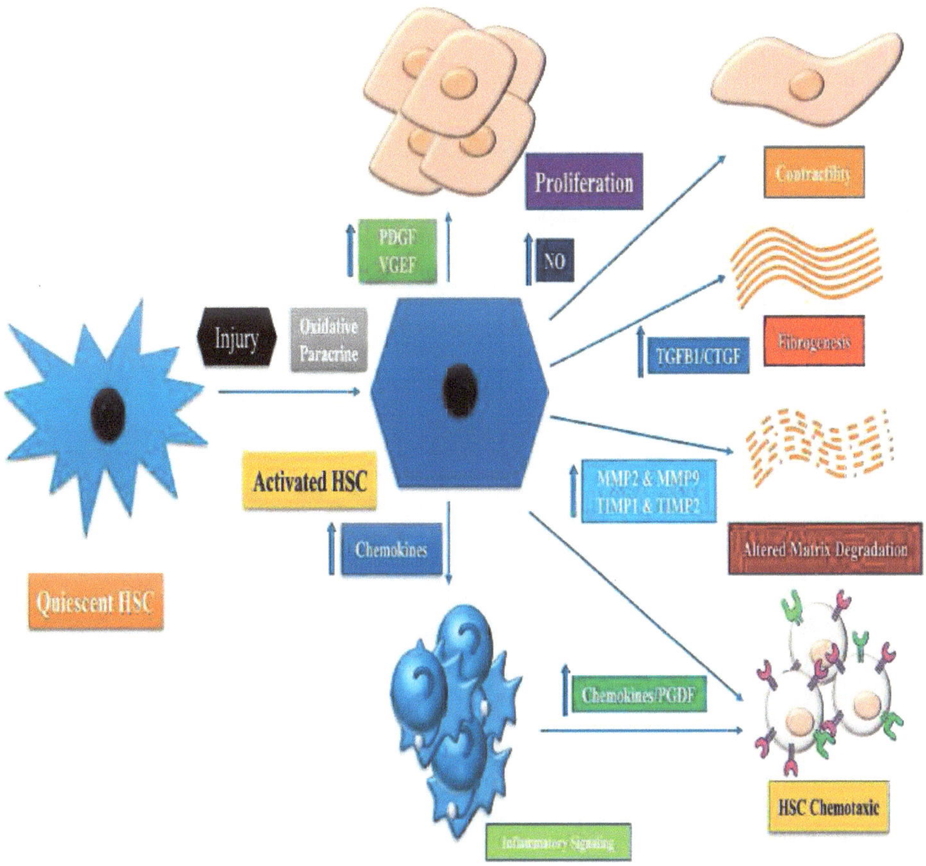

Fig. (2). Hepatic Stellate Cell (HSC) activation pathways: initiation and perpetuation phases.

HYBRID NANOCARRIERS FOR FATTY LIVER DISEASE

For treating FLD, the hybrid nanocarrier has emerged as a promising approach, particularly in NAFLD. The hybrid nanocarrier, in combination with different materials, improves drug delivery specificity and efficacy [20]. Hybrid nanomaterials have been used in the liver for targeted interleukin-22 gene delivery and show potential to enhance insulin resistance and alleviate hepatic steatosis. Moreover, compounds loaded onto lipid nanoparticles, *e.g.*, silibinin, have demonstrated enhanced therapeutic efficacy and bioavailability in the management of NAFLD by reducing insulin resistance and lipid accumulation. Hybrid systems offer a potential approach for developing novel treatments for the management of fatty liver disease by reducing side effects and improving drug delivery.

Types of Hybrid Systems

There are several types of hybrid systems, like dendrimers-lipid hybrids, liposome-polymer hybrids, etc. Hybrid combinations of different substances leverage their individual abilities to enhance functionality and performance.

- ***Dendrimers-Lipid Hybrids:*** The combination of dendrimers with lipids is beneficial; dendrimers are highly branched molecules with a well-defined structure [34]. Dendrimers have the ability to encapsulate molecules through their branches, while lipid properties enhance the stability of the hybrid and improve its biocompatibility. The dendrimer–lipid hybrid is beneficial for delivering nanomolecules and genetic compounds into cells, as it can effectively interact with cell membranes and promote endocytosis. For drug targeting and drug loading, dendrimers provide a high surface area, while the lipidic system is beneficial for cell uptake and interaction with the cell membrane.
- ***Liposome-polymer Hydrogels:*** These systems are designed to enhance the stability and long-term activity of liposomes in vesicle form, which are composed of lipid layers. These hybrid systems improve protection and drug encapsulation against degradation [35]. Within the liposome membrane, the polymer components are incorporated, which enhances the controlled release of drugs and their stability.
- ***Polymer-based Hybrids:*** These systems create nanoparticles by integrating polymer and lipid matrices, which then encapsulate hydrophilic and hydrophobic drugs [36]. The polymer matrices provide controlled drug release and structural integrity, while the lipidic system facilitates solubilization of hydrophobic drugs.
- ***Carbon Nanotube-lipid Hybrids:*** In the specific system of lipids and carbon nanotubes, the two components combine to form stable and beneficial hybrids. Lipids aid in the loading and uptake of medicines using this approach, while carbon nanotubes increase mechanical strength and electrical conductivity [37]. The hybrid system offers a unique strategy for drug administration and nanotechnology by combining the strengths of its components, making it more robust, safe, and effective than either component alone.

ADVANTAGES OF HYBRID NANOCARRIERS OVER TRADITIONAL NANOCARRIERS

The ability of hybrid nanocarriers to blend the benefits of different materials is their key edge over normal nanocarriers. Enhanced stability and biocompatibility are the major advantages [38]. Combining components, such as lipids and polymers, may yield a hybrid nanocarrier that enhances interactions with biological systems and prevents drug degradation, thereby reducing toxicities and unwanted effects. The multifunctionality of the hybrid nanocarriers is another important feature. It allows for the co-delivery of potentially useful drugs and blends a variety of medical components [39]. Combining different treatment methods may help control outcomes and manage drug resistance. The hybrid nanocarriers' changing size, shape, and surface chemistry may make them useful for a range of applications. The ability of the hybrid nanocarrier to strengthen and reduce effects, improve drug delivery efficiency, and provide a variety of options for healing and tracking are its major benefits over the ordinary nanocarrier [37].

CHALLENGES AND LIMITATIONS

For dendrimers and hybrid nanocarriers to be clinically effective and safe in the treatment of FLD, several problems and limitations must be addressed. A major concern is the potential toxicity of nanocarriers [40]. In addition to the several significant enhancements that dendrimers offer in terms of pharmacokinetic and pharmacodynamic characteristics, their toxicity profile has also been documented. According to studies, certain dendrimers, particularly PAMAM, may be dangerous due to their cationic surface charges, which may promote haemolysis and damage cell membranes [41]. This cytotoxicity may damage healthy cells, as they usually have poor hydro solubility and high overall toxicity. Numerous toxicity-reduction approaches have been developed because the toxicity of many dendrimers limits their biological application. Due to their complex chemical structure, dendrimers and hybrid nanocarriers are difficult to ensure safety. For instance, despite their advantages in drug delivery, lipid–polymer hybrid nanoparticles have drawbacks, including rapid drug release, drug leakage, and inappropriate release mechanisms [42]. These issues may compromise the efficiency and reliability of the nanocarriers.

Due to their unique physical properties, nanoparticles require specific research on their long-term safety, metabolism, and biodistribution. The lack of standardized testing standards may make the licensing process more complicated for regulatory bodies, which seek expert data to measure specific characteristics [43]. Furthermore, the large-scale production of high-quality solid nanocarriers is a major challenge that affects their value as commercial products. Advantages and challenges of dendrimers in FLD are presented in Table **1**.

Table 1. Advantages and challenges of dendrimers in fatty liver disease therapy.

Property	Advantages	Challenges	Reference
Targeted Drug Delivery	Surface modification allows hepatocyte-specific targeting	May require additional functionalization for liver-specific uptake	[44]
High Drug Loading Capacity	Encapsulation of hydrophilic and hydrophobic drugs improves solubility	Drug release may be affected by dendrimer size and core chemistry	[45]
Controlled Drug Release	Surface functionalization enables sustained drug release	Toxicity concerns due to residual functional groups	[46]
Biocompatibility	Functionalized dendrimers (*e.g.*, PEGylation) improve safety	Unmodified dendrimers may cause cytotoxicity and immune responses	[47]

RECENT DEVELOPMENTS IN HYBRID NANOCARRIERS FOR LIVER-TARGETED DRUG DELIVERY

Recent developments in hybrid nanocarriers for liver-targeted drug delivery have shown significant promise [48]. The traditional methods describe challenges associated with multiple drug resistance, high clearance rates, and severe side effects. A combination of different substances in a hybrid nanocarrier can enhance specificity and drug-delivery efficiency.

The development of multifunctional nanoparticles that combine diagnostic capabilities and therapeutics is called theranostics. Hybrid nanocarrier systems for drug delivery offer a descriptive approach to diagnosis and treatment. Overall, hybrid nanotechnology represents a strategy to enhance drug delivery to the liver, reduce adverse effects, and improve treatment efficacy [48, 49]. Preclinical studies on dendrimers and hybrid nanocarriers in FLD are presented in Table **2**.

Table 2. Preclinical studies on dendrimers and hybrid nanocarriers in fatty liver disease.

Study type	Nanocarrier Used/design	Therapeutic Agent	Key Findings	Ref.
In vitro/ In vivo	Galactose-functionalized dendrimers for ASGPR-mediated targeted drug delivery to hepatocytes. These dendrimers consist of hydroxyl-terminated PAMAM dendrimers linked to galactose moieties to improve hepatocyte selectivity.	Therapeutic agents targeting hepatocytes	*In vitro* studies demonstrated effective uptake in a hepatocyte cell line, indicating internalization via ASGPR. *In vivo* studies demonstrated remarkable liver accumulation in mouse models (20% of the dose administered within 1 hour) and preserved hepatocyte-specific targeting in disease models, for instance, NASH and acetaminophen-induced hepatic necrosis.	[46]
In vitro/ In vivo	Hybrid nanoparticles based on penetratin and polymetformin. Hybrid nanoparticles made using DSPE-PEG2000, penetratin (a cell-penetrating peptide), and the chitosan-metformin conjugation. Through electrostatic interactions, these constituents self-assemble to create stable nanocomplexes that encapsulate the IL-22 gene.	Interleukin-22 gene	*In vitro* studies demonstrated successful IL-22 transfection and expression in hepatocyte cell lines, which reduced inflammatory markers and the buildup of fat. The nanoparticles enabled targeted liver delivery of IL-22 in experimental animal models of NAFLD, leading to noteworthy changes in liver histology, reduced hepatic steatosis, and decreased pro-inflammatory cytokine levels.	[44]
In vitro/ In vivo	Lipid-polymer hybrid nanoparticles functionalized with chitosan	Silymarin	The studied hybrid nanoparticles in an *in vitro* model improved oral bioavailability and therapeutic efficacy in liver disease. They increased hepatocyte uptake and reduced fat accumulation in fatty liver cells. *In vivo* studies on mice showed that the oral bioavailability of the compound was 14.38 times higher than that of silymarin. There was a notable reduction in ALT, AST, and lipid levels.	[50]
In vitro	Nanoengineered natural cell membrane-derived nanoparticles incorporating rosuvastatin within their bilayer assembly.	Rosuvastatin	Use of rosuvastatin-loaded cell membrane-derived nanoparticles led to a remarkable decrease in hepatocyte lipid accumulation in a MASLD model, as evidenced by lower triglyceride and total cholesterol levels.	[51]

(Table 2) cont.....

Study type	Nanocarrier Used/design	Therapeutic Agent	Key Findings	Ref.
In vivo	Stiff-soft hybrid biomimetic nano drug	Dihydromyricetin	The oral bioavailability of the drug was increased, enhancing its potency by inhibiting lipid accumulation and reducing tissue inflammation in an early NAFLD model. The hybrid nano-emulsion improved the stability and controlled release of dihydromyricetin. Increased penetration through the gastrointestinal mucus layer and enhanced uptake by intestinal epithelial cells were observed. Studies demonstrated targeted delivery to the liver with significant therapeutic effects in early NAFLD models, including reduced lipid accumulation and improved liver function markers.	[52]
In vitro/ In vivo	Chondroitin sulfate-derived hybrid micelles	Celastrol	The micelles expressed prolonged release behavior, excellent drug loading capacity, and outstanding stability. Biodistribution investigation showed that the prepared micelles considerably enhanced liver targeting as compared to free celastrol. The micelles successfully decreased oxidative stress, inflammation, and hepatic steatosis in NAFLD mice. Serum biochemical indicators of liver injury (ALT, AST) and lipid levels (total cholesterol, triglycerides) showed marked improvement; histological analysis revealed reduced lipid accumulation and improved hepatic architecture. The micelle group exhibited appreciably less systemic toxicity than the free celastrol.	[53]

FUTURE PERSPECTIVES

The field of nanotechnology has been advancing rapidly, driven by the development of novel and more effective drug-delivery methods for the treatment of NAFLD [21]. The treatment for FLD has advanced due to breakthroughs in nanomedicine, including the development of dendrimers and hybrid nanocarriers. By reducing risk and improving liver-specific targeting, these improvements may enhance drug delivery. To achieve the greatest possible drug release and minimize widespread harmful effects, researchers are developing smart nanocarriers that respond to specific liver conditions, such as pH or changes in enzyme activity [54]. Adding proteins like mannose and galactose to the surface of these drugs increases their sensitivity [55].

One significant feature is personalized nanomedicine, in which treatments vary based on a patient's biological traits and DNA makeup [56]. This includes the efficient regulation of genes associated with inflammation and fat metabolism using nanocarriers for RNA interference and gene therapy. Patients with considerable FLD or NASH may benefit from these approaches [57].

Despite limited success, converting these technologies from experimental studies to clinical use is challenging. To demonstrate a drug's long-term safety and efficacy, substantial studies are important. To ensure that patients have access to FLD nanomedicine options, academics, healthcare workers, and regulatory agencies must work together to overcome these limitations.

CONCLUSION

By enhancing medical efficacy, stability, and targeting, dendrimers and hybrid nanocarriers are altering the therapy of FLD. They minimize adverse effects and enhance absorption. Additional research and technical advances will help these nanocarriers enter clinical trials, offering patients with FLD new therapeutic options despite many challenges. To assure efficacy and safety, more scientific and clinical evaluations are required.

LIST OF ABBREVIATIONS

NAFLD Non-Alcoholic Fatty Liver Disease

NASH Non-Alcoholic Steatohepatitis

TZDs Thiazolidinediones

GLP-1 Glucagon-like peptide-1

DPP-4 Dipeptidyl peptidase-4

FGF21 Fibroblast Growth Factor 21

FLD Fatty Liver Disease

MASLD Metabolic Dysfunction-Associated Steatotic Liver Diseases

ASGPR Asialoglycoprotein Receptors

HSC Hepatic Stellate Cells

PAMAM Poly(amidoamine)

ALT- Alanine Transaminase

AST	Aspartate Transaminase
DNA	Deoxyribonucleic Acid
RNA	Ribonucleic Acid

REFERENCES

[1] Tirosh O. Hypoxic signaling and cholesterol lipotoxicity in fatty liver disease progression. Oxid Med Cell Longev 2018; 2018(1)2548154
[http://dx.doi.org/10.1155/2018/2548154] [PMID: 29955245]

[2] Yki-Järvinen H. Non-alcoholic fatty liver disease as a cause and a consequence of metabolic syndrome. Lancet Diabetes Endocrinol 2014; 2(11): 901-10.
[http://dx.doi.org/10.1016/S2213-8587(14)70032-4] [PMID: 24731669]

[3] Ahmed MH, Barakat S, Almobarak AO. Nonalcoholic fatty liver disease and cardiovascular disease: has the time come for cardiologists to be hepatologists? J Obes 2012; 2012(1): 1-9.
[http://dx.doi.org/10.1155/2012/483135] [PMID: 23320150]

[4] Loomba R, Sanyal AJ. The global NAFLD epidemic. Nat Rev Gastroenterol Hepatol 2013; 10(11): 686-90.
[http://dx.doi.org/10.1038/nrgastro.2013.171] [PMID: 24042449]

[5] Sharma S, Sharma A, Gupta P, *et al.* The green path to liver health: Herbal solutions for non-alcoholic steatohepatitis. Cardiovasc Hematol Disord Drug Targets 2025; 25(3): 168-92.
[http://dx.doi.org/10.2174/011871529X360903250211101856] [PMID: 40108906]

[6] Calzadilla Bertot L, Adams L. The natural course of non-alcoholic fatty liver disease. Int J Mol Sci 2016; 17(5): 774.
[http://dx.doi.org/10.3390/ijms17050774] [PMID: 27213358]

[7] Abenavoli L, Di Renzo L, Boccuto L, Alwardat N, Gratteri S, De Lorenzo A. Health benefits of Mediterranean diet in nonalcoholic fatty liver disease. Expert Rev Gastroenterol Hepatol 2018; 12(9): 873-81.
[http://dx.doi.org/10.1080/17474124.2018.1503947] [PMID: 30033779]

[8] Saba A. A comparative study to evaluate safety and efficacy of dipeptidyl peptidase-4 (DPP-4) inhibitors versus α-glucosidase inhibitors as add-on therapy in type 2 diabetes mellitus in a tertiary care hospital [dissertation]. Bangalore (India): Rajiv Gandhi University of Health Sciences 2017.

[9] Mazza A, Fruci B, Garinis GA, Giuliano S, Malaguarnera R, Belfiore A. The role of metformin in the management of NAFLD. Exp Diabetes Res 2012; 2012(1): 1-13.
[http://dx.doi.org/10.1155/2012/716404] [PMID: 22194737]

[10] Lavine JE, Schwimmer JB, Van Natta ML, *et al.* Effect of vitamin E or metformin for treatment of nonalcoholic fatty liver disease in children and adolescents: the TONIC randomized controlled trial. JAMA 2011; 305(16): 1659-68.
[http://dx.doi.org/10.1001/jama.2011.520] [PMID: 21521847]

[11] Farzanegi P, Dana A, Ebrahimpoor Z, Asadi M, Azarbayjani MA. Mechanisms of beneficial effects of exercise training on non□alcoholic fatty liver disease (NAFLD): Roles of oxidative stress and inflammation. Eur J Sport Sci 2019; 19(7): 994-1003.
[http://dx.doi.org/10.1080/17461391.2019.1571114] [PMID: 30732555]

[12] Boye KS, Shinde S, Kennedy-Martin T, Robinson S, Thieu VT. Weight change and the association with adherence and persistence to diabetes therapy: a narrative review. Patient Prefer Adherence 2022; 16: 23-39.
[http://dx.doi.org/10.2147/PPA.S328583] [PMID: 35023906]

[13] Angulo P. NAFLD, obesity, and bariatric surgery. Gastroenterology 2006; 130(6): 1848-52.
[http://dx.doi.org/10.1053/j.gastro.2006.03.041] [PMID: 16697746]

[14] Rinella ME, Sanyal AJ. Management of NAFLD: a stage-based approach. Nat Rev Gastroenterol Hepatol 2016; 13(4): 196-205.
[http://dx.doi.org/10.1038/nrgastro.2016.3] [PMID: 26907882]

[15] Wei S, Wang L, Evans PC, Xu S. NAFLD and NASH: etiology, targets and emerging therapies. Drug Discov Today 2024; 29(3)103910
[http://dx.doi.org/10.1016/j.drudis.2024.103910] [PMID: 38301798]

[16] Ruman U, Fakurazi S, Masarudin MJ, Hussein MZ. Nanocarrier-based therapeutics and theranostics drug delivery systems for next generation of liver cancer nanodrug modalities. Int J Nanomed 2020; pp. 1437-56.

[17] Salahpour Anarjan F. Active targeting drug delivery nanocarriers: Ligands. Nano-Structures & Nano-Objects 2019; 19: 100370.
[http://dx.doi.org/10.1016/j.nanoso.2019.100370]

[18] Du AW, Stenzel MH. Drug carriers for the delivery of therapeutic peptides. Biomacromolecules 2014; 15(4): 1097-114.
[http://dx.doi.org/10.1021/bm500169p] [PMID: 24661025]

[19] Bartneck M, Warzecha KT, Tacke F. Therapeutic targeting of liver inflammation and fibrosis by nanomedicine. Hepatobiliary Surg Nutr 2014; 3(6): 364-76.
[PMID: 25568860]

[20] Abou Assi R, Abdulbaqi IM, Siok Yee C. The evaluation of drug delivery nanocarrier development and pharmacological briefing for metabolic-associated fatty liver disease (MAFLD): an update. Pharmaceuticals (Basel) 2021; 14(3): 215.
[http://dx.doi.org/10.3390/ph14030215] [PMID: 33806527]

[21] Moghtadaie A, Mahboobi H, Fatemizadeh S, Kamal MA. Emerging role of nanotechnology in treatment of non-alcoholic fatty liver disease (NAFLD). EXCLI J 2023; 22: 946-74.
[PMID: 38023570]

[22] Poste G, Bucana C, Raz A, Bugelski P, Kirsh R, Fidler IJ. Analysis of the fate of systemically administered liposomes and implications for their use in drug delivery. Cancer Res 1982; 42(4): 1412-22.
[PMID: 7060015]

[23] Verma G, Hassan PA. Self assembled materials: design strategies and drug delivery perspectives. Phys Chem Chem Phys 2013; 15(40): 17016-28.
[http://dx.doi.org/10.1039/c3cp51207j] [PMID: 23907560]

[24] Fattahi FS, Zamani T. Synthesis of polylactic acid nanoparticles for the novel biomedical applications: a scientific perspective. Nanochem Res 2020; 5(1): 1-13.

[25] Tirnaksiz F, Akkus S, Celebi N. Nanoemulsions as drug delivery systems. Colloids. Drug Deliv 2010; 1: 221-44.

[26] Moghimipour E, Handali S. Liposomes as drug delivery systems: Properties and Applications. Res J Pharm Biol Chem Sci 2013; 4(1): 169-85.

[27] Pérez-Ferreiro M, M Abelairas A, Criado A, Gómez IJ, Mosquera J. M. Abelairas A, Criado A, Gómez IJ, Mosquera J. Dendrimers: exploring their wide structural variety and applications. Polymers (Basel) 2023; 15(22): 4369.
[http://dx.doi.org/10.3390/polym15224369] [PMID: 38006093]

[28] Boas U, Christensen JB, Heegaard PMH. Dendrimers: design, synthesis and chemical properties. J Mater Chem 2006; 16(38): 3785-98.
[http://dx.doi.org/10.1039/b611813p]

[29] Colino CI, Lanao JM, Gutierrez-Millan C. Targeting of hepatic macrophages by therapeutic nanoparticles. Front Immunol 2020; 11: 218.

[http://dx.doi.org/10.3389/fimmu.2020.00218] [PMID: 32194546]

[30] Wu Y, Zhang J, He W, Li C, Wang Y. Nanomaterials for targeting liver disease: Research progress and future perspectives. Nano Biomed Eng 2023; 15(2): 199-224. [http://dx.doi.org/10.26599/NBE.2023.9290024]

[31] Palan F, Chatterjee B. Dendrimers in the context of targeting central nervous system disorders. J Drug Deliv Sci Technol 2022; 73103474 [http://dx.doi.org/10.1016/j.jddst.2022.103474]

[32] Pandita D, Madaan K, Kumar S, Poonia N, Lather V. Dendrimers in drug delivery and targeting: Drug-dendrimer interactions and toxicity issues. J Pharm Bioallied Sci 2014; 6(3): 139-50. [http://dx.doi.org/10.4103/0975-7406.130965] [PMID: 25035633]

[33] Palmerston Mendes L, Pan J, Torchilin V. Dendrimers as nanocarriers for nucleic acid and drug delivery in cancer therapy. Molecules 2017; 22(9): 1401. [http://dx.doi.org/10.3390/molecules22091401] [PMID: 28832535]

[34] Rastogi V, Yadav P, Porwal M, Sur S, Verma A. Dendrimer as nanocarrier for drug delivery and drug targeting therapeutics: a fundamental to advanced systematic review. Int J Polym Mater 2024; 73(4): 310-32. [http://dx.doi.org/10.1080/00914037.2022.2158334]

[35] Sanati M, Amin Yavari S. Liposome-integrated hydrogel hybrids: Promising platforms for cancer therapy and tissue regeneration. J Control Release 2024; 368: 703-27. [http://dx.doi.org/10.1016/j.jconrel.2024.03.008] [PMID: 38490373]

[36] Mandal B, Bhattacharjee H, Mittal N, *et al.* Core–shell-type lipid–polymer hybrid nanoparticles as a drug delivery platform. Nanomedicine 2013; 9(4): 474-91. [http://dx.doi.org/10.1016/j.nano.2012.11.010] [PMID: 23261500]

[37] Mehta S, Suresh A, Nayak Y, Narayan R, Nayak UY. Hybrid nanostructures: Versatile systems for biomedical applications. Coord Chem Rev 2022; 460214482 [http://dx.doi.org/10.1016/j.ccr.2022.214482]

[38] Garg J, Pathania K, Sah SP, Pawar SV. Nanostructured lipid carriers: a promising drug carrier for targeting brain tumours. Future J Pharm Sci 2022; 8(1): 25. [http://dx.doi.org/10.1186/s43094-022-00414-8]

[39] Madni A, Tahir N, Rehman M, Raza A, Mahmood MA, Khan MI, *et al.* Hybrid Nano-carriers for potential drug delivery. Adv Tech Deliv Ther 2017; pp. 54-87.

[40] Kesharwani P, Gothwal A, Iyer AK, Jain K, Chourasia MK, Gupta U. Dendrimer nanohybrid carrier systems: an expanding horizon for targeted drug and gene delivery. Drug Discov Today 2018; 23(2): 300-14. [http://dx.doi.org/10.1016/j.drudis.2017.06.009] [PMID: 28697371]

[41] Li X, Naeem A, Xiao S, Hu L, Zhang J, Zheng Q. Safety challenges and application strategies for the use of dendrimers in medicine. Pharmaceutics 2022; 14(6): 1292. [http://dx.doi.org/10.3390/pharmaceutics14061292] [PMID: 35745863]

[42] Gajbhiye KR, Salve R, Narwade M, Sheikh A, Kesharwani P, Gajbhiye V. Lipid polymer hybrid nanoparticles: a custom-tailored next-generation approach for cancer therapeutics. Mol Cancer 2023; 22(1): 160. [http://dx.doi.org/10.1186/s12943-023-01849-0] [PMID: 37784179]

[43] Alshawwa SZ, Kassem AA, Farid RM, Mostafa SK, Labib GS. Nanocarrier drug delivery systems: characterization, limitations, future perspectives and implementation of artificial intelligence. Pharmaceutics 2022; 14(4): 883. [http://dx.doi.org/10.3390/pharmaceutics14040883] [PMID: 35456717]

[44] Zai W, Chen W, Wu Z, *et al.* Targeted interleukin-22 gene delivery in the liver by polymetformin and penetratin-based hybrid nanoparticles to treat nonalcoholic fatty liver disease. ACS Appl Mater

Interfaces 2019; 11(5): 4842-57.
[http://dx.doi.org/10.1021/acsami.8b19717] [PMID: 30628769]

[45] Wang J, Li B, Qiu L, Qiao X, Yang H. Dendrimer-based drug delivery systems: history, challenges, and latest developments. J Biol Eng 2022; 16(1): 18.
[http://dx.doi.org/10.1186/s13036-022-00298-5] [PMID: 35879774]

[46] Sharma R, Porterfield JE, An HT, *et al.* Rationally designed galactose dendrimer for hepatocyte-specific targeting and intracellular drug delivery for the treatment of liver disorders. Biomacromolecules 2021; 22(8): 3574-89.
[http://dx.doi.org/10.1021/acs.biomac.1c00649] [PMID: 34324818]

[47] Cheng Y, Zhao L, Li Y, Xu T. Design of biocompatible dendrimers for cancer diagnosis and therapy: current status and future perspectives. Chem Soc Rev 2011; 40(5): 2673-703.
[http://dx.doi.org/10.1039/c0cs00097c] [PMID: 21286593]

[48] Ji G, Li Y, Zhang Z, Li H, Sun P. Recent advances of novel targeted drug delivery systems based on natural medicine monomers against hepatocellular carcinoma. Heliyon 2024; 10(2)e24667
[http://dx.doi.org/10.1016/j.heliyon.2024.e24667] [PMID: 38312669]

[49] Chen J, Yao Y, Mao X, Chen Y, Ni F. Liver-targeted delivery based on prodrug: passive and active approaches. J Drug Target 2024; 32(10): 1155-68.
[http://dx.doi.org/10.1080/1061186X.2024.2386416] [PMID: 39072411]

[50] Liang J, Liu Y, Liu J, *et al.* Chitosan-functionalized lipid-polymer hybrid nanoparticles for oral delivery of silymarin and enhanced lipid-lowering effect in NAFLD. J Nanobiotechnology 2018; 16(1): 64.
[http://dx.doi.org/10.1186/s12951-018-0391-9] [PMID: 30176941]

[51] Zahid AA, Chakraborty A, Shamiya Y, Wilson RB, Borradaile N, Paul A. Cell membrane-derived nanoparticles as biomimetic nanotherapeutics to alleviate fatty liver disease. ACS Appl Mater Interfaces 2024; 16(30): 39117-28.
[http://dx.doi.org/10.1021/acsami.4c08240] [PMID: 39022877]

[52] Li J, Yin M, Tian M, Fang J, Xu H. Stiff-soft hybrid biomimetic nano-emulsion for targeted liver delivery and treatment of early nonalcoholic fatty liver disease. Pharmaceutics 2024; 16(10): 1303.
[http://dx.doi.org/10.3390/pharmaceutics16101303] [PMID: 39458632]

[53] Pan Y, Zhang Y, Ouyang H, *et al.* Targeted delivery of celastrol via chondroitin sulfate derived hybrid micelles for alleviating symptoms in nonalcoholic fatty liver disease. ACS Appl Bio Mater 2023; 6(11): 4877-93.
[http://dx.doi.org/10.1021/acsabm.3c00612] [PMID: 37890075]

[54] Kalaydina R-V, Bajwa K, Qorri B, Decarlo A, Szewczuk MR. Recent advances in "smart" delivery systems for extended drug release in cancer therapy. Int J Nanomedicine 2018; 13: 4727-45.
[http://dx.doi.org/10.2147/IJN.S168053] [PMID: 30154657]

[55] Athanasopoulou F, Manolakakis M, Vernia S, Kamaly N. Nanodrug delivery systems for metabolic chronic liver diseases: advances and perspectives. Nanomedicine (Lond) 2023; 18(1): 67-84.
[http://dx.doi.org/10.2217/nnm-2022-0261] [PMID: 36896958]

[56] Ambre SG, Barchi JJ Jr. Carbohydrate nanotechnology and its applications for the treatment of cancer. In: Stine KJ, Ed. Carbohydrate Nanotechnology. Cambridge: Royal Society of Chemistry; 2015. p. 267-302.
[http://dx.doi.org/10.1002/9781118860212.ch13]

[57] Domingues I, Leclercq IA, Beloqui A. Nonalcoholic fatty liver disease: Current therapies and future perspectives in drug delivery. J Control Release 2023; 363: 415-34.
[http://dx.doi.org/10.1016/j.jconrel.2023.09.040] [PMID: 37769817]

CHAPTER 8

Novel Therapeutics for Fatty Liver Disease

Kirti Goel[1], **Sonia Kamboj**[2] and **Rajan Swami**[3,*]

[1] *Department of Pharmaceutics, Lala Ami Chand College of Pharmacy, Ambala, Haryana, India*

[2] *Department of Pharmaceutical Chemistry, Ch. Devi Lal College of Pharmacy, Jagadhri, Haryana, India*

[3] *Department of Pharmaceutics, Chitkara College of Pharmacy, Chitkara University, Rajpura, Punjab, India*

Abstract: Fatty liver disorders encompass both alcoholic fatty liver disorder (AFLD) and non-alcoholic fatty liver disorder (NAFLD) and have arisen as a substantial universal problem owing to their escalating occurrence and linkage with metabolic diseases. At advanced stages, fatty liver disease becomes more precarious as it can be converted into liver cirrhosis, fibrosis, steatohepatitis, and carcinoma in hepatic cells. The conventional pharmacotherapy for various liver diseases mainly focuses on lifestyle modifications to manage associated health concerns, but these approaches have limitations and side effects, prompting scientists to explore more modern approaches via novel therapeutics. This chapter provides insights into pioneering innovations in the management of fatty liver disease, accentuating novel drug delivery systems, molecular targets, and bioactive combinations. Advancements in new-era technologies, including lipid nanoparticles and novel polymeric formulations with enhanced bioavailability profiles, have emerged as cutting-edge approaches for delivering therapeutic agents to specific sites in the liver. Moreover, other evolving treatment strategies, including the roles of biomarkers, such as fibroblast growth factor analogues, peroxisome proliferator-activated receptor agonists, and gut microbiota modulators, are reviewed for their significant roles in modulating metabolic pathways, thereby decreasing hepatic lipid accretion and, in turn, improving patient safety. This chapter offers an inclusive overview of novel therapeutic strategies and other non-pharmacological strategies available, aiming to promote further investigation to address the medical needs in the management of fatty liver disorders.

Keywords: AFLD, Biomarkers, Fatty liver, NAFLD, Novel therapeutics.

* **Corresponding author Rajan Swami:** Department of Pharmaceutics, Chitkara College of Pharmacy, Chitkara University, Rajpura, Punjab, India; E-mail: drrjnswami@gmail.com

Anjali Sharma, Devkant Sharma, Ajmer Singh Grewal, Geeta Deswal & Ganga Reddy Velma (Eds.)

INTRODUCTION

Fatty liver disease (FLD) is a public health problem worldwide, characterized by excess hepatic fat. The disease, which affects about a quarter of the world population, is linked to metabolic disorders, including obesity, type 2 diabetes, and dyslipidaemia. FLD, when not treated, can progress to severe liver diseases, such as cirrhosis and hepatocellular carcinoma (HCC), leading to a significant burden on health care [1]. Sedentary lifestyles, poor dietary habits, and increases in the prevalence of obesity have led to the rising rate of FLD. Although awareness of the disease has increased, early diagnosis remains challenging because it is typically asymptomatic in its initial stages. As a result, a large cohort of patients receives a diagnosis only after progression to more advanced stages, creating an urgent need for improvements in both therapeutic and diagnostic approaches [2]. This disease is of two broad types: a) Alcoholic Fatty Liver Disease (AFLD), resulting from excess alcohol consumption, causing liver inflammation and fibrosis. b) Non-Alcoholic Fatty Liver Disease (NAFLD), which occurs in individuals who consume little or no alcohol and is mainly associated with metabolic disorders. NAFLD encompasses a spectrum of disease ranging from simple steatosis to non-alcoholic steatohepatitis (NASH), involving inflammation and fibrosis. Despite advancements in therapies, the treatment of FLD remains difficult due to the lack of Food and Drug Administration (FDA)-approved pharmacological therapies. The only available strategies are designed to modify lifestyle or to use existing medications off-label, which have limited efficacy for slowing disease progression [3].

PATHOPHYSIOLOGY AND DISEASE PROGRESSION

Severe liver damage is caused by the pathophysiology that comprises multiple molecular mechanisms associated with disease progression from simple steatosis. Increased de novo lipogenesis (DNL) mediated by SREBP-1c and ChREBP, combined with impaired fatty acid β-oxidation, leads to hepatic lipid accumulation. Insulin resistance also contributes to this phenomenon by stimulating lipogenesis and inhibiting fatty acid oxidation, thereby enhancing hepatic fat deposition. Impaired very-low-density lipoprotein secretion also leads to sterol build-up in the liver [4]. The mechanisms and risk factors are graphically represented in Fig. (**1**) and summarized in Table **1**.

The progression from a healthy liver to cirrhosis involves lipid accumulation, oxidative stress, glucose impairment, insulin resistance, and systemic chronic inflammation, ultimately leading to hepatocellular injury and fibrosis. Significant underlying molecular mechanisms, such as hepatic stellate cell activation, mitochondrial dysfunction, and cytokine release, further aggravate the disorder and result in irreversible cirrhosis and liver failure. HSC-Hepatic Stellate Cells, NAFLD - Non-Alcoholic Fatty Liver Disease, NASH- Non-Alcoholic Steatohepatitis, ECM-Extracellular Matrix Deposition [10, 11].

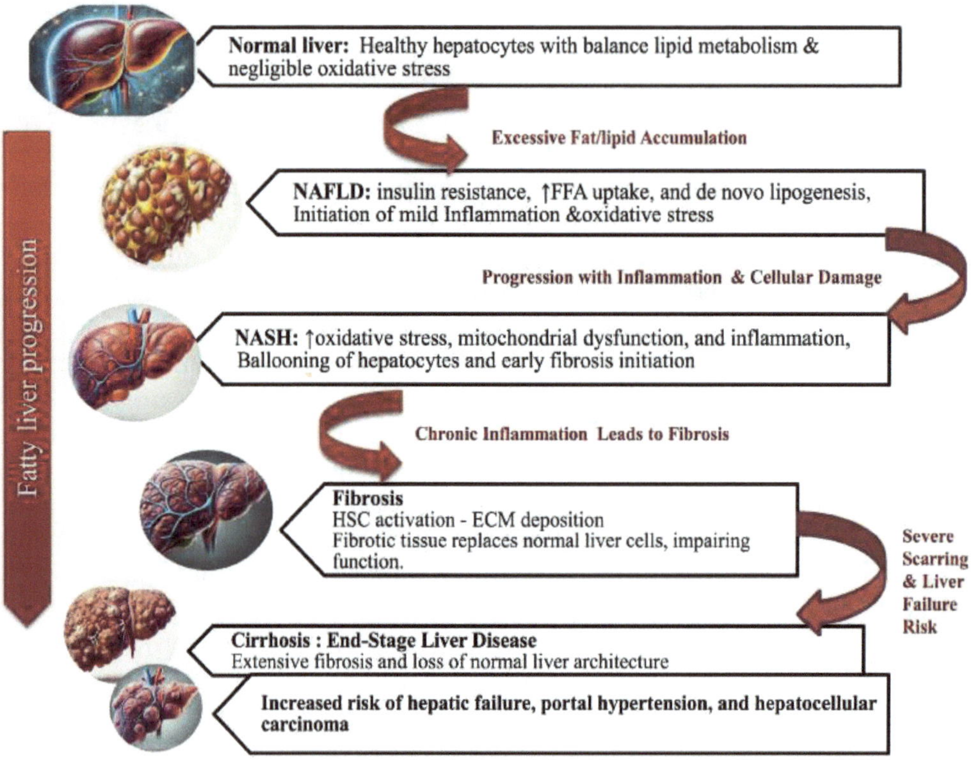

Fig. (1). Schematic overview of the pathophysiology and progression of NAFLD/NASH.

Table 1. Molecular mechanisms, risk factors, and progression of fatty liver disease.

Sr.no	Key Factors	Description	Reference
Molecular Mechanisms			
1.	**Hepatic Lipid Accumulation (Steatosis)**	Activation of de novo lipogenesis (DNL) via SREBP-1c and ChREBP, β-oxidation impaired, poor very-lo--density lipoprotein oozing, and excess free fatty acid influx from adipose tissue.	[12, 13]
2.	**Insulin Resistance and Metabolic Dysfunction**	Enhanced lipogenesis as a result of the hyperinsulinemic conditions. Diminished AMPK activation limits fatty acid oxidation and increases hepatic glucose output, exacerbating metabolic stress.	[14]

(Table 1) cont.....

Sr.no	Key Factors	Description	Reference
3.	**Oxidative Stress and Mitochondrial Dysfunction**	In the JNK pathway, lipotoxicity induces reactive oxygen species, mitochondrial dysfunction, lipid peroxidation, and hepatocyte apoptosis.	[15]
4.	**Endoplasmic Reticulum Stress**	Initiation of the unfolded protein response due to misfolded proteins, leading to apoptosis via the PERK-eIF2α-CHOP pathway.	[16]
5.	**Inflammation and Immune Activation**	Inflammatory cytokines (TNF-α, IL-6, IL-1β), secreted from Kupffer cells, activate the NLRP3 inflammasome in hepatocytes and lead to hepatocyte injury. Increased gut permeability and endotoxemia worsen inflammation.	[17]
6.	**Fibrosis and Cirrhosis Progression**	Upon a fibrogenic stimulus (such as TGF-β or PDGF), hepatic stellate cells (HSCs) deposit extracellular matrix (ECM), resulting in fibrosis, cirrhosis, and HCC.	[18]
		Risk Factors	
7.	**Metabolic Syndrome**	Obesity, type 2 diabetes, dyslipidemia, and hypertension.	[19]
8.	**Genetic Predisposition**	Susceptibility is increased by mutations in PNPLA3 and TM6SF2.	[20]
9.	**Unhealthy Diet and Lifestyle**	High-fat/fructose intake and a sedentary lifestyle aggravate the fat build-up.	[21]
10.	**Gut Microbiota Dysbiosis**	Increased intestinal permeability and lipopolysaccharide accumulation worsen liver inflammation.	[22]
11.	**Alcohol Consumption**	The prime aspect for alcoholic liver disease progression.	[23]
12.	**Environmental Toxins and Drugs**	Certain medications and pollutants are responsible for liver damage.	[24]
		Stages of Disease Progression	
13.	**Simple Steatosis (NAFL/ALD)**	Fat accumulation without significant inflammation.	[25]
14.	**(NASH)/Alcoholic Hepatitis**	Inflammation and hepatocyte injury (ballooning).	[26]
15.	**Fibrosis**	Excess extracellular matrix (ECM) deposition due to chronic liver injury.	[27]
16.	**Cirrhosis**	Advanced fibrosis leading to liver dysfunction.	[28]
17.	**Hepatocellular Carcinoma (HCC)**	Malignant transformation in cirrhotic livers.	[29]

Both mitochondrial dysfunction and oxidative stress contribute significantly to hepatocellular injury. The accumulation of free fatty acids, driven by increased reactive oxygen species (ROS) production, induces lipid peroxidation and activates the c-Jun N-terminal kinase (JNK) pathway, thereby fueling hepatocyte apoptosis [5]. Mechanistically, endoplasmic reticulum (ER) stress exacerbates liver injury by activating the unfolded protein response (UPR) and facilitating apoptosis via the PERK-eIF2α-CHOP pathway. Activated Kupffer cell-derived tumor necrosis factor-alpha (TNF-α), interleukin-6 (IL-6), and interleukin-1β (IL-1β) are involved in triggering inflammatory responses, ultimately leading to chronic hepatic inflammation [6]. The NLRP3 inflammasome also plays vital roles in inflammatory amplification, contributing to hepatocyte injury and fibrosis [7].

The progression of simple steatosis to fibrosis and cirrhosis is driven by activation of hepatic stellate cells (HSCs), which secrete extracellular matrix proteins in response to inflammatory and fibrogenic signals, such as TGF-β and platelet-derived growth factor (PDGF). Continued inflammation and fibrosis contribute to cirrhosis and hepatocellular carcinoma (HCC), the end stages of the disease [7].

There are multiple risk factors for the progression of fatty liver disease. A substantial driver of NAFLD is metabolic syndrome, including obesity, type 2 diabetes, dyslipidemia, and hypertension. Disease susceptibility is significantly determined by genetic predisposition, including mutations in genes, such as PNPLA3 and TM6SF2. Moreover, dysbiosis of the gut microbiota has been reported to be associated with metabolic disorders and disease progression and to contribute to unhealthy lifestyle factors, including a high-calorie diet, physical inactivity, and gut microbiota dysbiosis [8]. In ALD, increased alcohol consumption leads to liver injury progression due to oxidative stress and inflammation. Hepatotoxic chemicals, specific toxins, and certain medications can contribute to liver damage [9].

CONVENTIONAL THERAPEUTICS: LIMITATIONS AND CHALLENGES

There are no available pharmacological therapies that can effectively halt or reverse disease progression in fatty liver disease, including non-alcoholic fatty liver disease (NAFLD) and non-alcoholic steatohepatitis (NASH). Current management is primarily symptom-based and focuses on lifestyle modifications, including weight loss, diet, and physical activity, which remain the mainstay of therapy [30]. However, due to low patient adherence and the heterogeneous progression of the disease, pharmacological therapies are often required. No drug approved by the US Food and Drug Administration specifically targets NAFLD/NASH despite continued investigation, and available pharmacologic approaches are fraught with limitations relating to efficacy, safety, and prolonged usage [31].

EXISTING PHARMACOLOGICAL OPTIONS AND THEIR EFFICACY

Drugs investigated for NAFLD/NASH treatment generally target insulin resistance, lipid metabolism, oxidative stress, or inflammation. However, their action is usually restricted to specific components of the disease, and most do not confer broad therapeutic effects [32].

Insulin Sensitizers

Used for type 2 diabetes, metformin improves insulin resistance and hepatic glucose metabolism. However, clinical trials have not demonstrated appreciable histological improvements in NASH, impeding its use in fatty liver disease [33]. Thiazolidinediones (TZDs), including pioglitazone, stimulate PPAR-γ, enhancing insulin sensitivity and decreasing hepatic fat deposition. Although they show some benefits in NASH, their adverse effects, such as weight gain, fluid retention, and cardiovascular risk, limit long-term use [34].

Lipid-Lowering Agents

Statins have proven efficacious in decreasing cardiovascular risk, which is relevant among patients with non-alcoholic fatty liver disease (NAFLD), who frequently exhibit dyslipidaemia [35]. Direct effects on hepatic steatosis and fibrosis, however, are less clear, as is their use in patients with advanced liver disease. Fibrates and omega-3 fatty acids reduce triglyceride levels but have limited activity in reversing NASH-related fibrosis and inflammation [36].

Antioxidants and Anti-inflammatory Components

Vitamin E has the potential to ameliorate oxidative stress and has been shown to improve liver histology in patients with NASH without diabetes [37]. Pentoxifylline, an anti-TNF-α agent, has been studied for its anti-inflammatory properties, but clinical evidence is limited to support its broad application [38].

Bile Acid Modulators

Obeticholic acid (OCA; farnesoid X receptor (FXR) agonist) has demonstrated efficacy in the reduction of liver fibrosis and liver steatosis. However, due to their side effects, such as pruritus, increased LDL cholesterol, and cardiovascular events, there is a growing clinical dilemma about the use of these drugs [39].

While several pharmacotherapy candidates show promise for disease treatment, none to date has been 100% successful in addressing the multifaceted pathobiology of NAFLD/NASH, leaving a gap with respect to therapy, especially with regard to preventing disease progression.

CONS OF CURRENT TREATMENT APPROACHES

- **Lack of FDA-Approved Drugs:** Currently, no drug is formally approved for NAFLD/NASH treatment, forcing healthcare providers to rely on off-label therapeutic options, which provide only partial benefits [40].
- **Decreased Effectiveness in Reducing Fibrosis:** Fibrosis is the most important predictor of liver-related morbidity and mortality in patients with NAFLD/NASH. Current therapies generally do not substantially reverse fibrosis, exposing patients to the risk of cirrhosis and hepatocellular carcinoma (HCC) [41].
- **Long-term Safety Concerns:** For many traditional drugs, their adverse effects outweigh their benefits, especially for long-term usage. As TZDs can lead to weight gain, vitamin E can raise the risk for prostate cancer, and OCA can exert unfavorable actions on lipid profiles. These safety issues restrict their utility in clinical practice [42]
- **Early Diagnosis and Monitoring Challenges:** Liver biopsy is the gold standard for diagnosing NASH and assessing fibrosis, though it is invasive and impractical for routine evaluation. Despite efforts to develop non-invasive biomarkers and imaging, these tools are not yet widely used or standardized, making tracking disease progression challenging [43].

Current conventional therapeutics have significant limitations, such as adverse side effects, drug resistance, and others; therefore, there is an unmet need for new treatment strategies that target multiple aspects of disease progression while also being safe and efficacious [44]. Novel experimental therapies include nanotechnology-based drug-delivery systems, gene therapy, modulation of the gut microbiome, and herbal formulations with hepatoprotective effects. Since lipid metabolism, inflammation, and fibrosis are interconnected, combination therapies targeting these processes may lead to superior clinical outcomes [45].

EMERGING PHARMACOLOGICAL INTERVENTIONS

Existing therapies are limited, and newer drug candidates under development are specifically targeting NAFLD/NASH. These agents target multiple pathophysiologic processes, including insulin resistance, lipid metabolism, inflammation, fibrosis, and oxidative stress. Some drugs are in clinical trials;

others remain preclinical but show potential. The available pharmacological interventions for combating fatty liver disease are summarized in Fig. (**2**) and further discussed in the respective sections and Table **2**.

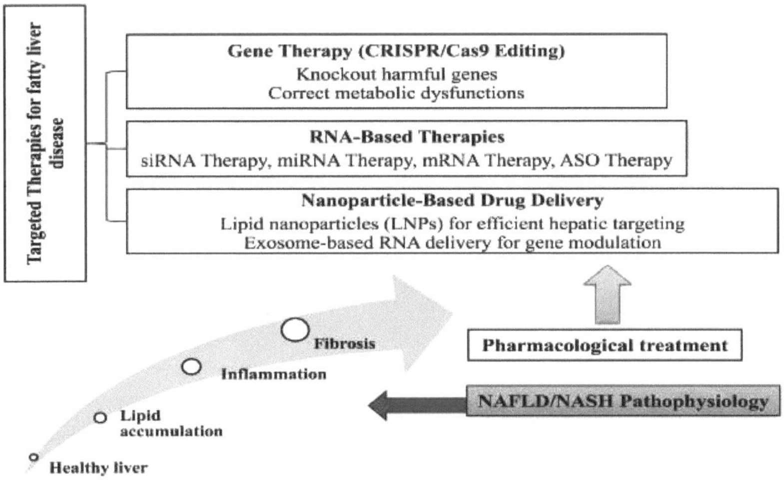

Fig. (2). Pharmacological interventions for fatty liver disease management.

Table 2. An overview of emerging drug applicants for NAFLD/NASH.

Drug Class	Examples	MOA	Clinical Status	Potential Benefits	Limitations	Ref.
FXR Agonists	Obeticholic Acid (OCA), Tropifexor, Cilofexor	Regulates bile acid metabolism, reduces hepatic inflammation and fibrosis	OCA - Phase 3, others in earlier trials	Targets multiple liver pathways, reduces fibrosis	Increases LDL cholesterol, pruritus	[46]
PPAR Agonists	Lanifibrano, Saroglitazar	Activates PPAR-$\alpha/\gamma/\delta$, improving lipid metabolism and insulin sensitivity	Lanifibranor-Phase 3, Saroglitazar approved in India	Improves fat oxidation, reduces hepatic steatosis	Weight gain (PPAR-γ activation), potential cardiovascular risks	[47]
THR-β Agonists	Resmetirom (MGL-3196)	Enhances hepatic lipid metabolism, promotes fat clearance	Phase 3	Reduces liver fat, with minimal systemic side effects	Limited impact on fibrosis	[48]

(Table 2) cont.....

Drug Class	Examples	MOA	Clinical Status	Potential Benefits	Limitations	Ref.
GLP-1 Receptor Agonists	Semaglutide, Tirzepatide	Enhances insulin secretion, induces weight loss, and reduces appetite	Phase 3	Addresses metabolic dysfunction, improves hepatic lipid accumulation	Primarily affects weight loss rather than fibrosis	[49]
ASK1 Inhibitors	Selonsertib	Inhibits oxidative stress-induced hepatocyte apoptosis	Failed Phase 3	Potential fibrosis reduction	Lack of efficacy in trials	[50]
CCR2/CCR5 Inhibitors	Cenicriviroc	Blocks inflammatory signaling, reducing liver inflammation	Phase 2/3	Anti-inflammatory, fibrosis reduction	Mixed clinical results	[51]
Galectin-3 Inhibitors	Belapectin	Targets fibrosis progression via galectin-3 inhibition	Phase 2	Anti-fibrotic potential	Needs further validation	[52]
FGF21 and FGF19 Analogues	Pegbelfermin (FGF21), Aldafermin (FGF19)	Enhances insulin sensitivity and reduces liver fat	Phase 2/3	Reduces inflammation and fibrosis	Requires frequent dosing; long-term effects are unknown	[53]
Gut Microbiome Modulators	Bile acid therapies, Probiotics	Modulates gut-liver axis and reduces inflammatory endotoxins	Preclinical/Early Clinical	Non-invasive approach; improves metabolism	Limited clinical validation	[54]

NANOTECHNOLOGY-BASED DRUG DELIVERY FOR NAFLD/NASH

Due to the rising prevalence of NAFLD and its progressive form, NASH, along with their substantial global health impact, there remains a significant unmet need for effective pharmacological treatment options. Conventional therapy suffers from limited bioavailability, systemic side effects, and unsatisfactory hepatic targeting, which increases the urgency for advanced drug formulation strategies [55]. Nanotechnology-based drug delivery systems, such as liposomes, hydrogels, polymeric nanoparticles, solid lipid nanoparticles, and exosome-based nanocarriers, are emerging with improved therapeutic efficacy, better drug solubility and stability, controlled release, and liver targeting [56]. These novel technologies may be combined to address existing treatment limitations and optimize therapeutic gains in NAFLD/NASH. Therefore, nanotechnology-based drug delivery systems, such as nanostructured lipid carriers (NLCs), solid lipid nanoparticles (SLNs), liposomes, dendrimers, hydrogels, and nanogels, enable liver-targeted treatment with reduced doses, reduced systemic toxicity, and enhanced pharmacokinetic profiles. A few nanoformulated drugs are currently in preclinical or clinical studies, and resmetirom was recently granted FDA approval for treating NASH [57].

- **NLC-based SCD1 Inhibitor: Aramchol (Galmed Pharmaceuticals)**

Aramchol is a novel nanostructured lipid carrier (NLC) formulation comprising an inhibitor of stearoyl-CoA desaturase 1 (SCD1), an important enzyme in hepatic lipogenesis. Orally administered aramchol markedly attenuates hepatic fat content and fibrosis markers by inhibiting de novo lipogenesis and enhancing fatty acid β-oxidation. In clinical trials, this has led to an apparent dose-dependent decrease in liver fat accumulation, making it a potential candidate for NAFLD treatment [58].

- **Azemiglitazone (CinnaGen, Huadong Medicine) – SLN-Based PPARγ Agonist**

Azemiglitazone, a PPARγ agonist that modulates lipid and glucose metabolism, is formulated as solid lipid nanoparticles (SLNs) and improves the condition of patients with NAFLD, particularly those with accompanying type 2 diabetes mellitus (T2DM) [4]. Moreover, based on the solubility and stability of the drugs, the SNL technology is utilized to improve insulin sensitivity and reduce hepatic steatosis [59].

- **Resmetirom (Madrigal Pharmaceuticals) – Lipid-Clearing TRβ Agonist**

Resmetirom is a liposomal nanoformulation of a selective TRβ agonist that activates hepatic TRβ to enhance mitochondrial activity and hepatic fat metabolism. This drug decreased liver fat by more than 25% in clinical trials and significantly improved fibrosis; therefore, it was recently approved by the FDA for NASH. Targeted hepatobiliary delivery from liposomal technology minimizes cardiovascular and metabolic off-target effects [60]

- **NLC-based Mitochondrial Uncoupler (HU6, Hepion Pharmaceuticals)**

Using this chemical library, we identified HU6, an NLC-formulated mitochondrial uncoupler that increases cellular energy expenditure and inhibits fat deposition in hepatocytes. HU6 decreases liver fat and enhances insulin resistance by stimulating thermogenesis and promoting metabolic activation. NLCs improve the bioavailability of HU6 and reduce mitochondrial stress due to toxicity. Preliminary studies reported a 30–50% reduction in liver fat in just 12 weeks of treatment and are thus a formidable candidate for advanced NASH therapeutics [61].

- **AXA1125 (Axcella Health) – Nanogel-Controlled Metabolic Modulator**

AXA1125 is a nanogel-based small-molecule metabolic modulator that targets multiple pathways associated with mitochondrial dysfunction and metabolic stress. This composition has shown improved ATP synthesis, decreased oxidative stress, and increased fatty acid β-oxidation, resulting in decreased hepatic lipid accumulation. Intestinal absorption improvement and sustained drug release in nanogel delivery Phase II trials showed marked increases in liver enzyme levels and fat metabolism [62].

- **BMS-986263 (Bristol-Myers Squibb) – Liposomal siRNA Targeted against Fibrosis**

BMS-986263 is a liposomal siRNA formulation targeting heat shock protein 47 (HSP47), a principal driver of extracellular collagen deposition and the development of NASH-related fibrosis. This therapy has the potential to reverse liver fibrosis by decreasing fibrotic tissue accumulation through HSP47 inhibition. Due to liposomal encapsulation, siRNA molecules are protected from degradation, facilitating their delivery to the liver. BMS-986263 reduced fibrosis markers in early clinical results. It is an anti-APOC3 antibody that has demonstrated early clinical results, suggesting a significant reduction in fibrosis markers in patients and has the potential to serve as an anti-fibrotic therapy for patients with NASH [63].

- **Survodutide (Boehringer Ingelheim, Zealand Pharma) – Dendrimer based GLP-1/Glucagon Dual Agonist**

Suovorutide is a dendrimer-based dual agonist of GLP-1 and glucagon, which results in increased energy expenditure, appetite suppression, and improved lipid metabolism. In clinical studies, this treatment has shown considerable decreases in body weight and liver fat (up to ~55%), making it a new potential therapeutic approach in the management of NASH-driven obesity. Dendrimeric systems enhance drug stability, controlled release, and liver targeting [64].

- **VK2809 (Viking Therapeutics) – Selenoether-based TRβ Agonist**

Resmetirom is also an SLN-formulated TRβ agonist, as is VK2809. VK2809 acts on thyroid hormone receptors to promote fat oxidation and lipid metabolism and to reduce liver fat by up to 60%. SLN technology offers superior hepatic accumulation and prolonged drug release, thereby enhancing its pharmacokinetic properties. Phase III trials are underway, with good efficacy in NASH patients with mild-to-moderate fibrosis [65].

- **Hydrogel-based FGF21 Analog — Efruxifermin (Akero Therapeutics)**

Efruxifermin (EFX), an FGF21 analogue formulated within a hydrogel, has biological properties that mimic those of fibroblast growth factor 21 (FGF21) and promote glucose and lipid metabolism whilst suppressing inflammation and fibrosis. This study also details a subcutaneous delivery method for the hydrogel that enables sustained bioactivity of FGF21, resulting in beneficial effects on liver function, insulin sensitivity, and fibrosis regression. According to PhaseIII trials, 39% of patients demonstrated a reversal of symptoms associated with cirrhosis, establishing EFX as a potential treatment option for patients with late-stage NASH [66].

The nanoformulated therapies emerging in the field of NAFLD/NASH significantly amplify progress in reversing/fighting liver fibrosis and its associated biochemistry, including lipid accumulation and metabolic dysfunction. Hepatic drug delivery with nanocarrier systems leads to preferential targeting, controlled release, increased efficacy with an optimal therapeutic window, and potentially reduced systemic toxicity. With Resmetirom's recent FDA approval and the ongoing development of multiple candidates, such as VK2809, Efruxifermin, and Survodutide, in late-stage clinical trials, nano-based drug delivery technologies are poised to transform the therapeutic paradigm for fatty liver disease. The future promise of nanobased treatments lies in investigating long-term safety, combination therapies, and personalized medicine approaches. Nano-formulations for fatty liver disease are depicted in Table **3**.

Table 3. Nano-formulations for fatty liver disease.

Formulation (Drug (Name+company Name)	Type/ Route	Animal Study/ Model Dosage	Mechanism of Action	Side Effects	Regulatory Status	Key Clinical Trial Findings	Ref.
NLC (Aramchol+**Galmed Pharmaceuticals)**	SCD1 Inhibitor/ Oral	Rodent models 600 mg/day	Inhibits the SCD1 enzyme to reduce hepatic lipogenesis	Mild GI symptoms	Phase II/III trials for NAFLD	Significant reduction in liver fat	[58]
SLN (Azemiglitazone+CinnaGen, Huadong Medicine)	PPARγ Agonist/ Oral	Mouse models 100 mg/day	Regulates glucose and lipid metabolism via PPARγ activation	Edema, weight gain	Phase II trials for NAFLD and diabetes	Improved insulin sensitivity, reduced liver fat	[67]
Liposomes (Resmetirom+ Madrigal Pharmaceuticals)	TRβ Agonist/ Oral	Not specified 80 mg/day	Activates thyroid hormone receptor-β to enhance liver fat metabolism	Mild GI symptoms	FDA-approved for NASH (2024)	25% reduction in liver fat and improvement in fibrosis	[68]
NLC (**HU6**+ Hepion Pharmaceuticals)	Mitochondrial Uncoupler/ Oral	Not specified 150 mg/day	Increases mitochondrial energy expenditure to reduce fat accumulation	Increased heart rate	Phase IIb trials are ongoing	30-50% liver fat reduction in 12 weeks	[61]
Nanogels (AXA1125+ **Axcella Health**)	Metabolic modulator/ oral	Not specified 24 g/day	Targets multiple pathways, including mitochondrial function	Mild GI discomfort	Phase II trials are ongoing	Reduced liver fat and improved energy metabolism	[69]
Liposomes (BMS-986263+ Bristol-Myers Squibb)	HSP47 siRNA in Lipid nanoparticles/i.v.	Not specified	Inhibits HSP47 to prevent collagen deposition and fibrosis	Not available	Phase II for hepatic fibrosis	Early promising results for fibrosis reduction	[70]
Dendrimers (Survodutide+ Boehringer Ingelheim, Zealand Pharma)	GLP-1/Glucagon Dual Agonist/ Subcutaneous	Not specified	Activates GLP-1 and glucagon receptors for weight loss and liver fat reduction	Nausea, vomiting	FDA breakthrough therapy, Phase III trials	55% liver fat reduction, weight loss	[71, 72]

(Table 3) cont.....

Formulation (Drug (Name+company Name)	Type/ Route	Animal Study/ Model Dosage	Mechanism of Action	Side Effects	Regulatory Status	Key Clinical Trial Findings	Ref.
SLN (VK2809+ Viking Therapeutics)	TRβ Agonist/ Oral	Not specified	Similar to resmetirom, targeting TRβ for lipid metabolism	Mild GI issues	Preparing for Phase III trials	Showed 60% reduction in liver fat	[68, 73]
Hydrogel Efruxifermin (EFX+ Akero Therapeutics)	FGF21 Analog/ Subcutaneous	Not specified	Mimics FGF21 effects, improving metabolism and fibrosis	Injection site reactions	Phase III trials	39% of patients experienced reversal of cirrhosis symptoms	[74]

GENE THERAPY AND RNA-BASED APPROACHES FOR NAFLD/NASH

The increase in global strain of NAFLD/NASH, together with the scarcity of FDA-approved medications, has made gene therapy and RNA-based therapeutics promising therapeutic strategies [75]. These strategies focus on fine-tuning gene expression, regulating metabolic networks, and even preventing disease outcomes, all at the molecular scale. Targeted interventions using CRISPR/Cas9 gene editing, siRNA, miRNA-based therapies, messenger RNA (mRNA) therapeutics, and antisense oligonucleotides (ASOs) have the potential to suppress lipid accumulation, reduce inflammation, and mitigate fibrosis [76]. Importantly, many RNA-based drugs are in preclinical or early clinical development, but the issues of delivery, specificity, and long-term safety remain problematic [77]. A summary of the main gene therapy and RNA-based strategies for NAFLD/NASH treatment is shown in Table **4**.

Table 4. Gene therapy and RNA-based approaches for NAFLD/NASH.

Therapeutic Approach	Mechanism of Action	Advantages	Challenges	Clinical Status	Ref.
CRISPR/Cas9 Gene Editing	Directly edits liver genes to correct mutations or suppress harmful pathways (*e.g.*, knocking out pro-fibrotic genes like TGF-β)	-Precise gene correction -Long-term effects -Potential one-time treatment	Off-target effects Delivery challenges (requires safe vectors) Ethical concerns	Preclinical	[78]

(Table 4) cont.....

Therapeutic Approach	Mechanism of Action	Advantages	Challenges	Clinical Status	Ref.
siRNA Therapy	Silences specific mRNAs to reduce the expression of disease-related proteins (*e.g.*, siRNA targeting **SREBP-1c** to decrease lipid accumulation)	-Highly specific gene silencing -Reversible and controlled **-Non-permanent modifications**	Short half-life, requires frequent dosing Potential immune responses Delivery to liver cells must be optimized	Phase 2/3 clinical trials (*e.g.*, Inclisiran for lipid regulation)	[77]
miRNA Therapy	Modulates microRNA levels to regulate metabolic and inflammatory pathways (*e.g.*, **miR-122 inhibition** to lower cholesterol and prevent fibrosis)	-Regulates multiple pathways simultaneously -Can be used for fibrosis and lipid metabolism **-Potential for combination therapy**	Off-target effects due to broad gene interactions Delivery and stability issues Limited clinical data	Preclinical/early clinical trial	[79]
mRNA Therapy	Introduces synthetic mRNA to restore beneficial protein expression (*e.g.*, encoding mitochondrial regulators to improve energy metabolism)	-Potential for liver regeneration -Can treat enzyme deficiencies **-Rapid response and adaptable technology**	Requires effective lipid nanoparticle (LNP) delivery Short-lived expression, requiring repeated doses High production costs	Preclinical	[80]
Antisense Oligonucleotides (ASOs)	Binds to specific mRNA sequences to degrade or modify gene expression (*e.g.*, ASOs targeting **DGAT2** to reduce triglyceride synthesis)	Targets specific disease-related RNA Prolonged effects compared to siRNA Potential for oral delivery	May require frequent administration Possible off-target effects Limited liver-specific delivery	Phase 1/2 clinical trials	[81]

Gene therapy and RNA-based modalities are paradigm shift approaches to treating NAFLD/NASH through specific molecular targeting to the drivers of disease progression. CRISPR/Cas9 gene editing as a long-term, precise therapeutic strategy seems promising, but further challenges with off-target effects and delivery must still be overcome prior to clinical translation [75]. RNA mechanisms include siRNA or antisense oligonucleotide–based therapeutics, the latter of which is among the most advanced (phase 2/3 clinical trials for lipid metabolism and inflammatory pathways). RNAi-based therapies are generally limited in their applicability, need to be optimized for specificity and safety, and can regulate multiple pathways (miRNA-mediated regulation). Conversely, mRNA therapeutics offer a compelling path toward restoring a missing hepatic protein but are limited by their instability and liver-targeted delivery [77]. The success of such therapies largely depends on advanced nanocarrier systems, including lipid nanoparticles (LNPs) and exosomes, which facilitate hepatic accumulation while minimizing systemic toxicity. As research progresses, these innovative approaches offer considerable promise to transform the therapeutic landscape for fatty liver disease and enable more effective, tailored treatment options [81].

NON-PHARMACOLOGICAL THERAPIES

There are non-pharmacological treatments available for fatty liver disease that are effective but take a much longer time and require patience; they are pictorially represented in Fig. (**3**).

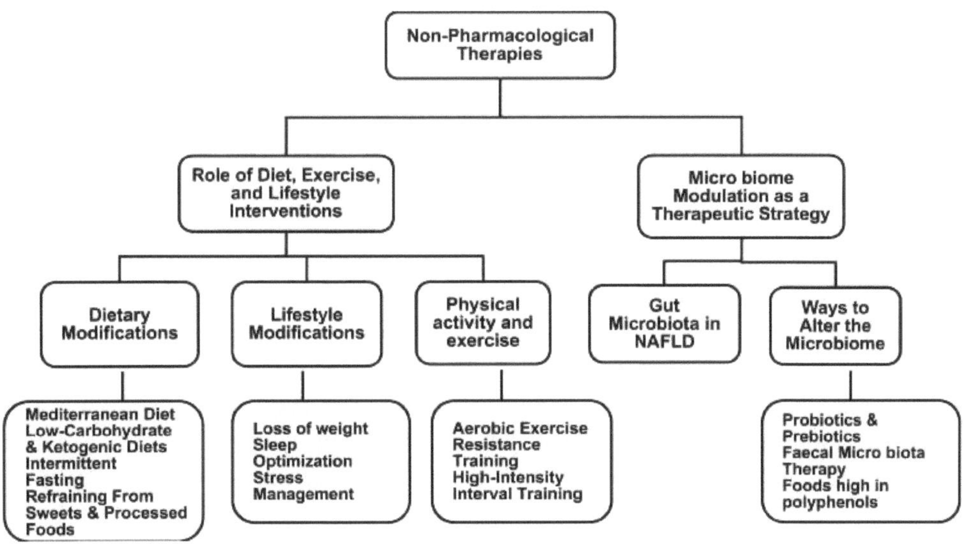

Fig. (3). Non-Pharmacological interventions for fatty liver disease.

Impact of Diet, Exercise, and Lifestyle Interventions

The modulation strategies for NAFLD and its progressive form, NASH, should primarily be directed towards metabolic dysfunction, as lifestyle plays a key role in both their pathogenesis. Unlike prescription medications, which mainly focus on symptoms, dietary changes, physical activity, and lifestyle adjustments tackle the underlying drivers, including insulin resistance, oxidative stress, and chronic inflammation [82]. Research indicates that structured diet, exercise, and lifestyle changes can greatly mitigate liver fat content, improve liver enzymes, and even reverse the progression of the disease. As such, personalized nutritional management, physical exercise, and lifestyle changes will still be the mainstay therapeutic alternatives for NAFLD/NASH [83].

A. Dietary Modifications

Dietary alterations help manage fatty liver disease by reducing hepatic fat accumulation and inflammation [84].

- **Mediterranean Diet:** Full of unsaturated fats (olive oil, nuts), fiber (vegetables, whole grains), and lean proteins (fish). For example, patients with NAFLD who adhered to the Mediterranean diet for 12 months showed significant declines in liver fat content [85].
- **Low-Carbohydrate and Ketogenic Diets:** Aids in reducing insulin resistance and enhancing fatty acid oxidation. Clinical trials of patients on a ketogenic diet reveal improved liver enzyme levels and less hepatic steatosis [86].
- **Intermittent Fasting:** Improves fat metabolism and downplays oxidative stress. Example: The 16:8 intermittent fasting regimen has been shown to modulate liver function markers in patients with NAFLD [87].
- **Refraining from Sweets and Processed Foods:** It lowers fructose-mediated lipogenesis. For example, a decrease in soft drink intake was found to be associated with reduced liver fat accumulation in adolescents with NAFLD [88].

B. Physical Activity and Exercise

Regular exercise is important for improving liver function and reducing hepatic fat.

- **Aerobic Exercise (*e.g.*, brisk walking, cycling):** Reduces liver enzymes and improves insulin sensitivity. Example: A 12-week walking program (≥150 minutes per week) demonstrated a 20% reduction in liver fat [89].
- **Resistance Training (weightlifting, bodyweight exercises, etc.):** Decreases accumulation of visceral and hepatic fat. For example, engaging in strength training for 2 days per week reduced liver fat percentage in overweight individuals [90].
- **High-Intensity Interval Training (HIIT):** Promotes mitochondrial function and fat metabolism. Example: 8 weeks of HIIT improve liver fat and insulin sensitivity in patients with NAFLD [91].

C. Lifestyle Modifications

- **Loss of weight** (≥7–10% of body weight): Weight loss may result in histological improvements in NASH. An example is a meta-analysis that demonstrated that weight loss of 10% or more led to regression of fibrosis in 45% [4].
- **Sleep Optimization**: Metabolic dysfunction and heightened hepatic inflammation are associated with poor sleep. Example: Some studies have found that people with sleep apnea had a higher prevalence of NAFLD, and treatment of sleep disorders improved liver health [92].
- **Stress Management (Meditation, Yoga):** It inhibits fat accumulation in the liver induced by cortisol. For example, mindfulness-based stress reduction techniques were associated with lower liver enzyme levels in patients with NAFLD [93].

Microbiome Modulation as a Therapeutic Strategy

The gut microbiome is closely linked to the development and progression of NAFLD/NASH. Emerging research indicates the importance of the gut-liver axis, which is precisely correlated with the intestinal microbiome. Gut microbial dysbiosis has been associated with increased intestinal permeability, endotoxemia, and chronic hepatic inflammation, leading to liver dysfunction [94]. Novel therapeutic approaches targeting the gut microbiome through probiotics, prebiotics, fecal microbiota transplantation (FMT), and diet modification have emerged as promising means of improving liver health. Given that restoring microbial imbalance, modulating inflammatory pathways, and increasing metabolic homeostasis, microbiome-based interventions may represent novel non-pharmacological therapeutic options for NAFLD/NASH management [95].

A. Gut Microbiota in NAFLD

Dysbiosis (change in gut bacteria balance) induces increased intestinal epithelial permeability, allowing the entry of bacterial endotoxins (lipopolysaccharides, etc.) into the liver, triggering inflammation. For example, patients with NAFLD have a lower abundance of beneficial gut bacteria (*Bifidobacterium, Akkermansia muciniphila*) [96].

B. Ways to Alter the Microbiome

- **Probiotics and Prebiotics**: Increase beneficial bacteria that decrease liver fat deposition. For example, in NAFLD patients, *Lactobacillus* and *Bifidobacterium* supplementation improved liver enzyme levels [97]

- **Fecal Microbiota Therapy (FMT):** Searching for a novel strategy for gut microbiome restoration. Preliminary evidence from small clinical studies indicates that FMT may improve insulin sensitivity and liver health in patients with NAFLD [98].
- **Foods High in Polyphenols** (such as green tea, berries, and dark chocolate): Enhance the diversity of gut microbiota and lower inflammation. For example, green tea extract reduces hepatic fat content and modulates gut microbiota in NAFLD [99].
- **Short-Chain Fatty Acids (SCFAs) and Postbiotics**: Increase insulin sensitivity and preserve the liver. For instance, butyrate (a type of SCFA) supplementation was shown to improve metabolic markers in NAFLD patients [100].

BIOMARKERS AND PRECISION MEDICINE

The advent of precision medicine has reshaped the management of NAFLD and NASH into patient-specific diagnosis and treatment. Due to the heterogeneous nature of fatty liver disease, conventional approaches to diagnosis and confirmation are often inadequate in differentiating between stages of disease or predicting treatment response on a patient-by-patient basis [101]. The growing importance of biomarkers and advanced diagnostic tools for patient stratification has enabled early detection, risk assessment, and personalized interventions in clinical practice. Precision medicine is a nascent field that aims to merge genetic/metabolic/molecular information to provide customized treatment approaches, thereby enhancing treatment effectiveness while reducing disease progression [102, 103]. The roles of biomarkers and precision medicine in fatty liver disease are presented in Table **5**.

Table 5. Biomarkers and precision medicine in fatty liver disease.

Category	Key Aspects	Examples	Ref.
Advancements in Diagnostic Tools for Patient Stratification			
Serum Biomarkers	Blood-based indicators of liver inflammation and fibrosis	FIB-4, NAFLD Fibrosis Score (NFS), Cytokeratin-18 (CK-18)	[104]
Genetic and Epigenetic Biomarkers	Genetic predisposition and DNA modifications linked to disease severity	PNPLA3 (rs738409) variant, DNA methylation of *SREBF1* and *PPARα*	[105]
Gut Microbiome Biomarkers	Dysbiosis-related markers for NAFLD severity	Increased *Escherichia coli*, reduced *Akkermansia muciniphila*	[106]

(Table 5) cont.....

Category	Key Aspects	Examples	Ref.
Advancements in Diagnostic Tools for Patient Stratification			
Advanced Imaging Techniques	Non-invasive assessment of liver fat, inflammation, and fibrosis	FibroScan® (elastography), Magnetic Resonance Elastography (MRE)	[107]
Metabolomics and Lipidomics	Metabolic signatures linked to disease progression	Increased ceramides and sphingolipids in NAFLD	[108]
Role of Personalized Treatment Strategies			
Pharmacogenomics-Guided Therapy	Genetic variations influencing drug response	PNPLA3-based lipid-lowering therapy; TM6SF2 variant effects on statins	[109]
Lifestyle and Nutritional Interventions	Tailored diet and exercise based on metabolic profile	Low-carb diets for insulin resistance; antioxidant-rich diets for oxidative stress	[110]
RNA-Based and Gene Editing Therapies	Molecular interventions for genetic risk factors	ASO therapy targeting APOC3, CRISPR/Cas9 for PNPLA3 correction	[75]
Gut Microbiome Modulation	Personalized probiotics and prebiotics for liver health	Balancing *Firmicutes/Bacteroidetes* ratio; Fecal Microbiota Transplantation (FMT)	[111]

Biomarkers and precision medicine are revolutionizing the landscape of NAFLD/NASH management. Advanced diagnostics enable early, accurate disease stratification, while personalized therapeutic strategies enable targeted, effective intervention. Building on the discovery of new biomarkers and novel therapeutic targets in previous research, precision medicine seeks to deliver tailored treatments, thereby improving patient outcomes and enabling disease prevention [103].

CHALLENGES IN TRANSLATIONAL RESEARCH IN NAFLD/NASH

Importantly, although the pathophysiology of NAFLD and NASH is becoming increasingly well understood, translating new therapeutics from preclinical studies into clinical practice remains challenging. Emerging therapies face many obstacles to their success, including scientific, logistical, regulatory, and ethical barriers. Overcoming these challenges is essential to ensure that innovative treatment strategies can be delivered safely and effectively to patients [112].

Barriers to Clinical Adoption of New Therapeutics

Translation from bench to bedside is not without significant challenges, including, but not limited to, disease heterogeneity, a dearth of predictive preclinical models, and difficulties in accruing patients to clinical trials [113]. Due to the intricate, multifactorial etiology of NAFLD/NASH, which is influenced by genetic, metabolic, and environmental factors, it is often difficult to develop a single, universal treatment-directed approach. Many drugs that show promise in animal models fail to advance to human trials because disease progression and drug responses differ between species, rendering them ineffective in humans. Moreover, differing endpoints have severely hampered the clinical trial evaluation of treatment efficacy, resulting in inadequate regulatory evaluation [114].

Patient recruitment and retention in clinical trials is yet another significant challenge in the industry. However, because NAFLD/NASH is asymptomatic in early stages, many patients remain undiagnosed and unaware of their condition, leading to a smaller pool of potential trial participants [115]. Moreover, achieving long-term lifestyle changes, which are often needed as adjuncts to pharmacological interventions, is difficult; thus, non-compliance with therapy remains a major challenge to therapy success [116].

However, the delivery of new therapeutic approaches also introduces a range of difficulties, including RNA-based therapies, gene-editing methodologies, and microbiome-related treatments. Safe and efficient hepatic delivery while minimizing off-target effects remains a critical challenge. Nanoparticle-based drug delivery systems hold great promise, yet their scalability for clinical use needs to be optimized to improve stability, bioavailability, and tissue specificity [117].

Regulatory and Ethical Implications

Developers of novel therapeutics will face challenges in obtaining approval due to the absence of disease-specific, approved pharmacological treatments in the current NAFLD/NASH landscape. Although regulatory organizations like the U.S. FDA and the European Medicines Agency acknowledge the need for a thorough evaluation of long-term effectiveness and safety, the studies required are often long-term clinical trials [118]. NAFLD/NASH is a slowly progressive disease, which renders the definitive demonstration of clinical outcomes challenging within conventional durations of clinical trials. Other reasons for regulatory hesitancy include the relevance of surrogate markers (including liver enzymes and imaging-based fibrosis assessment), which may not fully reflect long-term treatment benefit [40].

The ethical implications of new therapies, especially gene-editing technologies such as CRISPR/Cas9, only add another layer of complexity. This has raised serious safety concerns about unintended alterations of the genetic code and off-target effects. Access to advanced, often costly, therapies is also a burning issue (most crucially in low-resource settings, where NAFLD is reaching epidemic proportions) [119]. Ethical issues also apply to microbiome-based therapeutics (*e.g.*, FMT), which necessitate defining ethical stakeholder selection, evaluating long-term risks and benefits, and ascertaining potential unintended changes in microbial composition, diversity, and function. The pace of innovation in precision medicine also needs to be matched by the evolution of the regulatory framework. Precision-based therapy is further complicated by ethical considerations related to patient consent, genetic data privacy, and long-term monitoring [120].

The path to overcoming barriers to the translational research of NAFLD/NASH should be through a collaborative approach to generating more predictive preclinical models, optimizing clinical trials, and adopting a more flexible regulatory framework that can accommodate novel disease-modifying/redirection agents emerging with precision medicine [121]. Gene editing, microbiome therapies, and data privacy are just a few areas where ethical considerations must be explored on the path to responsible implementation. It is the duty of all parties, including researchers, regulators, and clinicians, to ensure that the strides in science translate into saving lives from NAFLD/NASH when the drug hits the market [122].

FUTURE DIRECTIONS AND CONCLUSION

NAFLD and NASH research landscape shifts toward innovative therapeutic developments. Future studies are focusing on precision medicine, novel biomarkers, and targeted therapies against the backdrop of the global epidemic of fatty liver diseases. Articles reflecting the current state of the art in the molecular mechanisms underlying these diseases highlight that they cannot be diagnosed and treated solely on a patient-by-patient basis. These studies discuss advancements, such as the development of biologics, novel gene-editing technologies like CRISPR/Cas9, RNA-based therapeutics, and microbiome-targeted therapies, all of which aim to modulate the metabolic and inflammatory pathways driving disease progression [123]. Moreover, various nanotechnology-based drug delivery systems are under consideration for improved hepatic targeting and drug efficacy. Further, deployment of artificial intelligence (AI) and machine learning (ML) in clinical decision-making, imaging analysis, and drug discovery is also anticipated to accelerate the pace of progress in NAFLD/NASH management [124].

Future developments in the field could address potential barriers to implementation, such as the need for novel, non-invasive biomarkers for early detection and disease stratification, the optimization of combination therapies (pharmacological and lifestyle-based), and improved methodologies for clinical trials to allow for greater precision and efficiency in assessing potential outcomes [125]. Indeed, genetic profiling and metabolic phenotyping will be critical for developing treatment approaches tailored to each individual patient based on his or her unique genetics and metabolism. Moreover, a focus on inequality and access barriers to advanced therapies, particularly in resource-poor settings, will be critical for equitable solutions in healthcare [126].

Importantly, advances in fundamental research have also accelerated the understanding of NAFLD/NASH pathophysiology, along with progress in diagnostic tools, precision medicine, and new therapeutics to improve patient outcomes [125]. Nevertheless, there are still barriers to clinical translation, regulatory issues, and ethical challenges that need to be addressed to allow a successful introduction of these innovative therapies. Bridging scientific discovery and clinical applications requires a collaborative, multidisciplinary approach among researchers, clinicians, regulators, and policymakers. As we continue to evolve in our understanding of this disease, the future of NAFLD/NASH management seems bright, with improved diagnostic and therapeutic approaches providing a personalised, more targeted, and more effective response to patients [127].

LIST OF ABBREVIATIONS

NAFLD	Non-Alcoholic Fatty Liver Disease
NASH	Non-Alcoholic Steatohepatitis
HCC	Hepatocellular Carcinoma
GLP-1	Glucagon-Like Peptide-1
TRβ	Thyroid Hormone Receptor Beta
SCD1	Stearoyl-CoA Desaturase 1
PPAR	Peroxisome Proliferator-Activated Receptor
FGF21 / FGF19	Fibroblast Growth Factor 21 / 19
FXR	Farnesoid X Receptor
ASK1	Apoptosis Signal-Regulating Kinase 1
CCR2/CCR5	C-C Motif Chemokine Receptor 2/5
FDA	Food and Drug Administration
EMA	European Medicines Agency
FMT	Fecal Microbiota Transplantation

SCFA	Short-Chain Fatty Acid
AI	Artificial Intelligence
ML	Machine Learning
siRNA	Small Interfering RNA
miRNA	MicroRNA
mRNA	Messenger RNA
ASO	Antisense Oligonucleotides
CRISPR/Cas9	Clustered Regularly Interspaced Short Palindromic Repeats / CRISPR-associated protein 9
LDL / HDL / VLDL	Low-Density Lipoprotein / High-Density Lipoprotein / Very-Low-Density Lipoprotein
TG	Triglyceride
MRE	Magnetic Resonance Elastography
CK-18	Cytokeratin-18
PNPLA3	Patatin-Like Phospholipase Domain-Containing Protein 3
SREBF1	Sterol Regulatory Element Binding Transcription Factor 1
TM6SF2	Transmembrane 6 Superfamily Member 2
APOC3	Apolipoprotein C3

REFERENCES

[1] Cohen JC, Horton JD, Hobbs HH. Human fatty liver disease: old questions and new insights. Science 2011; 332(6037): 1519-23.
[http://dx.doi.org/10.1126/science.1204265] [PMID: 21700865]

[2] Cotter TG, Rinella M. Nonalcoholic fatty liver disease 2020: the state of the disease. Gastroenterology 2020; 158(7): 1851-64.
[http://dx.doi.org/10.1053/j.gastro.2020.01.052] [PMID: 32061595]

[3] Younossi ZM, Golabi P, Paik JM, Henry A, Van Dongen C, Henry L. The global epidemiology of nonalcoholic fatty liver disease (NAFLD) and nonalcoholic steatohepatitis (NASH): a systematic review. Hepatology 2023; 77(4): 1335-47.
[http://dx.doi.org/10.1097/HEP.0000000000000004] [PMID: 36626630]

[4] Pouwels S, Sakran N, Graham Y, *et al.* Non-alcoholic fatty liver disease (NAFLD): a review of pathophysiology, clinical management and effects of weight loss. BMC Endocr Disord 2022; 22(1): 63.
[http://dx.doi.org/10.1186/s12902-022-00980-1] [PMID: 35287643]

[5] Pierantonelli I, Svegliati-Baroni G. Nonalcoholic fatty liver disease: basic pathogenetic mechanisms in the progression from NAFLD to NASH. Transplantation 2019; 103(1): e1-e13.
[http://dx.doi.org/10.1097/TP.0000000000002480] [PMID: 30300287]

[6] Galiero R, Caturano A, Vetrano E, *et al.* Pathophysiological mechanisms and clinical evidence of relationship between Nonalcoholic fatty liver disease (NAFLD) and cardiovascular disease. Rev Cardiovasc Med 2021; 22(3): 755-68.
[http://dx.doi.org/10.31083/j.rcm2203082] [PMID: 34565074]

[7] Sharma S, Sharma A, Gupta P, *et al.* The green path to liver health: herbal solutions for non-alcoholic

steatohepatitis. Cardiovasc Hematol Disord Drug Targets 2025; 25(3): 168-92.
[http://dx.doi.org/10.2174/011871529X360903250211101856] [PMID: 40108906]

[8] Simon G, Heckmann V, Tóth D, Pauka D, Petrus K, Molnár TF. The effect of hepatic steatosis and fibrosis on liver weight and dimensions. Leg Med (Tokyo) 2020; 47: 101781.
[http://dx.doi.org/10.1016/j.legalmed.2020.101781] [PMID: 32889367]

[9] Ayoub F, Trillo-Alvarez C, Morelli G, Lascano J. Risk factors for hepatic steatosis in adults with cystic fibrosis: Similarities to non-alcoholic fatty liver disease. World J Hepatol 2018; 10(1): 34-40.
[http://dx.doi.org/10.4254/wjh.v10.i1.34] [PMID: 29399276]

[10] Gjorgjieva M, Sobolewski C, Dolicka D, Correia de Sousa M, Foti M. miRNAs and NAFLD: from pathophysiology to therapy. Gut 2019; 68(11): 2065-79.
[http://dx.doi.org/10.1136/gutjnl-2018-318146] [PMID: 31300518]

[11] Peverill W, Powell L, Skoien R. Evolving concepts in the pathogenesis of NASH: beyond steatosis and inflammation. Int J Mol Sci 2014; 15(5): 8591-638.
[http://dx.doi.org/10.3390/ijms15058591] [PMID: 24830559]

[12] ten Hove M, Pater L, Storm G, *et al.* The hepatic lipidome: From basic science to clinical translation. Adv Drug Deliv Rev 2020; 159: 180-97.
[http://dx.doi.org/10.1016/j.addr.2020.06.027] [PMID: 32615143]

[13] Yan Z, Liu Z, Yang B, Zhu X, Song E, Song Y. Long-term exposure of molybdenum disulfide nanosheets leads to hepatic lipid accumulation and atherogenesis in apolipoprotein E deficient mice. NanoImpact 2023; 30: 100462.
[http://dx.doi.org/10.1016/j.impact.2023.100462] [PMID: 37059265]

[14] Bugianesi E, McCullough AJ, Marchesini G. Insulin resistance: a metabolic pathway to chronic liver disease. Hepatology 2005; 42(5): 987-1000.
[http://dx.doi.org/10.1002/hep.20920] [PMID: 16250043]

[15] Paradies G, Paradies V, Ruggiero FM, Petrosillo G. Oxidative stress, cardiolipin and mitochondrial dysfunction in nonalcoholic fatty liver disease. World J Gastroenterol 2014; 20(39): 14205-18.
[http://dx.doi.org/10.3748/wjg.v20.i39.14205] [PMID: 25339807]

[16] Liu X, Green RM. Endoplasmic reticulum stress and liver diseases. Liver Res 2019; 3(1): 55-64.
[http://dx.doi.org/10.1016/j.livres.2019.01.002] [PMID: 32670671]

[17] Ashraf NU, Sheikh TA. Endoplasmic reticulum stress and Oxidative stress in the pathogenesis of Non-alcoholic fatty liver disease. Free Radic Res 2015; 49(12): 1405-18.
[http://dx.doi.org/10.3109/10715762.2015.1078461] [PMID: 26223319]

[18] Singh S, Allen AM, Wang Z, Prokop LJ, Murad MH, Loomba R. Fibrosis progression in nonalcoholic fatty liver *vs* nonalcoholic steatohepatitis: a systematic review and meta-analysis of paired-biopsy studies. Clin Gastroenterol Hepatol. 2015; 13(4): 643-54. e9.
[http://dx.doi.org/10.1016/j.cgh.2014.04.014]

[19] Lonardo A, Ballestri S, Marchesini G, Angulo P, Loria P. Nonalcoholic fatty liver disease: A precursor of the metabolic syndrome. Dig Liver Dis 2015; 47(3): 181-90.
[http://dx.doi.org/10.1016/j.dld.2014.09.020] [PMID: 25739820]

[20] Sookoian S, Pirola CJ. Genetic predisposition in nonalcoholic fatty liver disease. Clin Mol Hepatol 2017; 23(1): 1-12.
[http://dx.doi.org/10.3350/cmh.2016.0109] [PMID: 28268262]

[21] Nseir W, Hellou E, Assy N. Role of diet and lifestyle changes in nonalcoholic fatty liver disease. World J Gastroenterol 2014; 20(28): 9338-44.
[PMID: 25071328]

[22] Boursier J, Mueller O, Barret M, *et al.* The severity of nonalcoholic fatty liver disease is associated with gut dysbiosis and shift in the metabolic function of the gut microbiota. Hepatology 2016; 63(3): 764-75.

[http://dx.doi.org/10.1002/hep.28356] [PMID: 26600078]

[23] Lieber CS. Alcoholic fatty liver: its pathogenesis and mechanism of progression to inflammation and fibrosis. Alcohol 2004; 34(1): 9-19.
[http://dx.doi.org/10.1016/j.alcohol.2004.07.008] [PMID: 15670660]

[24] Al-Eryani L, Wahlang B, Falkner KC, *et al.* Identification of environmental chemicals associated with the development of toxicant-associated fatty liver disease in rodents. Toxicol Pathol 2015; 43(4): 482-97.
[http://dx.doi.org/10.1177/0192623314549960] [PMID: 25326588]

[25] Mazzolini G, Sowa JP, Atorrasagasti C, Kücükoglu Ö, Syn WK, Canbay A. Significance of simple steatosis: an update on the clinical and molecular evidence. Cells 2020; 9(11): 2458.
[http://dx.doi.org/10.3390/cells9112458] [PMID: 33187255]

[26] Sharma P, Arora A. Clinical presentation of alcoholic liver disease and non-alcoholic fatty liver disease: spectrum and diagnosis. Transl Gastroenterol Hepatol 2020; 5: 19.
[http://dx.doi.org/10.21037/tgh.2019.10.02] [PMID: 32258523]

[27] Dulai PS, Singh S, Patel J, *et al.* Increased risk of mortality by fibrosis stage in nonalcoholic fatty liver disease: Systematic review and meta-analysis. Hepatology 2017; 65(5): 1557-65.
[http://dx.doi.org/10.1002/hep.29085] [PMID: 28130788]

[28] Farrell GC, Larter CZ. Nonalcoholic fatty liver disease: from steatosis to cirrhosis. Hepatology 2006; 43 (Suppl. 1): S99-S112.
[http://dx.doi.org/10.1002/hep.20973] [PMID: 16447287]

[29] Suresh D, Srinivas AN, Kumar DP. Etiology of hepatocellular carcinoma: special focus on fatty liver disease. Front Oncol 2020; 10: 601710.
[http://dx.doi.org/10.3389/fonc.2020.601710] [PMID: 33330100]

[30] Angulo P, Lindor KD, Eds. Treatment of nonalcoholic fatty liver: present and emerging therapies. Semin Liver Dis 2001; 21(1): 81-.
[http://dx.doi.org/10.1055/s-2001-12931] [PMID: 11296699]

[31] Younossi ZM, Loomba R, Rinella ME, *et al.* Current and future therapeutic regimens for nonalcoholic fatty liver disease and nonalcoholic steatohepatitis. Hepatology 2018; 68(1): 361-71.
[http://dx.doi.org/10.1002/hep.29724] [PMID: 29222911]

[32] Abdel-Rahman RF. Non-alcoholic fatty liver disease. Asian Pac J Trop Biomed 2022; 12(3): 99-114.
[http://dx.doi.org/10.4103/2221-1691.338919]

[33] Ozturk ZA, Kadayifci A. Insulin sensitizers for the treatment of non-alcoholic fatty liver disease. World J Hepatol 2014; 6(4): 199-206.
[http://dx.doi.org/10.4254/wjh.v6.i4.199] [PMID: 24799988]

[34] Ndakotsu A, Vivekanandan G. The role of thiazolidinediones in the amelioration of nonalcoholic fatty liver disease: a systematic review. Cureus 2022; 14(5): e25380.
[http://dx.doi.org/10.7759/cureus.25380] [PMID: 35765391]

[35] Tzanaki I, Agouridis AP, Kostapanos MS. Is there a role of lipid-lowering therapies in the management of fatty liver disease? World J Hepatol 2022; 14(1): 119-39.
[http://dx.doi.org/10.4254/wjh.v14.i1.119] [PMID: 35126843]

[36] Tziomalos K. Lipid-lowering agents in the management of nonalcoholic fatty liver disease. World J Hepatol 2014; 6(10): 738-44.
[http://dx.doi.org/10.4254/wjh.v6.i10.738] [PMID: 25349644]

[37] Nagashimada M, Ota T. Role of vitamin E in nonalcoholic fatty liver disease. IUBMB Life 2019; 71(4): 516-22.
[http://dx.doi.org/10.1002/iub.1991] [PMID: 30592129]

[38] Du J, Ma Y-Y, Yu C-H, Li Y-M. Effects of pentoxifylline on nonalcoholic fatty liver disease: A meta-

analysis. World J Gastroenterol 2014; 20(2): 569-77.
[http://dx.doi.org/10.3748/wjg.v20.i2.569] [PMID: 24574727]

[39] Mudaliar S, Henry RR, Sanyal AJ, Morrow L, Marschall HU, Kipnes M, *et al.* Efficacy and safety of the farnesoid X receptor agonist obeticholic acid in patients with type 2 diabetes and nonalcoholic fatty liver disease. Gastroenterology. 2013; 145(3): 574-82. e1.
[http://dx.doi.org/10.1053/j.gastro.2013.05.042]

[40] Harvey BE. NASH: regulatory considerations for clinical drug development and U.S. FDA approval. Acta Pharmacol Sin 2022; 43(5): 1210-4.
[http://dx.doi.org/10.1038/s41401-021-00832-z] [PMID: 35110697]

[41] Linares I, Hamar M, Selzner N, Selzner M. Steatosis in liver transplantation: current limitations and future strategies. Transplantation 2019; 103(1): 78-90.
[http://dx.doi.org/10.1097/TP.0000000000002466] [PMID: 30418431]

[42] Akhter A, Pulla A, Said A. Review of current and potential future pharmacological treatments in nonalcoholic steatohepatitis. Clin Liver Dis (Hoboken) 2016; 7(1): 11-4.
[http://dx.doi.org/10.1002/cld.523] [PMID: 31041018]

[43] Ofosu A, Ramai D, Reddy M. Non-alcoholic fatty liver disease: controlling an emerging epidemic, challenges, and future directions. Ann Gastroenterol 2018; 31(3): 288-95.
[http://dx.doi.org/10.20524/aog.2018.0240] [PMID: 29720854]

[44] Crabb DW, Im GY, Szabo G, Mellinger JL, Lucey MR. Diagnosis and treatment of alcohol-associated liver diseases: 2019 practice guidance from the american association for the study of liver diseases. Hepatology 2020; 71(1): 306-33.
[http://dx.doi.org/10.1002/hep.30866] [PMID: 31314133]

[45] Harrison SA, Di Bisceglie AM. Advances in the understanding and treatment of nonalcoholic fatty liver disease. Drugs 2003; 63(22): 2379-94.
[http://dx.doi.org/10.2165/00003495-200363220-00001] [PMID: 14609346]

[46] Fiorucci S, Biagioli M, Baldoni M, *et al.* The identification of farnesoid X receptor modulators as treatment options for nonalcoholic fatty liver disease. Expert Opin Drug Discov 2021; 16(10): 1193-208.
[http://dx.doi.org/10.1080/17460441.2021.1916465] [PMID: 33849361]

[47] Siddiqui MS, Parmar D, Sheikh F, Sarin SK, Cisneros L, Gawrieh S, *et al.* Saroglitazar, a dual PPAR α/γ agonist, improves atherogenic dyslipidemia in patients with non-cirrhotic nonalcoholic fatty liver disease: a pooled analysis. Clinical Gastroenterology and Hepatology. 2023; 21(10): 2597-605. e2.

[48] Harrison SA, Bashir MR, Guy CD, *et al.* Resmetirom (MGL-3196) for the treatment of non-alcoholic steatohepatitis: a multicentre, randomised, double-blind, placebo-controlled, phase 2 trial. Lancet 2019; 394(10213): 2012-24.
[http://dx.doi.org/10.1016/S0140-6736(19)32517-6] [PMID: 31727409]

[49] Adeniran O, Nieto LM, Kwentoh IP, *et al.* Tirzepatide *vs* semaglutide in obese patients with MAFLD or MASH: a comparative analysis of cardiovascular and gastrointestinal outcomes, and the risk of progression to fibrosis or hepatocellular carcinoma. Am J Gastroenterol. 2024;119(10 Suppl):S1221-S1222.
[http://dx.doi.org/10.14309/01.ajg.0001036068.77159.99]

[50] Nelson CH, Etchevers K, Yi S, *et al.* Pharmacokinetics, safety, and tolerability of selonsertib, an apoptosis signal-regulating kinase 1 (ASK1) inhibitor, following first-in-human single and multiple ascending doses in healthy subjects. Clin Pharmacokinet 2020; 59(9): 1109-17.
[http://dx.doi.org/10.1007/s40262-020-00878-y] [PMID: 32333325]

[51] Tacke F. Cenicriviroc for the treatment of non-alcoholic steatohepatitis and liver fibrosis. Expert Opin Investig Drugs 2018; 27(3): 301-11.
[http://dx.doi.org/10.1080/13543784.2018.1442436] [PMID: 29448843]

[52] Chalasani N, Abdelmalek MF, Garcia-Tsao G, Vuppalanchi R, Alkhouri N, Rinella M, *et al.* Effects of belapectin, an inhibitor of galectin-3, in patients with nonalcoholic steatohepatitis with cirrhosis and portal hypertension. Gastroenterology. 2020; 158(5): 1334-45. e5. [http://dx.doi.org/10.1053/j.gastro.2019.11.296]

[53] Tian H, Zhang S, Liu Y, Wu Y, Zhang D. Fibroblast growth factors for nonalcoholic fatty liver disease: opportunities and challenges. Int J Mol Sci 2023; 24(5): 4583. [http://dx.doi.org/10.3390/ijms24054583] [PMID: 36902015]

[54] Chen J, Thomsen M, Vitetta L. Interaction of gut microbiota with dysregulation of bile acids in the pathogenesis of nonalcoholic fatty liver disease and potential therapeutic implications of probiotics. J Cell Biochem 2019; 120(3): 2713-20. [http://dx.doi.org/10.1002/jcb.27635] [PMID: 30443932]

[55] Moghtadaie A, Mahboobi H, Fatemizadeh S, Kamal MA. Emerging role of nanotechnology in treatment of non-alcoholic fatty liver disease (NAFLD). EXCLI J 2023; 22: 946-74. [PMID: 38023570]

[56] Tang R, Li R, Li H, *et al.* Design of hepatic targeted drug delivery systems for natural products: insights into nomenclature revision of nonalcoholic fatty liver disease. ACS Nano 2021; 15(11): 17016-46. [http://dx.doi.org/10.1021/acsnano.1c02158] [PMID: 34705426]

[57] Sargazi S, Toudeshkchouei MG, Rahdar A, *et al.* Emerging nano-theranostic strategies against non-alcoholic fatty liver disease: a review. Iran J Mater Sci Eng 2023; 20(1) [http://dx.doi.org/10.22068/ijmse.2861]

[58] Ratziu V, Yilmaz Y, Lazas D, *et al.* Aramchol improves hepatic fibrosis in metabolic dysfunction–associated steatohepatitis: Results of multimodality assessment using both conventional and digital pathology. Hepatology 2025; 81(3): 932-46. [http://dx.doi.org/10.1097/HEP.0000000000000980] [PMID: 38916482]

[59] Kamata S, Honda A, Ishii I. Current clinical trial status and future prospects of PPAR-targeted drugs for treating nonalcoholic fatty liver disease. Biomolecules 2023; 13(8): 1264. [http://dx.doi.org/10.3390/biom13081264] [PMID: 37627329]

[60] Keam SJ. Resmetirom: First Approval. Drugs 2024; 84(6): 729-35. [http://dx.doi.org/10.1007/s40265-024-02045-0] [PMID: 38771485]

[61] Harrison SA, Loomba R, Dubourg J, Ratziu V, Noureddin M. Clinical trial landscape in NASH. Clin Gastroenterol Hepatol 2023; 21(8): 2001-14. [http://dx.doi.org/10.1016/j.cgh.2023.03.041] [PMID: 37059159]

[62] Harrison SA, Baum SJ, Gunn NT, *et al.* Safety, tolerability, and biologic activity of AXA1125 and AXA1957 in subjects with nonalcoholic fatty liver disease. Official journal of the American College of Gastroenterology| ACG. 2021; 116(12): 2399-409. [http://dx.doi.org/10.14309/ajg.0000000000001375]

[63] Qosa H, de Oliveira CHMC, Cizza G, *et al.* Pharmacokinetics, safety, and tolerability of BMS-986263, a lipid nanoparticle containing HSP47 siRNA, in participants with hepatic impairment. Clin Transl Sci 2023; 16(10): 1791-802. [http://dx.doi.org/10.1111/cts.13581] [PMID: 37654022]

[64] Lawitz EJ, Fraessdorf M, Neff GW, *et al.* Efficacy, tolerability and pharmacokinetics of survodutide, a glucagon/glucagon-like peptide-1 receptor dual agonist, in cirrhosis. J Hepatol 2024; 81(5): 837-46. [http://dx.doi.org/10.1016/j.jhep.2024.06.003] [PMID: 38857788]

[65] Dahiya K, Palkar M, Sharma S. Unlocking the potential of THR-β agonist therapies: resmetirom's chemistry, biology, and patent insights. Naunyn Schmiedebergs Arch Pharmacol 2025; 398(8): 9703-20. [http://dx.doi.org/10.1007/s00210-025-03880-y] [PMID: 40067441]

[66] Carvalho T. Efruxifermin combined with a GLP-1 receptor agonist reduces liver fat in NASH. Nat Med 2023; 29(8): 1881.
[http://dx.doi.org/10.1038/d41591-023-00055-1] [PMID: 37340082]

[67] Khare T, Liu K, Chilambe LO, Khare S. NAFLD and NAFLD related HCC: Emerging treatments and clinical trials. Int J Mol Sci 2025; 26(1): 306.
[http://dx.doi.org/10.3390/ijms26010306] [PMID: 39796162]

[68] Kokkorakis M, Boutari C, Hill MA, *et al.* Resmetirom, the first approved drug for the management of metabolic dysfunction-associated steatohepatitis: Trials, opportunities, and challenges. Metabolism 2024; 154: 155835.
[http://dx.doi.org/10.1016/j.metabol.2024.155835] [PMID: 38508373]

[69] Harrison SA, Gunn NT, Baum SJ, Younes ZH, Kohli A, Patil R, *et al.* Multifactorial effects of AXA1125 and AXA1957 observed on markers of metabolism, inflammation and fibrosis: A 16-week randomized placebo-controlled study in subjects with nonalcoholic fatty liver disease (NAFLD) with and without type 2 diabetes (T2D). Metabolism. 2020;7:0.88.

[70] Lawitz EJ, Shevell DE, Tirucherai GS, *et al.* BMS-986263 in patients with advanced hepatic fibrosis: 36-week results from a randomized, placebo-controlled phase 2 trial. Hepatology 2022; 75(4): 912-23.
[http://dx.doi.org/10.1002/hep.32181] [PMID: 34605045]

[71] le Roux CW, Steen O, Lucas KJ, Startseva E, Unseld A, Hennige AM. Glucagon and GLP-1 receptor dual agonist survodutide for obesity: a randomised, double-blind, placebo-controlled, dose-finding phase 2 trial. Lancet Diabetes Endocrinol 2024; 12(3): 162-73.
[http://dx.doi.org/10.1016/S2213-8587(23)00356-X] [PMID: 38330987]

[72] Blüher M, Rosenstock J, Hoefler J, Manuel R, Hennige AM. Dose–response effects on HbA_{1c} and bodyweight reduction of survodutide, a dual glucagon/GLP-1 receptor agonist, compared with placebo and open-label semaglutide in people with type 2 diabetes: a randomised clinical trial. Diabetologia 2024; 67(3): 470-82.
[http://dx.doi.org/10.1007/s00125-023-06053-9] [PMID: 38095657]

[73] Viking Therapeutics Inc. VKTX [Internet]. United States. Available from: https://www.vikingtherapeutics.com/

[74] Harrison SA, Ruane PJ, Freilich BL, *et al.* Efruxifermin in non-alcoholic steatohepatitis: a randomized, double-blind, placebo-controlled, phase 2a trial. Nat Med 2021; 27(7): 1262-71.
[http://dx.doi.org/10.1038/s41591-021-01425-3] [PMID: 34239138]

[75] Yan Q, Li D, Jia S, Yang J, Ma J. Novel gene-based therapeutic approaches for the management of hepatic complications in diabetes: Reviewing recent advances. J Diabetes Complications 2024; 38(2): 108688.
[http://dx.doi.org/10.1016/j.jdiacomp.2024.108688] [PMID: 38281457]

[76] Anwar AA, Jalan-Sakrikar N, Huebert RC, Eds. LncRNAs, RNA therapeutics, and emerging technologies in liver pathobiology. Semin Liver Dis 2025; 45(1): 1-14.
[http://dx.doi.org/10.1055/a-2490-1921] [PMID: 39603269]

[77] Mahmoudi A, Rostami M, Mahdi Hajihasani M, Sukhorukov VN, Kesharwani P, Sahebkar A. siRNA-mediated gene silencing for non-alcoholic fatty liver disease: A comprehensive review of molecular targets. Eur Polym J 2024; 208: 112866.
[http://dx.doi.org/10.1016/j.eurpolymj.2024.112866]

[78] Li J, Arest S, Olszowy B, Gordon J, Barrero CA, Perez-Leal O. CRISPR/Cas9-based screening of FDA-approved drugs for NRF2 activation: a novel approach to discover therapeutics for non-alcoholic fatty liver disease. Antioxidants 2023; 12(7): 1363.
[http://dx.doi.org/10.3390/antiox12071363] [PMID: 37507903]

[79] Sun Y, Shen Y, Liang X, Zheng H, Zhang Y. MicroRNAs as biomarkers and therapeutic targets for nonalcoholic fatty liver disease: A narrative review. Clin Ther 2023; 45(3): 234-47.

[http://dx.doi.org/10.1016/j.clinthera.2023.02.001] [PMID: 36841739]

[80] Di Ciaula A, Passarella S, Shanmugam H, *et al.* Nonalcoholic fatty liver disease (NAFLD). Mitochondria as players and targets of therapies? Int J Mol Sci 2021; 22(10): 5375. [http://dx.doi.org/10.3390/ijms22105375] [PMID: 34065331]

[81] Li S, Xiong F, Zhang S, *et al.* Oligonucleotide therapies for nonalcoholic steatohepatitis. Mol Ther Nucleic Acids 2024; 35(2): 102184. [http://dx.doi.org/10.1016/j.omtn.2024.102184] [PMID: 38665220]

[82] Semmler G, Datz C, Reiberger T, Trauner M. Diet and exercise in NAFLD/NASH: Beyond the obvious. Liver Int 2021; 41(10): 2249-68. [http://dx.doi.org/10.1111/liv.15024] [PMID: 34328248]

[83] Hallsworth K, Adams LA. Lifestyle modification in NAFLD/NASH: Facts and figures. JHEP Reports 2019; 1(6): 468-79. [http://dx.doi.org/10.1016/j.jhepr.2019.10.008] [PMID: 32039399]

[84] Glass O, Filozof C, Noureddin M, *et al.* Standardisation of diet and exercise in clinical trials of NAFLD-NASH: Recommendations from the Liver Forum. J Hepatol 2020; 73(3): 680-93. [http://dx.doi.org/10.1016/j.jhep.2020.04.030] [PMID: 32353483]

[85] Procopio AC, Paravati MR, Scarlata GGM, *et al.* Is the Mediterranean diet a good preventive measure for NASH? Hepatoma Res 2024; 10: 9.

[86] Dyńka D, Rodzeń Ł, Rodzeń M, *et al.* Beneficial effects of the ketogenic diet on nonalcoholic fatty liver disease (NAFLD/MAFLD). J Clin Med 2024; 13(16): 4857. [http://dx.doi.org/10.3390/jcm13164857] [PMID: 39200999]

[87] Marjot T, Tomlinson JW, Hodson L, Ray DW. Timing of energy intake and the therapeutic potential of intermittent fasting and time-restricted eating in NAFLD. Gut 2023; 72(8): 1607-19. [http://dx.doi.org/10.1136/gutjnl-2023-329998] [PMID: 37286229]

[88] Armandi A, Schattenberg JM. Beyond the paradigm of weight loss in non-alcoholic fatty liver disease: from pathophysiology to novel dietary approaches. Nutrients 2021; 13(6): 1977. [http://dx.doi.org/10.3390/nu13061977] [PMID: 34201382]

[89] Houttu V, Bouts J, Vali Y, *et al.* Does aerobic exercise reduce NASH and liver fibrosis in patients with non-alcoholic fatty liver disease? A systematic literature review and meta-analysis. Front Endocrinol (Lausanne) 2022; 13: 1032164. [http://dx.doi.org/10.3389/fendo.2022.1032164] [PMID: 36407307]

[90] Zelber-Sagi S, Buch A, Yeshua H, *et al.* Effect of resistance training on non-alcoholic fatty-liver disease a randomized-clinical trial. World J Gastroenterol 2014; 20(15): 4382-92. [http://dx.doi.org/10.3748/wjg.v20.i15.4382] [PMID: 24764677]

[91] Fredrickson G, Barrow F, Dietsche K, *et al.* Exercise of high intensity ameliorates hepatic inflammation and the progression of NASH. Mol Metab 2021; 53: 101270. [http://dx.doi.org/10.1016/j.molmet.2021.101270] [PMID: 34118476]

[92] Bu LF, Xiong CY, Zhong JY, *et al.* Non-alcoholic fatty liver disease and sleep disorders. World J Hepatol 2024; 16(3): 304-15. [http://dx.doi.org/10.4254/wjh.v16.i3.304] [PMID: 38577533]

[93] Manteghian M. Advancements in Non-Alcoholic Fatty Liver Disease and Nonalcoholic Steatohepatitis Treatment: From Lifestyle Interventions to Novel Therapies. Univ Toronto Med J 2024; 101(2) [http://dx.doi.org/10.33137/utmj.v101i2.41857]

[94] Liu Q, Liu S, Chen L, *et al.* Role and effective therapeutic target of gut microbiota in NAFLD/NASH (Review). Exp Ther Med 2019; 18(3): 1935-44. [http://dx.doi.org/10.3892/etm.2019.7781] [PMID: 31410156]

[95] Hu H, Lin A, Kong M, *et al.* Intestinal microbiome and NAFLD: molecular insights and therapeutic

perspectives. J Gastroenterol 2020; 55(2): 142-58.
[http://dx.doi.org/10.1007/s00535-019-01649-8] [PMID: 31845054]

[96] Kobayashi T, Iwaki M, Nakajima A, Nogami A, Yoneda M. Current research on the pathogenesis of NAFLD/NASH and the gut–liver Axis: gut microbiota, dysbiosis, and leaky-gut syndrome. Int J Mol Sci 2022; 23(19): 11689.
[http://dx.doi.org/10.3390/ijms231911689] [PMID: 36232990]

[97] Fernández-Martínez E, Rodríguez-Pastén A, Pérez-Hernández N, Soria-Jasso LE, Cariño-Cortés R. Prebiotics and probiotics: effects on dyslipidemia and NAFLD/NASH and the associated mechanisms of action. Curr Pharm Biotechnol 2023; 24(5): 633-46.
[http://dx.doi.org/10.2174/1389201023666220818145350] [PMID: 35984030]

[98] Abenavoli L, Maurizi V, Rinninella E, *et al.* Fecal Microbiota Transplantation in NAFLD Treatment. Medicina (Kaunas) 2022 Oct 30; 58(11): 1559.
[http://dx.doi.org/10.3390/medicina58111559] [PMID: 36363516]

[99] Ji L, Deng H, Xue H, *et al.* Research progress regarding the effect and mechanism of dietary phenolic acids for improving nonalcoholic fatty liver disease via gut microbiota. Compr Rev Food Sci Food Saf 2023; 22(2): 1128-47.
[http://dx.doi.org/10.1111/1541-4337.13106] [PMID: 36717374]

[100] Wang LJ, Sun JG, Chen SC, Sun YL, Zheng Y, Feng JC. The role of intestinal flora in metabolic dysfunction-associated steatotic liver disease and treatment strategies. Front Med (Lausanne) 2025; 11: 1490929.
[http://dx.doi.org/10.3389/fmed.2024.1490929] [PMID: 39839647]

[101] Lonardo A, Arab JP, Arrese M. Perspectives on precision medicine approaches to NAFLD diagnosis and management. Adv Ther 2021; 38(5): 2130-58.
[http://dx.doi.org/10.1007/s12325-021-01690-1] [PMID: 33829368]

[102] Duan J, Wu Y, Liu J, *et al.* Genetic biomarkers for hepatocellular carcinoma in the era of precision medicine. J Hepatocell Carcinoma 2019; 6: 151-66.
[http://dx.doi.org/10.2147/JHC.S224849] [PMID: 31696097]

[103] Sookoian S, Pirola CJ. Precision medicine in nonalcoholic fatty liver disease: New therapeutic insights from genetics and systems biology. Clin Mol Hepatol 2020; 26(4): 461-75.
[http://dx.doi.org/10.3350/cmh.2020.0136] [PMID: 32906228]

[104] Wong VWS, Adams LA, de Lédinghen V, Wong GLH, Sookoian S. Noninvasive biomarkers in NAFLD and NASH — current progress and future promise. Nat Rev Gastroenterol Hepatol 2018; 15(8): 461-78.
[http://dx.doi.org/10.1038/s41575-018-0014-9] [PMID: 29844588]

[105] Eslam M, Valenti L, Romeo S. Genetics and epigenetics of NAFLD and NASH: Clinical impact. J Hepatol 2018; 68(2): 268-79.
[http://dx.doi.org/10.1016/j.jhep.2017.09.003] [PMID: 29122391]

[106] Plaza-Díaz J, Solis-Urra P, Aragón-Vela J, Rodríguez-Rodríguez F, Olivares-Arancibia J, Álvarez-Mercado AI. Insights into the impact of microbiota in the treatment of NAFLD/NASH and its potential as a biomarker for prognosis and diagnosis. Biomedicines 2021; 9(2): 145.
[http://dx.doi.org/10.3390/biomedicines9020145] [PMID: 33546191]

[107] Ajmera V, Loomba R. Imaging biomarkers of NAFLD, NASH, and fibrosis. Mol Metab 2021; 50: 101167.
[http://dx.doi.org/10.1016/j.molmet.2021.101167] [PMID: 33460786]

[108] Masoodi M, Gastaldelli A, Hyötyläinen T, *et al.* Metabolomics and lipidomics in NAFLD: biomarkers and non-invasive diagnostic tests. Nat Rev Gastroenterol Hepatol 2021; 18(12): 835-56.
[http://dx.doi.org/10.1038/s41575-021-00502-9] [PMID: 34508238]

[109] Lorbek G, Urlep Ž, Rozman D. Pharmacogenomic and personalized approaches to tackle nonalcoholic

fatty liver disease. Pharmacogenomics 2016; 17(11): 1273-88.
[http://dx.doi.org/10.2217/pgs-2016-0047] [PMID: 27377717]

[110] Montemayor S, Bouzas C, Mascaró CM, *et al.* Effect of dietary and lifestyle interventions on the amelioration of NAFLD in patients with metabolic syndrome: the FLIPAN study. Nutrients 2022; 14(11): 2223.
[http://dx.doi.org/10.3390/nu14112223] [PMID: 35684022]

[111] Maestri M, Santopaolo F, Pompili M, Gasbarrini A, Ponziani FR. Gut microbiota modulation in patients with non-alcoholic fatty liver disease: Effects of current treatments and future strategies. Front Nutr 2023; 10: 1110536.
[http://dx.doi.org/10.3389/fnut.2023.1110536] [PMID: 36875849]

[112] Chen JYS, Chua D, Lim CO, Ho WX, Tan NS. Lessons on drug development: a literature review of challenges faced in nonalcoholic fatty liver disease (NAFLD) clinical trials. Int J Mol Sci 2022; 24(1): 158.
[http://dx.doi.org/10.3390/ijms24010158] [PMID: 36613602]

[113] Tanaka N, Kimura T, Fujimori N, Nagaya T, Komatsu M, Tanaka E. Current status, problems, and perspectives of non-alcoholic fatty liver disease research. World J Gastroenterol 2019; 25(2): 163-77.
[http://dx.doi.org/10.3748/wjg.v25.i2.163] [PMID: 30670907]

[114] Ocker M. Challenges and opportunities in drug development for nonalcoholic steatohepatitis. Eur J Pharmacol 2020; 870: 172913.
[http://dx.doi.org/10.1016/j.ejphar.2020.172913] [PMID: 31926994]

[115] Berardo C, Di Pasqua LG, Cagna M, Richelmi P, Vairetti M, Ferrigno A. Nonalcoholic fatty liver disease and non-alcoholic steatohepatitis: current issues and future perspectives in preclinical and clinical research. Int J Mol Sci 2020; 21(24): 9646.
[http://dx.doi.org/10.3390/ijms21249646] [PMID: 33348908]

[116] Gottlieb A, Mosthael W, Sowa JP, Canbay A. Nonalcoholic-fatty-liver-disease and nonalcoholic steatohepatitis: successful development of pharmacological treatment will depend on translational research. Digestion 2019; 100(2): 79-85.
[http://dx.doi.org/10.1159/000493259] [PMID: 30537758]

[117] Roeb E. Non-alcoholic fatty liver diseases: current challenges and future directions. Ann Transl Med 2021; 9(8): 726.
[http://dx.doi.org/10.21037/atm-20-3760] [PMID: 33987424]

[118] Geier A, Tiniakos D, Denk H, Trauner M. From the origin of NASH to the future of metabolic fatty liver disease. Gut 2021; 70(8): 1570-9.
[http://dx.doi.org/10.1136/gutjnl-2020-323202] [PMID: 33632710]

[119] Harvey BE. How improvements in US FDA regulatory process and procedures led to the drug approval for first ever treatment of a common liver disease. Acta Pharmacol Sin 2025; 46(3): 515-24.
[PMID: 39511464]

[120] Fleming GA, Harvey BE. Regulatory considerations for early clinical development of drugs for diabetes, obesity, nonalcoholic steatohepatitis (NASH) and other cardiometabolic disorders. In: LeRoith D, Taylor SI, Olefsky JM, Eds. Translational research methods in diabetes, obesity, and nonalcoholic fatty liver disease. Cham (CH): Springer; 2019. p.487-515.
[http://dx.doi.org/10.1007/978-3-030-11748-1_19]

[121] Sergi CM. NAFLD (MASLD)/NASH (MASH): does it bother to label at all? A comprehensive narrative review. Int J Mol Sci 2024; 25(15): 8462.
[http://dx.doi.org/10.3390/ijms25158462] [PMID: 39126031]

[122] Pirola CJ, Salatino A, Quintanilla MF, Castaño GO, Garaycoechea M, Sookoian S. The influence of host genetics on liver microbiome composition in patients with NAFLD. EBioMedicine 2022; 76: 103858.
[http://dx.doi.org/10.1016/j.ebiom.2022.103858] [PMID: 35092912]

[123] Wei S, Wang L, Evans PC, Xu S. NAFLD and NASH: etiology, targets and emerging therapies. Drug Discov Today 2024; 29(3): 103910.
[http://dx.doi.org/10.1016/j.drudis.2024.103910] [PMID: 38301798]

[124] Di Bartolomeo A, George J. Future directions for fatty liver disease In: Metabolic steatotic liver disease: current knowledge, therapeutic treatments, and future directions. 2024; pp. 297-317.
[http://dx.doi.org/10.1016/B978-0-323-99649-5.00016-9]

[125] Eeda V, Patil NY, Joshi AD, Awasthi V. Advancements in metabolic□associated steatotic liver disease research: Diagnostics, small molecule developments, and future directions. Hepatol Res 2024; 54(3): 222-34.
[http://dx.doi.org/10.1111/hepr.14008] [PMID: 38149861]

[126] Mak LY, Liu K, Chirapongsathorn S, *et al.* Liver diseases and hepatocellular carcinoma in the Asia-Pacific region: burden, trends, challenges and future directions. Nat Rev Gastroenterol Hepatol 2024; 21(12): 834-51.
[http://dx.doi.org/10.1038/s41575-024-00967-4] [PMID: 39147893]

[127] Geng W, Liao W, Cao X, Yang Y. Therapeutic targets and approaches to manage inflammation of NAFLD. Biomedicines 2025; 13(2): 393.
[http://dx.doi.org/10.3390/biomedicines13020393] [PMID: 40002806]

CHAPTER 9

Nanocarrier-based Imaging Agents for Fatty Liver Disease Diagnosis

Hadi Sardarabadi[1], **Saeedeh Zare Jalise**[2], **Piao Yang**[3] and **Mohsen Sheykhhasan**[4,*]

[1] *Department of Pharmacology and Medical Physics, Faculty of Medicine, Qom University of Medical Sciences, Qom, Iran*

[2] *Department of Tissue Engineering and Applied Cell Sciences, School of Medicine, Qom University of Medical Sciences, Qom, Iran*

[3] *Department of Molecular Genetics, College of Arts and Sciences, The Ohio State University, Columbus, OH, USA*

[4] *Cellular and Molecular Research Center, Qom University of Medical Sciences, Qom, Iran*

Abstract: Given the disadvantages of liver transplantation, including chronic immunosuppression, invasiveness, and a lack of donor livers, prompt diagnosis of fatty liver diseases is crucial. Nanocarriers have emerged as a transformative technology in the diagnosis and management of fatty liver diseases, which encompass a range of metabolic disorders characterized by abnormal fatty acid metabolism. This chapter explores the innovative applications of biocompatible nanocarriers to enhance diagnostic accuracy and efficiency in fatty acid diseases. By encapsulating diagnostic agents, including contrast agents and biomarkers, nanocarriers facilitate delivery to affected tissues through active and passive targeting, thereby improving the sensitivity and specificity of detection methods. Furthermore, their unique physicochemical properties enable real-time monitoring of metabolic processes, providing invaluable insights into disease progression and treatment responses. This chapter also discusses the integration of nanocarrier-based diagnostics with advanced imaging techniques, such as magnetic resonance imaging (MRI) and computed tomography (CT), to visualize fatty acid metabolism *in vivo*. Additionally, we address the challenges and future perspectives in the development of nanocarriers for clinical application, including biocompatibility, regulatory hurdles, and scalability. By harnessing the potential of nanocarriers, researchers and clinicians can pave the way for more effective diagnostic tools, ultimately leading to improved patient outcomes in fatty acid diseases.

Keywords: Fatty liver disease, Imaging agents, Nanocarriers, Real-time monitoring, Targeting.

[*] **Corresponding author Mohsen Sheykhhasan:** Cellular and Molecular Research Center, Qom University of Medical Sciences, Qom, Iran; E-mail: msheykhhasan@muq.ac.ir

Anjali Sharma, Devkant Sharma, Ajmer Singh Grewal, Geeta Deswal & Ganga Reddy Velma (Eds.)

INTRODUCTION

Fatty liver disease is characterized by excessive fat accumulation in liver cells. It is categorized into two main types: alcoholic fatty liver disease (AFLD) and non-alcoholic fatty liver disease (NAFLD). NAFLD is a generic term that encompasses the spectrum of non-alcoholic fatty liver (NAFL), non-alcoholic steatohepatitis (NASH), and NASH-related cirrhosis [1]. Simple steatosis is generally benign, while NASH can lead to significant liver damage and complications. The pathophysiology of NAFLD involves insulin resistance, oxidative stress, inflammation, and dysregulation of hepatic lipid metabolism. Accurate and early diagnosis is crucial for effective management and treatment of the disease. Traditional imaging techniques such as ultrasound, computed tomography (CT), and magnetic resonance imaging (MRI) have limitations in sensitivity and specificity for diagnosing fatty liver disease. Recent advancements in nanotechnology have opened new avenues for developing novel imaging agents that enhance diagnostic accuracy (Fig. **1**).

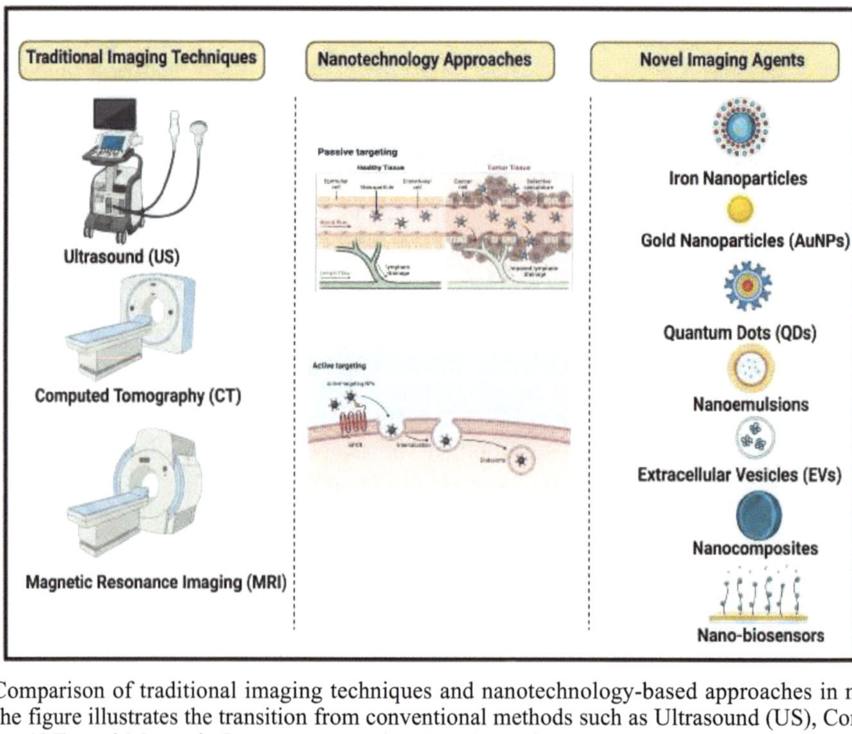

Fig. (1). Comparison of traditional imaging techniques and nanotechnology-based approaches in medical imaging. The figure illustrates the transition from conventional methods such as Ultrasound (US), Computed Tomography (CT), and Magnetic Resonance Imaging (MRI) to advanced nanotechnology-driven imaging agents, including Iron Nanoparticles, Gold Nanoparticles (AuNPs), Quantum Dots (QDs), Nanoemulsions, Extracellular Vesicles (EVs), Nanocomposites, and Nano-biosensors. These novel imaging agents offer enhanced precision and functionality in diagnostic applications.

Numerous methods have been employed to diagnose fatty liver disease, each with its own advantages and limitations. Ultrasound is commonly the first-line imaging technique used for detecting fatty liver due to its safety, widespread availability, and cost-effectiveness. However, its sensitivity in detecting and grading steatosis can be compromised, particularly in patients with larger body habitus. In such cases, steatosis may be overestimated due to beam attenuation caused by surrounding adipose tissue rather than liver fat itself. Additionally, ultrasound provides relatively imprecise qualitative classifications of steatosis, ranging from mild to severe, and can struggle to differentiate between steatosis and fibrosis in patients with chronic liver disease. Factors such as shadowing from ribs or gas can obscure portions of the liver, further complicating assessment, as ultrasound measurements serve as indirect indices of fat content [2]. Machine learning-based ultrasound imaging is increasingly recognized for its effectiveness in detecting and quantifying non-alcoholic fatty liver disease (NAFLD). Techniques such as transient elastography, acoustic radiation force impulse, and magnetic resonance elastography provide accurate measurements of liver stiffness, a key indicator of fibrosis. However, these methods often entail high costs, limited availability, and a need for skilled operators, hindering widespread adoption [3]. Computed tomography (CT) scans offer rapid acquisition, straightforward analysis, and quantitative results; however, they are limited in accurately diagnosing mild steatosis and expose patients to ionizing radiation. CT scan calibration can vary significantly across scanners, manufacturers, and reconstruction algorithms, leading to variability in results. Moreover, the attenuation of X-ray beams is not specific to steatosis [4]. Magnetic Resonance Imaging (MRI) is superior in distinguishing fat from water and quantifying fat content more accurately than ultrasound or CT. MRI assesses the proton density fat fraction (PDFF), a fundamental tissue property that does not require internal calibration or reference standards. This allows for volumetric assessments of steatosis. Nonetheless, MRI is often more expensive and less accessible than other imaging modalities. Additionally, motion artifacts and parallel imaging can negatively affect measurement accuracy, and magnitude data-based MRI struggles to differentiate fat fractions above and below 50%. Current MRI techniques also face challenges with $R2^*$ correction [5]. While liver biopsy remains the gold standard for diagnosing non-alcoholic fatty liver disease (NAFLD) and evaluating its severity, it is an invasive procedure prone to observer bias and lacks standardization. Non-invasive testing methods can be categorized into blood-based biomarker tests and imaging techniques. Blood-based tests, particularly multi-biomarker panels, can effectively measure biological processes within the liver and are often more accessible and cost-effective than imaging methods. For instance, the Fibrosis-4 index and enhanced liver fibrosis panel show promise in detecting advanced fibrosis and predicting disease progression. However, these tests may be influenced by factors such as age and gender, limiting their efficacy in staging liver disorders. Recently, efforts have been made to diagnose NASH using various biomarkers, scoring systems, and imaging techniques such as elastography. The NAFIC score, derived from the levels of ferritin, fasting insulin, and type IV collagen 7S, has shown promise in diagnosing NASH. Meanwhile, the NAFLD fibrosis score and the FIB-4 index are effective tools for ruling out NASH in patients with advanced fibrosis [6].

Consequently, researchers are exploring innovative imaging techniques, including nanotechnology applications. Nanotechnology involves manipulating materials at the nanoscale (1-100 nm) to develop new properties and functionalities. In medical imaging, nanoparticles can function as contrast agents, enhancing the visibility of tissues and lesions. Their small size facilitates improved tissue penetration and offers increased surface area for drug delivery, enabling targeted imaging. While contrast agents can be considered under the definition of drugs, they may also pose toxicity risks to healthy cells, necessitating minimal interaction with them. For instance, gadolinium-based contrast agents commonly used in MRI are known for their cytotoxicity and can lead to adverse effects such as injection-site discomfort, nausea, and headaches [7]. To mitigate these risks, researchers are investigating methods such as encapsulating contrast agents within carriers to optimize delivery. The carrier's size is critical; it must be appropriately sized based on the targeted delivery site. The kidneys may rapidly clear small carriers, while larger carriers risk vascular blockage. Studies indicate that nanoscale carriers exhibit unique properties that enhance their effectiveness in medical applications.

Nanocarriers are nanoscale delivery systems designed to transport therapeutic or diagnostic agents to specific sites within the body (Fig. **2**). They can be composed of various materials, including lipids, polymers, metals, or silica. The choice of nanocarrier affects the stability, release profile, and biodistribution of the loaded agents. In this section, we will explore a range of advanced imaging techniques for evaluating fatty liver disease, highlighting the unique strengths and limitations of each. Furthermore, we will unveil a groundbreaking nanotechnology solution that promises to enhance diagnosis and treatment, making it a pivotal tool for effectively managing this condition.

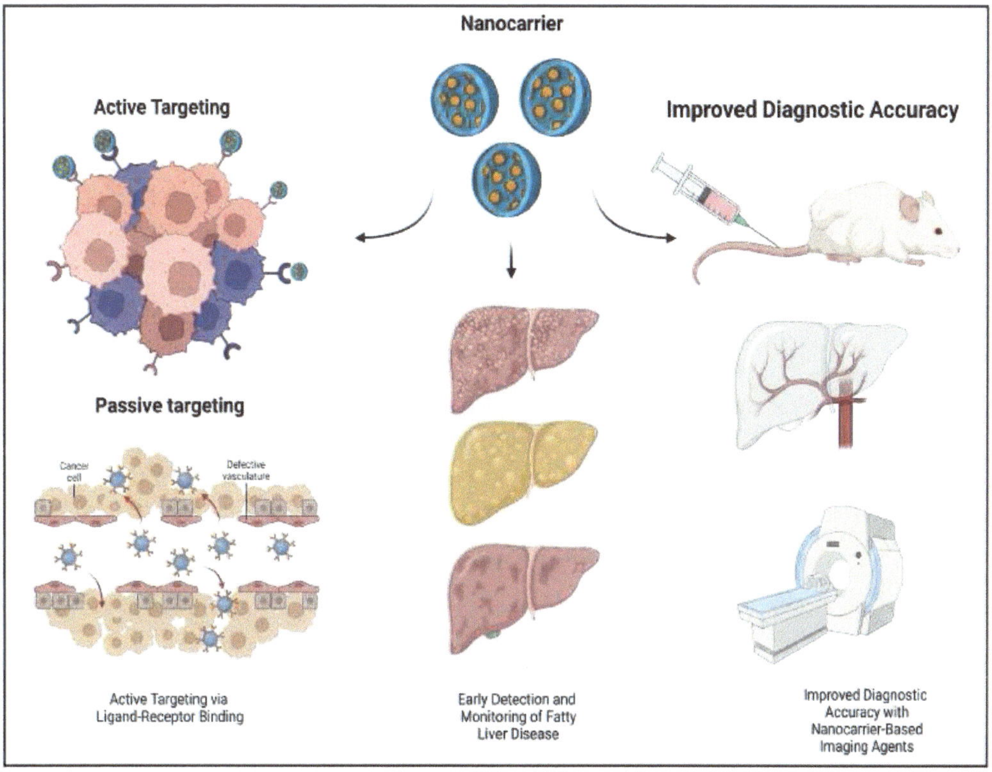

Fig. (2). Schematic illustration of a nanocarrier system for targeted drug delivery. The diagram highlights active targeting mechanisms, including ligand-receptor binding, and passive targeting through the enhanced permeability and retention (EPR) effect in cancer cells with defective vasculature. Additionally, the figure emphasizes the role of nanocarriers in improving diagnostic accuracy, particularly in early detection and monitoring of diseases such as fatty liver disease, using nanocarrier-based imaging agents.

NANOCARRIERS TO TARGETED DELIVERY OF IMAGING AGENTS

The Main Physicochemical Properties of Nanocarriers

Due to their small size and distinctive properties, these nanoparticles are highly effective for the targeted delivery of drugs and biological compounds. This section discusses the physicochemical properties of nanocarriers and examines how these properties influence the performance of the medications delivered. The physicochemical properties of nanocarriers, such as size, shape, surface characteristics, electrical charge, and optical properties, significantly influence their behavior and effectiveness. Understanding these properties is crucial for optimizing nanocarrier performance in various applications.

Size and Shape

The size of nanocarriers is crucial for their biological effectiveness. Although the optimal diameter varies by application, ligand-coated spherical nanoparticles ranging from 30 to 60 nm effectively bind to cellular receptors, facilitating the membrane-wrapping process necessary for endocytosis without receptor shortages [8]. However, many nanoparticles fail to reach their intended targets and are often sequestered by the liver and spleen if larger than 6 nm, or eliminated via the kidneys if smaller than 6 nm. Additionally, the shape of nanoparticles significantly affects their distribution and absorption in the body [9]. Generally, spherical nanoparticles are more readily taken up by cells compared to non-spherical ones. For imaging purposes, rod-shaped nanocarriers, which possess a high aspect ratio, may offer longer circulation times due to their resistance to phagocytic cell uptake, making them advantageous over spherical counterparts in certain applications [10].

Surface Characteristics

The surface properties of nanocarriers are critical to their effectiveness and include surface chemistry, surface area, surface roughness, and the ability to agglomerate, which play a main role in determining their stability and toxicity [11]. The electrical charge of nanoparticles significantly influences their interaction with target cells. For instance, positively charged nanoparticles demonstrate a stronger attraction to negatively and neutral charged surfaces, enhancing their targeting efficiency [12]. Surface charge can affect cell membrane permeability and overall cell health [13]. Furthermore, optimal surface functionalization not only improves solubility but also boosts the stability of nanocarriers, making them even more effective in various applications [14]. Nanocarriers with appropriate coatings generally exhibit greater stability and can retain drugs for longer periods. The results have shown that functionalizing nanocarriers with cell-penetrating peptides can affect their intracellular fate, such that a nanocarrier may be degraded by secondary endosomes after entering the cell [15].

In vivo Imaging Capabilities of Biocompatible Targeted Nanocarriers

Fatty liver disease, which encompasses both alcoholic and non-alcoholic forms (NAFLD), has become an urgent global health challenge due to its rising prevalence and link to metabolic disorders. This condition involves harmful fat buildup in liver cells (hepatocytes), leading to inflammation and fibrosis, and it can progress to severe consequences like cirrhosis or liver cancer (hepatocellular carcinoma). It is vital to prioritize early diagnosis and ongoing monitoring of fatty liver disease for effective management and intervention. Unfortunately, traditional imaging techniques, such as ultrasound and computed tomography (CT), often fall short in sensitivity for early detection. Therefore, leveraging advanced imaging technologies that incorporate biocompatible targeted nanocarriers offers a promising solution to enhance diagnostic accuracy and ultimately improve patient outcomes.

Biocompatible targeted nanocarriers represent a revolutionary advancement in drug delivery and imaging technologies. These innovative nanoscale systems are crafted to deliver therapeutic agents precisely to specific cells or tissues, maximizing the efficacy of treatments. Composed of diverse materials, including lipids, polymers, and inorganic substances, these carriers are designed with safety in mind. Their biocompatibility ensures minimal adverse reactions when administered *in vivo*, making them a reliable choice for next-generation medical applications [16].

Targeting mechanisms are crucial in modern medicine and can be categorized into two powerful approaches: passive targeting and active targeting (Fig. **2**) [17]. Passive targeting leverages the enhanced permeability and retention (EPR) effect, which enables nanoparticles to accumulate in tumor tissues by exploiting the leaky blood vessels (Fig. **2**). This method significantly enhances the delivery of treatments to cancer sites while minimizing damage to healthy tissues. In contrast, active targeting elevates this concept by functionalizing nanocarriers with ligands that specifically bind to receptors overexpressed on cancer cells. Active targeting involves interactions between specific biological systems, such as antigen-antibody, ligand-receptor, and enzyme-substrate [18]. This precision not only improves the effectiveness of therapies but also paves the way for more personalized treatment options, ensuring that patients receive the most targeted and efficient care possible.

In vivo imaging involves the visualization of biological processes occurring within a living organism. This technique offers essential insights into disease progression, treatment effectiveness, and interactions at the cellular and molecular levels. Biocompatible targeted nanocarriers improve *in vivo* imaging through various mechanisms.

NOVEL IMAGING AGENTS FOR MONITORING FATTY LIVER DISEASE STATES

Drawbacks of Traditional Imaging Agents and Nanotechnology Approaches

Fatty liver disease, which ranges from simple steatosis to nonalcoholic steatohepatitis (NASH), has become an urgent global health crisis. The alarming rise in obesity, diabetes, and metabolic syndrome has caused a surge in fatty liver disease cases, highlighting the pressing need for reliable diagnostic tools for early detection and ongoing monitoring. While traditional imaging techniques such as ultrasound (US), computed tomography (CT), and magnetic resonance imaging (MRI) are commonly used to assess liver fat content and diagnose fatty liver disease (Fig. **1**), they have significant limitations that can limit their effectiveness. This section aims to shed light on the shortcomings of these traditional imaging approaches in the context of fatty liver disease, emphasizing the need for improved diagnostic strategies via the application of nanomaterials.

Optical Imaging

Optical imaging techniques, such as fluorescence and bioluminescence imaging, use fluorescent or luminescent probes attached to nanocarriers. Once these advanced nanocarriers are introduced into the body, they can be precisely tracked using sophisticated imaging technologies. For instance, near-infrared (NIR) fluorescent dyes can be conjugated to targeted nanocarriers, enabling real-time imaging with extended excitation and emission wavelengths in the NIR range, thereby ensuring adequate tissue penetration depth *in vivo* [19]. The exceptional sensitivity and resolution of optical imaging render it an invaluable tool for monitoring cellular uptake and biodistribution, facilitating significant advancements in medical diagnostics and therapeutics. Fluorescent probes that exhibit excellent optical performance, high sensitivity, and real-time monitoring capabilities have become essential for detecting lipid droplets, particularly for diagnosing fatty liver disease [20]. Unlike other imaging modalities such as X-ray or magnetic resonance imaging (MRI), optical imaging benefits from a diverse array of contrast mechanisms. Endogenous contrasts present in many biological systems include the varying absorption characteristics of oxy- and deoxyhemoglobin, lipids, and water, as well as the intrinsic fluorescence of substances like keratin, elastin, collagen cross-links, phospholipids, tryptophan, retinol, lipofuscin, and key metabolites such as nicotinamide adenine dinucleotide and flavin adenine dinucleotide. Moreover, *in vivo* imaging reduces variability in inter-animal comparisons and enables real-time observation of physiological processes rather than relying solely on static post-mortem histological analyses

[21]. Compared to traditional small-molecule probes, nanoprobe technology demonstrates higher selectivity for early indicators of liver injury, such as peroxynitrite (ONOO−), longer liver retention times, and broader dynamic response ranges to glutathione (GSH) following oxidation by ONOO. Adenosine triphosphate (ATP) is a crucial biomolecule that serves as the primary energy source for cells and acts as a marker for diseases such as cancer and fatty liver. A study presents a novel near-infrared fluorescent nanoprobe, ZIF-90@SiR, developed from a zeolitic imidazole framework. The nanoprobe is synthesized by encapsulating the dye SiR within the ZIF-90 framework. When ATP is introduced, the structure of ZIF-90@SiR is disrupted, releasing SiR and generating near-infrared fluorescence at 670 nm. The ZIF-90@SiR nanoprobe demonstrates high sensitivity and selectivity for ATP detection, along with excellent biocompatibility due to its low toxicity. It enables fluorescence imaging of ATP in living cells, effectively distinguishing between normal, cancer, and fatty liver cells in mice [22, 23]. Hydrogen polysulfides (H2Sn, $n > 1$) are recognized as important signaling mediators in various physiological processes. However, their roles and signaling pathways in complex diseases like nonalcoholic fatty liver disease (NAFLD) remain unclear due to the lack of selective detection tools for intracellular H2Sn. In a study, researchers developed a ratiometric fluorescent nanoprobe, PPG-Np-RhPhCO, via recognition-site screening and nanoparticle self-assembly, thereby enhancing selectivity, photostability, and biocompatibility. This probe successfully imaged H2Sn in NAFLD for the first time, elucidating H2Sn-generating pathways and offering insights into future drug development [24]. However, despite its numerous advantages, *in vivo* optical imaging faces significant challenges, with light scattering being the most prominent obstacle to its implementation [25].

Ultrasound (US)

Ultrasound stands out as the primary imaging technique for evaluating fatty liver disease, due to its wide availability, affordability, and safety, as it does not expose patients to ionizing radiation. Nevertheless, it is essential to acknowledge that certain limitations can influence its diagnostic precision. Currently, two intravascular ultrasound contrast agents, Lumason and Definity, are clinically available in the USA for liver imaging [26]. However, there are two critical considerations regarding these agents. First, size is a crucial factor when targeting specific body regions. The vascular environment imposes an upper size limit of approximately 12 micrometers to prevent blood flow obstructions [27]. In contrast, there is no theoretical lower size limit for these agents. Second, the functionalization and stability of the contrast agents are vital. Research indicates that nanodroplets exhibit significantly higher stability than microbubbles, with half-lives of around 11 minutes compared to 3.5 minutes for microbubbles [28]. This enhanced stability has led to increased interest in nanobubbles as both imaging and drug delivery agents, offering potential advantages over traditional microbubble contrast agents [29]. Researchers developed a novel multifunctional nanobubble using poly(lactic-co-glycolic acid) (PLGA) as an ultrasound imaging contrast agent, doxorubicin carrier, and enhancer of ultrasound-mediated drug delivery. The doxorubicin nanobubble (DOX-NB), encapsulating carbon tetrafluoride gas, has prepared via a double emulsion method. *In vivo* evaluations demonstrated enhanced ultrasonic functionality and confirmed its antitumor effects. The nanobubble measured 500 nm in diameter, with a potential of -23 mV, achieving drug-loading and encapsulation efficiencies of 78.6% and 7.4%, respectively, thereby significantly improving ultrasound imaging and antitumor efficacy [30].

Computed Tomography (CT)

Computed tomography (CT) provides high-resolution images that accurately identify liver lesions. However, it is crucial to acknowledge its limitations when evaluating fatty liver disease, as these limitations can impede accurate diagnosis and treatment options. Contrast-enhanced CT, which assesses the liver-minu--spleen difference of 19 Hounsfield Units (HU) or less, has shown modest sensitivity and high specificity for diagnosing moderate to severe steatosis during the portal venous phase post-contrast. Despite this, contrast-enhanced CT is not typically used for clinical evaluation of steatosis due to overlap in HU values between normal and abnormal liver tissue, as well as variability in HU values based on scan delay and contrast protocols [31]. Several types of contrast materials are used in imaging studies, including iodine-based and barium sulfate compounds. Iodinated contrast media, which contain iodine atoms, are commonly used in X-ray-based imaging modalities, such as CT. While these agents can enhance image quality, they are not without risks. Late adverse reactions following the administration of intravascular iodinated contrast media may include symptoms such as nausea, vomiting, headaches, itching, skin rashes, musculoskeletal pain, and fever [32]. In contrast, adverse reactions associated with barium sulfate during radiological examinations of the digestive tract are relatively rare, and the procedures are generally considered low risk. Most side effects from barium sulfate administration tend to be mild and self-limiting, such as constipation, diarrhea, or cramping, often resolving without medical intervention within a few days. Nonetheless, more serious adverse reactions can occur, ranging from mild symptoms like urticaria and pruritus to severe complications such as edema of the head or neck, difficulty breathing, or even anaphylactic shock, which can be fatal. The likelihood of experiencing various adverse reactions and iatrogenic injuries is influenced by several factors, including the patient's clinical history and overall health status. Understanding these risks is essential for healthcare providers when considering the use of contrast agents in imaging studies, particularly for patients with known sensitivities or pre-existing conditions that may heighten their risk of complications [33].

Magnetic Resonance Imaging (MRI)

Magnetic resonance imaging (MRI) is recognized for its effective, non-invasive, and quantitative evaluation of liver fat content. However, it is essential to acknowledge the limitations of this imaging modality. Ideally, contrast agents should have low limits of detection (LOD) at lower doses. In MRI, only a minimal amount of contrast agent (in the micromolar range) is required; however, the doses administered in practice can be relatively high, raising concerns about safety and potential secondary toxicity. Gadolinium-based magnetic resonance contrast agents (MRCAs) have been linked to nephrogenic systemic fibrosis (NSF) and may pose risks to various body systems [34]. Consequently, only a limited number of MRCAs have received approval from the U.S. Food and Drug Administration (FDA) [35]. Another drawback of conventional MRI contrast agents is their low signal-to-noise ratios, which are attributed to relaxivity issues [36]. Furthermore, the routine application of MRI for liver fat quantification faces challenges due to variability in results stemming from differences in MRI systems, scanning parameters, and analytical methods [37]. The limited clinical adoption of liver-specific MR contrast agents can be attributed to several factors, including logistical challenges in integrating them into standard workflows, safety concerns, and a lack of commercial viability. These issues have contributed to the scarcity of liver-specific MRCAs in clinical practice, ultimately hindering their widespread application for accurate assessment of liver fat content. Addressing these limitations is crucial for enhancing the reliability and safety of MRI as a tool for evaluating hepatic steatosis [38]. Among these, magnetic resonance imaging (MRI) stands out for its non-invasive nature, high resolution, and excellent soft-tissue contrast. Recent developments in MRI, including magnetic resonance spectroscopy (MRS) and magnetic resonance elastography (MRE), have improved the detection and grading of hepatic fat and fibrosis [39, 40].

Nanomaterial-based Contrast Agents to Cover the Imaging Limitations

Nanomaterial-based contrast agents revolutionize imaging techniques by dramatically enhancing signal intensity and contrast resolution. With the ability to be specifically designed to target liver tissues or key cellular components linked to fatty liver disease, these agents offer a groundbreaking approach to diagnosis (Fig. 1). For instance, by functionalizing nanoparticles with ligands or antibodies that bind receptors overexpressed in fatty liver tissues, we can achieve exceptional targeted imaging, enabling earlier detection and improved patient outcomes.

Iron Nanoparticles

Magnetic resonance imaging (MRI) stands out as a vital non-invasive imaging technique, offering exceptionally high-resolution images of soft tissues. By designing biocompatible, targeted nanocarriers infused with superparamagnetic nanoparticles like iron oxide, we can revolutionize MRI contrast agents. These advanced carriers significantly enhance contrast between tumors and surrounding healthy tissues, enabling clearer, more accurate visualization of tumors during MRI scans. This innovation not only enhances diagnostic capabilities but also paves the way for better-targeted treatments in clinical settings. Due to their large surface area-to-volume ratio, magnetic nanoparticles often agglomerate and adsorb plasma proteins. As a result, the body's reticuloendothelial system (RES), particularly the Kupffer cells in the liver, typically takes up these nanoparticles due to their hydrophobic surfaces [41].

Molecular imaging for liver fibrosis is often constrained by the scarcity of biomarkers that reliably correlate with fibrosis grades. Researchers have evaluated the potential of fibroblast activation protein alpha (FAPα) as a grading biomarker for liver fibrosis through transcriptional analysis and biological assays on clinical liver samples. Findings revealed strong linear correlations between FAPα protein and mRNA expression and fibrosis grade ($R^2 = 0.89$ and 0.91, respectively). A FAPα-responsive MRI molecular nanoprobe was developed for the quantitative assessment of liver fibrosis, comprising superparamagnetic amorphous iron nanoparticles (AFeNPs) and paramagnetic gadoteric acid (Gd-DOTA) linked by FAPα-responsive peptide chains (ASGPAGPA). As liver fibrosis progressed, increased FAPα cleaved more ASGPAGPA, resulting in a heightened T1-MRI signal from Gd-DOTA. In contrast, the signal remained suppressed due to the distance-dependent magnetic resonance tuning (MRET) effect between AFeNPs and Gd-DOTA. The nanoprobe effectively differentiated fibrosis stages F1, F2, F3, and F4 in patient samples, achieving area under the curve values of 99.8%, 66.7%, 70.4%, and 96.3%, respectively. This approach demonstrated significant potential for early detection and grading of liver fibrosis in clinical settings [42].

While various imaging techniques, including dynamic computed tomography and enhanced MRI, are used in practice, SPION-enhanced MRI remains crucial for diagnosing hepatocellular carcinoma (HCC). Following intravenous administration, SPIONs are rapidly taken up by Kupffer cells, thereby enhancing tumor-to-liver contrast, as tumors lack these cells. This method has proven effective for identifying hypovascular HCC not visible on standard Gd-contrast imaging and for differentiating benign lesions from HCC. However, limitations include challenges in assessing lesion vascularity and the minimal signal intensity reduction in cirrhotic versus normal liver tissue. Clinically approved SPIONs for liver cancer imaging include Ferumoxide (Endorem, Ferridex) and Ferucarbotran (Resovist). Recently, UltraSPIONs have been utilized to create a "nanotheragnostic" system that integrates anticancer therapy with imaging capabilities by embedding them within squalenoyl-drug conjugate nanoparticles [43].

The pathogenesis of non-alcoholic fatty liver disease (NAFLD) remains poorly understood. Kupffer cells (KCs), liver-resident macrophages, typically protect against the translocation of endotoxins into systemic circulation. However, it is unclear whether their phagocytic function is compromised in NAFLD. Superparamagnetic iron oxide (SPIO) magnetic resonance imaging, which relies on KC function, was employed alongside abdominal CT and histological examination of liver biopsies to assess steatosis in NAFLD patients and chronic hepatitis C controls. Additionally, SPIO-MRI was conducted on normal rats fed a methionine-choline-deficient diet to induce non-alcoholic steatohepatitis (NASH) and on obese Zucker fa/fa rats. Results indicated that relative signal enhancement (RSE) was inversely related to KC function and correlated with steatosis severity, revealing impaired phagocytic uptake rather than reduced KC numbers in NAFLD [44].

While omics analyses offer non-invasive insights, they often require extensive sample collection and meticulous operational protocols, which can delay data interpretation. In contrast, the rapid and intuitive capabilities of MRI make it an appealing alternative for NASH diagnosis, particularly with the use of MRI contrast agents. Magnetic nanoparticles (MNPs), particularly superparamagnetic iron oxide nanoparticles (SPIOs), have shown promise due to their enhanced contrast and reduced cytotoxicity compared to traditional agents. Recent modifications to SPIOs have improved their stability and biocompatibility, making them effective for MRI applications in NASH diagnosis [45]. Additionally, cationized ferritin (CF) has emerged as a sensitive contrast agent, revealing alterations in liver microstructure associated with NASH through T2-weighted MRI [46, 47]. Collectively, these advancements suggest that MRI and novel contrast agents could serve as valuable tools in the non-invasive diagnosis of chronic liver diseases like NASH. In addition to T2-weighted imaging, integrated T1 and T2-weighted imaging using superparamagnetic iron oxide (SPIO) nanoparticles enhances diagnostic accuracy for non-alcoholic steatohepatitis (NASH).

Nanoemulsion

Nanoemulsions are highly effective, kinetically stable liquid-in-liquid dispersions characterized by droplet sizes of approximately 100 nm. Their minute size enables remarkable properties, including an impressive surface area per unit volume, exceptional stability, a visually appealing transparent appearance, and customizable rheological behavior, making them an ideal choice for various applications. In a study, researchers investigated the use of an intravenously delivered perfluorocarbon (PFC) nanoemulsion and fluorine-19 (F-19) MRI to detect inflammation in a non-alcoholic fatty liver disease (NAFLD) mouse model. C57BL/6 mice were fed either a standard or high-fat diet (HFD) for six weeks to induce NAFLD. Baseline hydrogen-1 (H-1) MRI measurements of proton density fat fraction (PDFF) and T-1 relaxation times were taken before administering the PFC nanoemulsion, allowing for subsequent F-19 MRI imaging of liver PFC uptake. Longitudinal assessments were conducted at 2, 21, and 42 days post-administration. Results showed significant increases in liver volume, PDFF, and total PFC uptake in HFD mice, alongside decreased liver fluorine density and T-1 relaxation times, indicating F-19 MRI's potential as a biomarker for liver pathology [48].

Gold Nanoparticles

Gold nanoparticles (AuNPs) are a promising advancement in imaging technologies due to their excellent biocompatibility and functionalization versatility. They can be tailored to detect key biomarkers linked to fatty liver disease. Recently, AuNPs have attracted attention for computed tomography (CT) applications due to their high X-ray attenuation, ease of synthesis, and straightforward surface chemistry. By attaching targeting molecules, AuNPs can specifically engage with particular cell types and disease conditions [49].

Quantum Dots

Quantum dots (QDs) are groundbreaking semiconductor nanoparticles with remarkable optical properties, making them a powerful tool for fluorescence imaging. By conjugating QDs with ligands that specifically target hepatic cells or markers of fatty liver disease, we unlock new possibilities for precision diagnostics. Their size-tunable emission spectra provide exceptional multiplexing capabilities, enabling simultaneous imaging of multiple targets within the liver and ultimately enhancing our understanding and treatment of liver conditions. Lipid droplets are dynamic subcellular organelles crucial for understanding the cellular origins of various diseases. However, existing imaging probes often fail to effectively monitor their activity over extended periods. To address this limitation, researchers developed a quantum-dot-based fluorescent nanoprobe for prolonged lipid droplet imaging. This nanoprobe features a quantum dot core, a polymer shell with a zwitterionic surface charge, and optimal lipophilic properties. With a hydrodynamic size of 30–40 nm and near-zero surface charge at physiological pH, it interacts modularly with cell membranes and enters cells primarily through lipid-raft endocytosis, effectively labeling lipid droplets. This innovative nanoprobe enables the investigation of lipid droplet function across various cellular processes, enhancing our understanding of their roles in health and disease [50].

Nonalcoholic fatty liver disease (NAFLD) can progress to liver failure, making early detection crucial for improving treatment outcomes. In situ imaging of overexpressed miR-21 offers a promising diagnostic strategy; however, high signals in living cells often complicate this approach due to the complexity of biological systems. To address this issue, researchers have developed a one-donor-two-acceptor nanoprobe by assembling gold nanoparticles (AuNPs) with BHQ2 (AuBHQ) and quantum dots (QDs) through DNA hybridization for enhanced imaging of miR-21 in living cells. The fluorescence of QDs has been quenched by up to 82.8% via nanometal surface energy transfer and fluorescence resonance energy transfer, significantly reducing background signals. This low-background nanoprobe effectively imaged miR-21 in nonalcoholic fatty liver cells by catalyzing QD disassembly and fluorescence recovery. Additionally, the probe exhibited enhanced sensitivity for miR-21 detection, with a detection limit of 0.22 nM, providing a novel approach for early warning and management of NAFLD [51].

Extracellular Vesicles (EVs)

Currently, the only reliable method for diagnosing and staging non-alcoholic fatty liver disease (NAFLD) is through invasive liver biopsy. However, emerging evidence suggests that components found in circulating extracellular vesicles (EVs), such as RNAs and proteins, may serve as valuable biomarkers for diagnosing NAFLD and non-alcoholic steatohepatitis (NASH) [52]. This indicates the potential of liquid biopsy as a noninvasive and accurate diagnostic tool [53]. For instance, EVs enriched with miR-135a-3p have demonstrated high sensitivity and specificity for NAFLD detection. Studies have shown a significant increase in circulating EVs after an 8-week L-amino acid-defined diet, with miRNA-122 and miR-192 levels elevated in NAFLD patients. These findings suggest that changes in EV levels can serve as early indicators of fatty liver disease, facilitating timely diagnosis [54]. Moreover, the composition of EVs varies dynamically across different stages of NAFLD progression, offering opportunities to identify biomarkers to monitor disease progression. Research by Newman et al. demonstrated that total cell-free RNA and EV-derived miR-128-3p can reliably distinguish between healthy individuals, NAFLD patients, and NASH patients, reflecting the severity of NAFLD [55]. Beyond NAFLD, EVs are also being explored as biomarkers in cancer diagnostics and monitoring [56]. Recent studies have shown that circulating exosome composition changes significantly in obese patients post-bariatric surgery, suggesting their potential as serological markers for evaluating surgical outcomes. Overall, the analysis of peripheral exosome content could become an essential tool for assessing the efficacy of bariatric surgery and monitoring NAFLD progression [57].

Nanocomposites

Nanocomposites are hybrid materials that, when combined, exhibit significantly different properties from their individual components. Researchers developed a NASH probe utilizing ultrasmall iron oxide (USIO) nanoparticles as adjustable magnetic relaxation switches. Sequential modifications with dopamine (DA), polyethylene glycol (PEG), and 5-hydroxytryptamine (5HT) resulted in a nanocomposite (USIO-DA-PEG-5HT) that exhibited spherical morphology and myeloperoxidase (MPO)-sensitive aggregation at inflammatory sites. The 5HT on the USIO surface acts as an MPO substrate, leading to oxidation and dimerization in the presence of H2O2 and MPO. In NASH models, T2 imaging showed significant darkening post-injection, indicating effective nanoparticle aggregation, while T1 imaging brightened in healthy controls, confirming the probe's diagnostic potential for NASH [58].

In a study, researchers successfully synthesized innovative magnetofluorescent hybrid nanoparticles by combining iron oxide nanoparticles with carbon nanoparticles. This advancement not only facilitates in vivo fluorescence imaging but also possesses the critical properties needed for an effective Magnetic Resonance Imaging (MRI) contrast agent. To create dual-functional imaging capabilities, alginate- and pullulan-coated superparamagnetic iron oxide nanoparticles (ASPION and PSPION) were synthesized separately, along with carbon dots (Cdts). The subsequent chemical conjugation of ASPIONs and PSPIONs with Cdts has yielded the remarkable dual-functional nanohybrid particles, ASPION-Cdts and PSPION-Cdts. The potential of these nanohybrids was demonstrated through *in vivo* fluorescence imaging of liver fibrosis in a rodent model, which revealed a strikingly high fluorescence signal in the harvested liver, underscoring the effectiveness of this dual-imaging approach [59].

Polymeric Nanocarriers

A study proposed a dual, non-invasive method for detecting elevated metal levels in patients suffering from liver disease. Researchers successfully synthesized a highly sensitive small-molecule 'pincer' scavenger, specifically designed for the detection and quantification of copper in serum and for monitoring its systemic presence *in vivo*. This innovative technique for in vitro diagnostics offers a significant advantage: it requires only a routine capillary blood sample or venipuncture, thereby eliminating the need for invasive, uncomfortable biopsies. The organic scavenger molecule exhibits impressive specificity for copper ions, boasting a detection sensitivity of 1.35 x 10^(-2) μg/L in mouse serum. Moreover, polymeric nanopincers were meticulously designed for systemic copper detection in the liver. These small-molecule scavengers were effectively incorporated into stable polymeric micelles via their long acyl chains, demonstrating their reliability as carriers when injected intravenously into mice. This remarkable organic scavenger molecule is not only highly fluorescent but also specifically targets Cu^2+, presenting an exciting opportunity to combat diseases associated with copper accumulation in critical organs. The results of this study pave the way for a revolutionary, non-invasive dual nanomedicine approach that enhances early detection and treatment of excessive metal deposits in human organs and ultimately improves patient outcomes [60].

Nano-biosensors for *in vitro* and *in vivo* Sensing of Fatty Liver Diseases

Early-stage nonalcoholic fatty liver disease (NAFLD) often remains undiagnosed, posing a risk of progression to liver cirrhosis and cancer. Developing a non-invasive, cost-effective detection method for early-stage NAFLD is essential for public health. A study presented an innovative on-skin soft adhesive sensor for early-stage NAFLD detection, featuring low electrode-skin contact impedance. Researchers synthesized platinum nanoparticles and reduced graphene quantum dots, then deposited them onto the sensor, thereby enhancing the double-layer capacitance and improving detection accuracy. Additionally, they employed an attention-based deep learning algorithm to differentiate impedance signals from high-fat diet-fed low-density lipoprotein receptor knockout (Ldlr−/−) mice and healthy controls. The combination of the advanced on-skin sensor and the deep learning algorithm achieved a detection accuracy exceeding 97.5%, with an area under the receiver operating characteristic curve (AUC) of 1.0. These findings highlight a promising non-invasive strategy for early-stage NAFLD detection using on-skin electronics and machine learning techniques [61].

The human fatty liver (HFL) volume was assessed using a specialized HFL device that incorporates a nanographene polyvinyl (NGP) sensor and a microcontroller unit (MCU). The NGP sensor detected electromagnetic radiation emitted by fatty liver tissue, which is characterized by its dielectric properties. Unlike traditional medical imaging methods that expose patients to radiation, the HFL device offers continuous monitoring for fatty liver disease, similar to devices used for diabetes and blood pressure management. The NGP sensor is fabricated via spray pyrolysis and consists of materials such as nano graphene, polyacrylic acid, methylenebisacrylamide (MBAAm), and 2,2-dimethoxy-2-phenyl acetophenone (DMPAP) polyvinyl acetate. Positioned on the liver surface, it captures scattering dielectric radiation, which is processed using nonnegative matrix filtering to eliminate noise and extract fatty liver signals. The instantaneous frequency derived from these signals is analyzed with a Gaussian regression model, achieving approximately 85% accuracy when validated against ultrasound-based volume measurements [62].

Intestinal microorganisms play a crucial role in regulating glucose and lipid metabolism, influencing the development of fatty liver. To investigate the relationship between intestinal flora distribution and fatty liver occurrence, researchers extracted fecal DNA from healthy individuals (group C) and fatty liver patients (group D). Using graphene oxide (GO) nano-solid nanopores, they sequenced the V3 and V4 regions of 16S rRNA. The sequencing data were processed with UPARSE 9 software to cluster operational taxonomic units (OTUs). Analysis revealed that the normal group had 512 OTUs, while the fatty liver group had 541, with 262 shared species. Notably, alpha diversity decreased in fatty liver patients, with increased abundance of *Pachytene* and *Proteus* and decreased *Clostridium*. *Fusicantibacter* emerged as the dominant flora associated with enhanced fat metabolism in patients with fatty liver. These results highlight the potential of GO nanopores for effective DNA sequencing [63].

Researchers developed a microwave-assisted, one-pot synthesis of monodispersed iron-gold bimetallic nanoparticles (BNPAu-Fe) using glucose as a reducing agent in just 90 seconds. The synthesized BNPAu-Fe were characterized by UV-Vis, XRD, TEM, EDX, elemental mapping, and Raman spectroscopy. These nanoparticles were then combined with reduced graphene oxide (rGO) and coated onto a glassy carbon electrode (GCE) to create a sensor for label-free electrochemical detection of acetaminophen, a key biomarker for non-alcoholic fatty liver disease. The sensor demonstrated a wide dynamic range (50-800 nM) and a detection limit of 0.14 nM, with effective recovery rates in human urine samples [64].

During living donor liver transplantation, the intricate process of connecting various blood vessels and bile ducts takes place as both the liver and gallbladder are surgically removed from the donor and recipient. Timely detection and intervention of post-surgery complications are crucial, as they rely on assessment of blood vessel and biliary tract function. A study introduced a bio-sensing chip that monitors patient health by analyzing bile excreted during recovery. This innovative solution employs surface-enhanced Raman sensing technology. By examining bile samples from mouse models with normal bile duct ligation and gallbladder damage induced by a cautery device, the research identified and analyzed critical signals. The findings revealed that the surface-enhanced Raman chip, featuring a nanometer-scale porous structure, can effectively isolate nanometer-sized biomarkers and accurately measure their Raman signals. By detecting these biomarkers in bile and conducting thorough histopathological comparisons, the Raman signals from the damaged gallbladder were clearly distinguished from those resulting from liver damage due to bile duct ligation [65].

Recent research highlights the remarkable capabilities of the Fatty Liver Sensor (FLS) for effectively measuring human fatty liver. This innovative technology enables continuous monitoring and is fabricated using screen-printing techniques with advanced materials such as graphene and polyacrylic. The FLS is designed to be placed around the liver surface, ensuring real-time measurement of fatty liver levels. The data collected by the FLS undergoes a sophisticated processing method known as blind source separation, which effectively filters out random noise, ensuring accurate results. This refined signal is then analyzed using the tunable Q wavelet transform (TQWT), enhancing the precision of fatty liver volume assessments. By leveraging Long Short-Term Memory (LSTM) networks and the Internet of Medical Things (IoMT), this technology stands at the forefront of continuous fatty liver monitoring, making it an essential tool in advancing liver health management [66].

In the field of clinical diagnosis of liver injury, a pressing health issue, serum aminotransferase assays have long been the standard method worldwide. However, these assays come with limitations, particularly in disease and enzyme specificity, which can hinder accurate diagnosis. A study employing nano liquid chromatography-tandem mass spectrometry (LC/MS/MS) introduced an innovative approach to simultaneously measure six liver proteins that hold great promise as biomarkers for liver injury. These key proteins are glutamic-pyruvic transaminase 1 (GPT1), glutamic-oxaloacetic transaminase 1 (GOT1), methionine adenosyltransferase 1A (MAT1A), glutathione peroxidase 1 (GPX1), cytokeratin 18 (KRT18), and apolipoprotein E (APOE). Remarkably, this advanced method has demonstrated excellent selectivity and sensitivity, with detection limits down to the picogram per milliliter (pg/mL) level. By providing a more precise diagnostic tool, this method sets the stage for significantly improving the reliability of liver injury indicators and enhancing patient care [67].

REAL-TIME MONITORING *VIA* INTEGRATION OF NANOCARRIERS AND ADVANCED IMAGING TECHNIQUES

The development of non-invasive assays for the accurate diagnosis of progressive liver diseases, such as fatty liver and hepatocellular carcinoma (HCC), is clinically significant yet challenging. Researchers reported the synthesis of strawberry-like Fe3O4-Au hybrid nanoparticles at room temperature, which exhibited fluorescence, enhanced X-ray attenuation, and magnetic properties. In vitro assays demonstrated their remarkable photostability and ability to evade endosomal degradation within cells. *In vivo* imaging in normal mice revealed a 34.61-fold contrast enhancement under magnetic resonance (MR) guidance 15 minutes post-administration. Computed tomography (CT) measurements indicated a peak Hounsfield Unit (HU) of 174 at 30 minutes after injection. Evaluations in rat models with various liver diseases showed nearly homogeneous contrast enhancement in the fatty liver model under MR (contrast ratio of 47.33) and CT (from 19 HU to 72 HU) without focal nodules or dysfunction. Pathological and biochemical analyses confirmed the biocompatibility of these nanoparticles, highlighting their potential for multi-modality bioimaging applications [68].

In a study evaluating various contrast agents for longitudinal imaging of the liver and spleen in a mouse model of liver metastasis, researchers reported compelling results. Mice with liver metastases underwent longitudinal micro-computed tomography imaging after receiving injections of Fenestra LC, ExiTron nano 6000, or ExiTron nano 12000. Remarkably, all contrast agents demonstrated peak liver contrast at approximately 4 hours and peak spleen contrast at 48 hours post-injection. Significantly, a single injection of just 100 μL of either ExiTron nano 6000 or 12000 yielded prolonged enhancement of liver and spleen tissue for more than 3 weeks. In contrast, Fenestra LC required multiple injections of 400 μL to achieve adequate contrast levels, allowing for imaging of the liver and spleen for just 2 and 9 days, respectively. These results clearly demonstrate that both ExiTron nano agents provide superior contrast enhancement of the liver and spleen compared to Fenestra LC, while using 75% less injection volume in mice [69].

The use of contrast agents (CAs) is pivotal for enhancing differentiation between normal and pathological tissues, thereby significantly improving diagnostic accuracy. Among these, Ferric oxide, recognized for its high magnetic moment, has emerged as a leading component in T2-weighted MRI contrast agents. In an innovative study, oil-soluble nanomaterials (Fe@Fe3O4) were synthesized, featuring surface modifications with both large and small-molecule ligands, and were conjugated to the F56 peptide. This approach led to the development of the MRI-specific bimodal contrast agent (Fe-Fe NPs/HYA/F56). The results are promising, indicating that this novel material can play a crucial role in the clinical assessment of liver function. Importantly, the nanoparticles (Fe@Fe3O4) with functional groups showed no significant changes in their structure or particle size. Furthermore, cellular tests demonstrated that the nanoparticles (Fe-Fe NPs/HYA/F56) possess lower cytotoxicity and enhanced targeting capabilities, as validated in mouse tumor models. Moreover, a comprehensive quantitative analysis of the absolute enhancement value (AEV) and contrast enhancement rate (CER) for MRI-enhanced liver cancer highlights their relevance. The results clearly illustrate a correlation between the pathology grade of liver functions, distinguishing pathological from cirrhotic tissue, and these critical indicators, underscoring the potential of this advanced contrast agent in medical diagnostics [70].

Acute liver injury (ALI) is a serious condition characterized by rapid loss of liver function that can progress to liver failure without timely intervention. Recent advances have introduced a novel silybin nano-prodrug, PTS@IR, designed for precise diagnosis and targeted therapy. PTS@IR integrates microenvironment-activatable near-infrared II (NIR-II) fluorescence imaging with therapeutic delivery. It is constructed through the self-assembly of a reactive oxygen species (ROS)-cleavable thioketal linker that connects polyethylene glycol to silybin, a clinically proven hepatoprotective drug, and encapsulates the NIR-II dye IR-1061. Under oxidative stress, NIR-II fluorescence is quenched, but it is restored, enabling sensitive visualization of liver injury. In models of ischemia-reperfusion and drug-induced injury, intravenous PTS@IR selectively illuminates damaged regions while releasing silybin in situ. This dual antioxidant and anti-inflammatory action, supported by inhibition of ferroptosis via the Nrf2/GPX4 axis, markedly alleviates ALI. Importantly, PTS@IR fully degrades into non-toxic molecules, minimizing metabolic burden and potential adverse effects [71].

Recent research highlights the potential of peroxynitrite (ONOO-) as a key indicator for the early diagnosis of drug-induced liver injury (DILI), underscoring the urgent need for a reliable assay to detect and monitor ONOO- in DILI cases. A groundbreaking study has introduced a highly selective and sensitive FRET-based ratiometric nano fluorescent probe, known as CD-N-I, specifically designed to detect ONO-. This innovative probe integrates carbon dots with a naphthalimide-isatin sensing system for peroxynitrite, utilizing electrostatic interactions for optimal performance. With CD-N-I, researchers successfully identified exogenous ONOO- in live cells, as well as endogenous ONOO- in APAP-induced liver injury in HepG2 cells. This significant advancement marks a crucial step forward in the detection and understanding of DILI and its underlying mechanisms [72].

The combination of Fe_3O_4 nanoparticles and indocyanine green (ICG), paired with the targeting ligand integrin αvβ3, specifically arginine–glycine–aspartic acid (RGD), represents a significant advancement in the detection of hepatic fibrosis (HF). In both *in vivo* and *in vitro* studies, the SPIO@SiO2–ICG–RGD complex demonstrated remarkable stability and safety, exhibiting low cytotoxicity. Notably, the biodistribution analysis highlighted striking differences between HF-affected mice and healthy controls. The imaging results clearly illustrated the presence of integrin αvβ3 on activated hepatic stellate cells (HSCs), reinforcing the potential of this approach. These compelling findings suggest that the SPIO@SiO2–ICG–RGD probe could serve as a groundbreaking diagnostic tool for early-stage hepatic fibrosis. This innovative nanoprobe, utilizing a dual-modality imaging strategy, offers tremendous promise for enhancing the diagnosis and classification of HF, paving the way for better patient outcomes [73].

The accurate diagnosis of liver fibrosis remains a significant challenge, particularly in a noninvasive context. A groundbreaking study introduced small (4 nm) heterogeneous iron oxide/dysprosium oxide nanoparticles (IO-DyO NPs) as an innovative contrast agent for magnetic resonance imaging (MRI). These nanoparticles enable precise in vivo diagnosis of liver fibrosis at both 7.0 and 9.4 T field strengths. The IO-DyO NPs are designed to target the liver specifically and exhibit increased T2 relaxivity with increasing magnetic field strength. At ultrahigh magnetic fields, these nanoparticles markedly enhance the spatial and temporal resolution of images and improve the signal-to-noise ratio, allowing for accurate differentiation between early and moderate stages of liver fibrosis. Notably, the diagnostic results obtained with this IO-DyO NP-based MRI closely align with biopsy findings, which are considered the gold standard in clinical practice, while eliminating the need for an invasive procedure. Additionally, the IO-DyO NPs have shown impressive biosafety in both in vitro and in vivo studies. This research represents a significant advancement in T2 contrast agents for ultrahigh-field MRI (UHFMRI), paving the way for more effective and noninvasive liver fibrosis diagnosis [74].

Timely detection of liver fibrosis through X-ray computed tomography (CT) is crucial in preventing its progression to severe liver diseases. However, this detection remains a complex challenge, as conventional CT primarily identifies differences in tissue density rather than distinct X-ray attenuation characteristics. An innovative solution presented in a study involves an X-ray energy-dependent attenuation strategy using bismuth (Bi)-based nanoprobes (BiF3 @PDA@HA), which could revolutionize the diagnosis of liver fibrosis. The unique properties of the Bi element in BiF3 @PDA@HA enable it to exhibit specific attenuation patterns based on varying X-ray energy levels—something conventional CT methods cannot achieve. This study revealed that targeting BiF3 @PDA@HA nanoprobes to regions affected by hepatic fibrosis resulted in a remarkable 40 Hounsfield unit increase in CT values at 70 keV monochromatic images. This capability allows for a clear distinction between healthy and fibrotic liver tissues. Furthermore, the enhancement from the BiF3 @PDA@HA nanoprobes increased as the monochromatic energy decreased from 70 to 40 keV, greatly enhancing the detection of diseased areas. This cutting-edge approach demonstrates that these specially designed nanoprobes not only expand the application of CT technology but also hold significant potential for accurate, imaging-based diagnosis of liver fibrosis [75].

CONCLUSION AND FUTURE PERSPECTIVES

The use of biocompatible, targeted nanocarriers for in vivo imaging in fatty liver disease represents an exciting frontier with transformative potential. Such systems could provide earlier detection, more accurate staging, and dynamic monitoring of disease progression, addressing major limitations of current imaging tools. However, to move from laboratory promise to clinical application, several opportunities and barriers must be critically examined. Among the most clinically advanced platforms are superparamagnetic iron oxide nanoparticles (SPIONs). Clinically approved formulations such as Ferumoxide (Ferridex) and Ferucarbotran (Resovist) have already been used for liver imaging, which provides valuable safety data and regulatory precedent. This legacy offers SPION-based probes a distinct advantage over newer, less characterized nanomaterials. Recent innovations in ultrasmall iron oxides (USIOs) that act as T_1-weighted agents, along with molecularly engineered probes such as fibroblast activation protein-α (FAPα)-responsive constructs for fibrosis grading, have demonstrated not only enhanced diagnostic sensitivity but also potential clinical utility in grading disease severity. These refinements help address the toxicity and imaging limitations observed with earlier formulations. Ultrasound contrast agents represent another translationally promising avenue. Commercially available microbubbles such as Lumason and Definity are already widely used in liver imaging, and their nanoscale derivatives, nanobubbles and nanodroplets, offer longer circulation times, smaller size, and the ability to serve as both imaging and drug-delivery carriers. Their established clinical precedent and straightforward adaptation accelerate their path toward regulatory approval. Other nanocarriers remain at earlier stages. Perfluorocarbon (PFC) nanoemulsions for F-19 MRI have generated strong preclinical data, particularly for longitudinal tracking of inflammation in nonalcoholic fatty liver disease (NAFLD). F-19 MRI provides background-free signal and inherently quantitative readouts, attributes that support clinical adoption if safety, clearance, and manufacturing hurdles can be addressed. Gold nanoparticles, with their high X-ray attenuation and flexible surface chemistry, have also shown strong potential for CT imaging. However, concerns regarding heavy metal safety, cost of raw materials, and reproducibility at scale remain significant barriers. By contrast, quantum dots and extracellular vesicles (EVs) illustrate both the promise and the challenges. Quantum dots exhibit exceptional optical brightness and multiplexing capabilities but face toxicity concerns from cadmium or other heavy-metal cores, as well as long-term tissue persistence. EVs, by comparison, are biologically derived, circulate naturally, and may carry liver-specific signals, making them attractive as both biomarkers and delivery vehicles. However, reproducibility, scalable GMP-compliant isolation, and standardization of characterization remain major obstacles to their translation. Across all nanocarrier systems, several overarching barriers recur. Toxicity is a key concern, particularly for non-degradable or heavy-metal-based particles that accumulate in the reticuloendothelial system (RES) organs such as the liver and spleen. Manufacturing scale-up poses another critical challenge; while academic labs often achieve precise control in small batches, translating these processes into reproducible, sterile, large-scale production with consistent physicochemical properties is complex. Furthermore, regulatory precedent is limited, and entirely novel materials face lengthy, costly safety evaluations. Economic feasibility is also a major concern, as material costs, multi-step syntheses, and uncertain reimbursement models may undermine commercialization. Encouragingly, a number of innovations are emerging to address these barriers. Ultrasmall iron oxides and biodegradable linkers enable renal clearance or breakdown into non-toxic metabolites, reducing concerns about long-term retention. Advanced surface chemistries, including PEGylation, zwitterionic polymers, polysaccharide coatings, and biomimetic strategies, minimize protein corona formation, enhance stability, and prolong circulation. Stimuli-responsive designs, such as ROS-cleavable linkers and enzyme-activated probes, improve both specificity and safety by releasing payloads only in diseased tissue. Multi-modal constructs, exemplified by Fe_3O_4–Au hybrids that combine MR, CT, and fluorescence imaging, can reduce per-modality dosing while increasing diagnostic accuracy. EV-inspired coatings and the potential use of autologous EVs also hold promise for personalized, immune-compatible nanocarriers, though reproducibility hurdles persist. To translate these advances effectively, research priorities must include selecting platforms with proven clinical track records, optimizing clearance and biodegradability, standardizing characterization, and assembling comprehensive toxicology packages tailored to nanomaterials. Economic considerations and scalable GMP manufacturing strategies must be integrated from the outset to ensure viability beyond proof-o-

-concept studies. Looking ahead, the convergence of nanocarrier imaging with artificial intelligence and machine learning (AI/ML) offers compelling opportunities. AI-driven analysis of multiparametric signals, such as MRI relaxometry, F-19 quantification, CT attenuation, and ultrasound kinetics, could generate robust, reproducible biomarkers for fibrosis and inflammation. Theranostic platforms that combine imaging with antifibrotic therapy exemplify another promising direction. Systems like the ROS-activated silybin nano-prodrug PTS@IR, which provides NIR-II imaging alongside therapeutic action, enable real-time monitoring of treatment delivery and response. Finally, personalized approaches leveraging patient-derived EVs as imaging carriers or liquid-biopsy biomarkers may reduce immunogenicity while improving disease stratification.

In summary, biocompatible nanocarriers represent a transformative opportunity for imaging in fatty liver disease. While SPIONs, nanobubbles, and PFC nanoemulsions are closest to translation, innovations in design, clearance, and integration with AI/ML and theranostics are expanding the horizon. Overcoming toxicity, scalability, and regulatory hurdles will be essential, but with strategic prioritization, these platforms could redefine how fatty liver disease is diagnosed, monitored, and treated.

LIST OF ABBREVIATIONS

NAFLD	Non-Alcoholic Fatty Liver Disease
NAFL	Non-Alcoholic Fatty Liver
NASH	Non-Alcoholic Steatohepatitis
CT	Computed Tomography
MRI	Magnetic Resonance Imaging
US	Ultrasound
PDFF	Proton Density Fat Fraction
EPR	Enhanced Permeability and Retention
ATP	Adenosine Triphosphate
$ONOO^-$	Peroxynitrite
GSH	Glutathione
NIR	Near-Infrared
SiR	Silicon Rhodamine dye
H2Sn	Hydrogen Polysulfides
PLGA	Poly(lactic-co-glycolic acid)
DOX-NB	Doxorubicin Nanobubble
MRCAs	Magnetic Resonance Contrast Agents
FDA	Food and Drug Administration

MRS	Magnetic Resonance Spectroscopy
MRE	Magnetic Resonance Elastography
ASGPR	Asialoglycoprotein Receptor
RGD	Arginine–Glycine–Aspartic Acid peptide
TNF-α	Tumor Necrosis Factor-alpha
IL-6	Interleukin-6
FAPα	Fibroblast Activation Protein alpha
ROS	Reactive Oxygen Species
SPION	Superparamagnetic Iron Oxide Nanoparticle
SPIO	Superparamagnetic Iron Oxide
HCC	Hepatocellular Carcinoma
CF	Cationized Ferritin
PFC	Perfluorocarbon
F-19 MRI	Fluorine-19 Magnetic Resonance Imaging
AuNPs	Gold Nanoparticles
QDs	Quantum Dots
EVs	Extracellular Vesicles
MPO	Myeloperoxidase
USIO	Ultra-Small Iron Oxide
DA	Dopamine
PEG	Polyethylene Glycol
5HT	5-Hydroxytryptamine
MCU	Microcontroller Unit
NGP	Nano Graphene Polyvinyl
MBAAm	Methylenebisacrylamide
DMPAP	2,2-Dimethoxy-2-phenyl acetophenone
OTUs	Operational Taxonomic Units
BNPAu-Fe	Bimetallic Nanoparticles (Au-Fe)
rGO	Reduced Graphene Oxide
GCE	Glassy Carbon Electrode

REFERENCES

[1] Han SK, Baik SK, Kim MY. Non-alcoholic fatty liver disease: Definition and subtypes. Clin Mol Hepatol 2023; 29 (Suppl.): S5-S16.
[http://dx.doi.org/10.3350/cmh.2022.0424] [PMID: 36577427]

[2] Zhang YN, Fowler KJ, Hamilton G, *et al.* Liver fat imaging—a clinical overview of ultrasound, CT, and MR imaging. Br J Radiol 2018; 91(1089): 20170959.

[http://dx.doi.org/10.1259/bjr.20170959] [PMID: 29722568]

[3] Li G, Zhang X, Lin H, Liang LY, Wong GLH, Wong VWS. Non-invasive tests of non-alcoholic fatty liver disease. Chin Med J (Engl) 2022; 135(5): 532-46. [http://dx.doi.org/10.1097/CM9.0000000000002027] [PMID: 35089884]

[4] Johnston RJ, Stamm ER, Lewin JM, Hendrick RE, Archer PG. Diagnosis of fatty infiltration of the liver on contrast enhanced CT: limitations of liver-minus-spleen attenuation difference measurements. Abdom Imaging 1998; 23(4): 409-15. [http://dx.doi.org/10.1007/s002619900370] [PMID: 9663278]

[5] Reeder SB, Cruite I, Hamilton G, Sirlin CB. Quantitative assessment of liver fat with magnetic resonance imaging and spectroscopy. J Magn Reson Imaging 2011; 34(4): 729-49. [http://dx.doi.org/10.1002/jmri.22580] [PMID: 22025886]

[6] Sumida Y, Nakajima A, Itoh Y. Limitations of liver biopsy and non-invasive diagnostic tests for the diagnosis of nonalcoholic fatty liver disease/nonalcoholic steatohepatitis. World J Gastroenterol 2014; 20(2): 475-85. [http://dx.doi.org/10.3748/wjg.v20.i2.475] [PMID: 24574716]

[7] Asadollahzade E, Ghadiri F, Ebadi Z, Moghadasi AN. The benefits and side effects of gadolinium-based contrast agents in multiple sclerosis patients. Rev Assoc Med Bras 2022; 68(8): 979-81. [http://dx.doi.org/10.1590/1806-9282.20220643] [PMID: 36134822]

[8] Zhang S, Li J, Lykotrafitis G, Bao G, Suresh S. Size-dependent endocytosis of nanoparticles. Adv Mater 2009; 21(4): 419-24. [http://dx.doi.org/10.1002/adma.200801393] [PMID: 19606281]

[9] Sun T, Zhang YS, Pang B, Hyun DC, Yang M, Xia Y. Engineered nanoparticles for drug delivery in cancer therapy. Nanomater Neoplasms 2021; pp. 31-142. [http://dx.doi.org/10.1201/9780429027819-2]

[10] Augustine R, Hasan A, Primavera R, Wilson RJ, Thakor AS, Kevadiya BD. Cellular uptake and retention of nanoparticles: Insights on particle properties and interaction with cellular components. Mater Today Commun 2020; 25: 101692. [http://dx.doi.org/10.1016/j.mtcomm.2020.101692]

[11] Gatoo MA, Naseem S, Arfat MY, Mahmood Dar A, Qasim K, Zubair S. Physicochemical properties of nanomaterials: implication in associated toxic manifestations. BioMed Res Int 2014; 2014: 1-8. [http://dx.doi.org/10.1155/2014/498420] [PMID: 25165707]

[12] De Jong WH, Hagens WI, Krystek P, Burger MC, Sips AJAM, Geertsma RE. Particle size-dependent organ distribution of gold nanoparticles after intravenous administration. Biomaterials 2008; 29(12): 1912-9. [http://dx.doi.org/10.1016/j.biomaterials.2007.12.037] [PMID: 18242692]

[13] Kohli AK, Alpar HO. Potential use of nanoparticles for transcutaneous vaccine delivery: effect of particle size and charge. Int J Pharm 2004; 275(1-2): 13-7. [http://dx.doi.org/10.1016/j.ijpharm.2003.10.038] [PMID: 15081134]

[14] Vardharajula S, Ali SZ, Tiwari PM, *et al.* Functionalized carbon nanotubes: biomedical applications. Int J Nanomedicine 2012; 7: 5361-74. [PMID: 23091380]

[15] Prater AR, Pellois JP. Endosomal escape. In: Oba M, Demizu Y, editors. Cell-penetrating peptides. Weinheim: Wiley□VCH; 2022 [http://dx.doi.org/10.1002/9783527835997.ch10]

[16] Dhilip Kumar SS, Abrahamse H. Recent advances in the development of biocompatible nanocarriers and their cancer cell targeting efficiency in photodynamic therapy. Front Chem 2022; 10: 969809. [http://dx.doi.org/10.3389/fchem.2022.969809] [PMID: 36046728]

[17] Himri I, Guaadaoui A. Cell and organ drug targeting: types of drug delivery systems and advanced

targeting strategies.Nanostructures for the Engineering of Cells, Tissues and Organs. Elsevier 2018; pp. 1-66.
[http://dx.doi.org/10.1016/B978-0-12-813665-2.00001-6]

[18] Li J, Wang Q, Xia G, *et al.* Recent advances in targeted drug delivery strategy for enhancing oncotherapy. Pharmaceutics 2023; 15(9): 2233.
[http://dx.doi.org/10.3390/pharmaceutics15092233] [PMID: 37765202]

[19] Chao JJ, Liao QT, Hu L, *et al.* Near-infrared fluorescent probe for the imaging of viscosity in fatty liver mice and valuation of drug efficacy. Talanta 2024; 276: 126227.
[http://dx.doi.org/10.1016/j.talanta.2024.126227] [PMID: 38733935]

[20] He L, Li H, Tang Y, Ren TB, Yuan L. Recent advances in fluorescent probes for fatty liver imaging by detecting lipid droplets. J Mater Chem B Mater Biol Med 2024; 12(40): 10149-62.
[http://dx.doi.org/10.1039/D4TB01741B] [PMID: 39282742]

[21] Hillman EMC, Amoozegar CB, Wang T, *et al. In vivo* optical imaging and dynamic contrast methods for biomedical research. Philos Trans- Royal Soc, Math Phys Eng Sci 2011; 369(1955): 4620-43.
[http://dx.doi.org/10.1098/rsta.2011.0264] [PMID: 22006910]

[22] Liu X, He L, Gong X, *et al.* Engineering of reversible luminescent probes for real-time intravital imaging of liver injury and repair. CCS Chemistry 2022; 4(1): 356-68.
[http://dx.doi.org/10.31635/ccschem.021.202000679]

[23] Chen JT, Chen SS, Wang ZQ, *et al.* Near-infrared fluorescent nanoprobes for adenosine triphosphate-guided imaging in cancer and fatty liver mice. Anal Chem 2023; 95(3): 2119-27.
[http://dx.doi.org/10.1021/acs.analchem.2c05235] [PMID: 36622664]

[24] Li W, Wang L, Yin S, Lai H, Yuan L, Zhang X. Engineering a highly selective probe for ratiometric imaging of H_2S_n and revealing its signaling pathway in fatty liver disease. Chem Sci (Camb) 2020; 11(30): 7991-9.
[http://dx.doi.org/10.1039/D0SC03336G] [PMID: 34094167]

[25] Wilson BC, Jacques SL. Optical reflectance and transmittance of tissues: principles and applications. IEEE J Quantum Electron 1990; 26(12): 2186-99.
[http://dx.doi.org/10.1109/3.64355]

[26] Lyshchik A, Kono Y, Dietrich CF, *et al.* Contrast-enhanced ultrasound of the liver: technical and lexicon recommendations from the ACR CEUS LI-RADS working group. Abdom Radiol (NY) 2018; 43(4): 861-79.
[http://dx.doi.org/10.1007/s00261-017-1392-0] [PMID: 29151131]

[27] Späth M, Hohmann M, Rohde M, Lengenfelder B, Stelzle F, Klämpfl F. Determination of the diameter of simulated human capillaries using shifted position□diffuse reflectance imaging. J Biophotonics 2021; 14(4): e202000465.
[http://dx.doi.org/10.1002/jbio.202000465] [PMID: 33432711]

[28] Shakya G, Cattaneo M, Guerriero G, Prasanna A, Fiorini S, Supponen O. Ultrasound-responsive microbubbles and nanodroplets: A pathway to targeted drug delivery. Adv Drug Deliv Rev 2024; 206: 115178.
[http://dx.doi.org/10.1016/j.addr.2023.115178] [PMID: 38199257]

[29] Exner AA, Kolios MC. Bursting microbubbles: How nanobubble contrast agents can enable the future of medical ultrasound molecular imaging and image-guided therapy. Curr Opin Colloid Interface Sci 2021; 54: 101463.
[http://dx.doi.org/10.1016/j.cocis.2021.101463] [PMID: 34393610]

[30] Meng M, Gao J, Wu C, *et al.* Doxorubicin nanobubble for combining ultrasonography and targeted chemotherapy of rabbit with VX2 liver tumor. Tumour Biol 2016; 37(7): 8673-80.
[http://dx.doi.org/10.1007/s13277-015-4525-5] [PMID: 26738862]

[31] Kodama Y, Ng CS, Wu TT, *et al.* Comparison of CT methods for determining the fat content of the

liver. AJR Am J Roentgenol 2007; 188(5): 1307-12.
[http://dx.doi.org/10.2214/AJR.06.0992] [PMID: 17449775]

[32] Webb JA, Stacul F, Thomsen HS, Morcos SK. Late adverse reactions to intravascular iodinated contrast media. Eur Radiol 2003; 13(1): 181-4.
[http://dx.doi.org/10.1007/s00330-002-1650-5] [PMID: 12541128]

[33] Périard MA. Adverse effects and complications related to the use of barium sulphate contrast media for radiological examinations of the gastrointestinal tract: a literature review. Can J Med Radiat Technol 2003; 34(3): 3-9.
[http://dx.doi.org/10.1016/S0820-5930(09)60005-0]

[34] Lersy F, Boulouis G, Clément O, *et al.* Consensus guidelines of the French Society of Neuroradiology (SFNR) on the use of gadolinium-based contrast agents (GBCAs) and related MRI protocols in neuroradiology. J Neuroradiol 2020; 47(6): 441-9.
[http://dx.doi.org/10.1016/j.neurad.2020.05.008] [PMID: 32565280]

[35] Wei H, Bruns OT, Kaul MG, *et al.* Exceedingly small iron oxide nanoparticles as positive MRI contrast agents. Proc Natl Acad Sci USA 2017; 114(9): 2325-30.
[http://dx.doi.org/10.1073/pnas.1620145114] [PMID: 28193901]

[36] Gutierrez JE, Koenig S, Breuer J. Overview on the efficacy and safety of gadobutrol: an MRI contrast agent for the CNS, body and vessels. Imaging Med 2012; 4(1): 25-40.
[http://dx.doi.org/10.2217/iim.11.70]

[37] Ma X, Holalkere NS, R AK, Mino-Kenudson M, Hahn PF, Sahani DV. Imaging-based quantification of hepatic fat: methods and clinical applications. Radiographics 2009; 29(5): 1253-77.
[http://dx.doi.org/10.1148/rg.295085186] [PMID: 19755595]

[38] Oudkerk M, Torres CG, Song B, *et al.* Characterization of liver lesions with mangafodipir trisodium-enhanced MR imaging: multicenter study comparing MR and dual-phase spiral CT. Radiology 2002; 223(2): 517-24.
[http://dx.doi.org/10.1148/radiol.2232010318] [PMID: 11997562]

[39] Yoon SH, Goo JM, Lee SM, Park CM, Seo HJ, Cheon GJ. Positron emission tomography/magnetic resonance imaging evaluation of lung cancer: current status and future prospects. J Thorac Imaging 2014; 29(1): 4-16.
[http://dx.doi.org/10.1097/RTI.0000000000000062] [PMID: 24296699]

[40] Dadfar SM, Roemhild K, Drude NI, *et al.* Iron oxide nanoparticles: Diagnostic, therapeutic and theranostic applications. Adv Drug Deliv Rev 2019; 138: 302-25.
[http://dx.doi.org/10.1016/j.addr.2019.01.005] [PMID: 30639256]

[41] Gupta AK, Wells S. Surface-modified superparamagnetic nanoparticles for drug delivery: preparation, characterization, and cytotoxicity studies. IEEE Trans Nanobiosci 2004; 3(1): 66-73.
[http://dx.doi.org/10.1109/TNB.2003.820277] [PMID: 15382647]

[42] Gao J, Wang Y, Meng X, *et al.* A FAPα-activated MRI nanoprobe for precise grading diagnosis of clinical liver fibrosis. Nat Commun 2024; 15(1): 8036.
[http://dx.doi.org/10.1038/s41467-024-52308-3] [PMID: 39271701]

[43] Reddy LH, Couvreur P. Nanotechnology for therapy and imaging of liver diseases. J Hepatol 2011; 55(6): 1461-6.
[http://dx.doi.org/10.1016/j.jhep.2011.05.039] [PMID: 21801699]

[44] Asanuma T, Ono M, Kubota K, *et al.* Super paramagnetic iron oxide MRI shows defective Kupffer cell uptake function in non-alcoholic fatty liver disease. Gut 2010; 59(2): 258-66.
[http://dx.doi.org/10.1136/gut.2009.176651] [PMID: 19919948]

[45] Luo X, Song X, Zhu A, *et al.* Development of poly(vinyl acetate-methylacrylic acid)/chitosan/Fe_3O_4 nanoparticles for the diagnosis of non-alcoholic steatohepatitis with magnetic resonance imaging. J Mater Sci Mater Med 2012; 23(12): 3075-82.

[http://dx.doi.org/10.1007/s10856-012-4763-7] [PMID: 22976475]

[46] Beeman SC, Mandarino LJ, Georges JF, Bennett KM. Cationized ferritin as a magnetic resonance imaging probe to detect microstructural changes in a rat model of non-alcoholic steatohepatitis. Magn Reson Med 2013; 70(6): 1728-38.
[http://dx.doi.org/10.1002/mrm.24619] [PMID: 23390010]

[47] Gupta A, Eral HB, Hatton TA, Doyle PS. Nanoemulsions: formation, properties and applications. Soft Matter 2016; 12(11): 2826-41.
[http://dx.doi.org/10.1039/C5SM02958A] [PMID: 26924445]

[48] Lister D, Blizard G, Hosseini M, *et al.* Imaging non-alcoholic fatty liver disease model using 1H and 19F MRI. Mol Imaging Biol 2023; 25(3): 443-9.
[http://dx.doi.org/10.1007/s11307-022-01798-y] [PMID: 36575339]

[49] Cole LE, Ross RD, Tilley JMR, Vargo-Gogola T, Roeder RK. Gold nanoparticles as contrast agents in x-ray imaging and computed tomography. Nanomedicine (Lond) 2015; 10(2): 321-41.
[http://dx.doi.org/10.2217/nnm.14.171] [PMID: 25600973]

[50] Mandal S, Jana NR. Quantum dot-based designed nanoprobe for imaging lipid droplet. J Phys Chem C 2017; 121(42): 23727-35.
[http://dx.doi.org/10.1021/acs.jpcc.7b07571]

[51] Chai SQ, Lv WY, He JH, *et al.* Dual energy transfer-based fluorescent nanoprobe for imaging miR-21 in nonalcoholic fatty liver cells with low background. Anal Chem 2019; 91(10): 6761-8.
[http://dx.doi.org/10.1021/acs.analchem.9b00841] [PMID: 31020834]

[52] Jiang WY, Xun YH. [Value of detection of extracellular vesicles in the diagnosis of nonalcoholic fatty liver disease]. Zhonghua Gan Zang Bing Za Zhi 2020; 28(1): 92-6.
[PMID: 32023709]

[53] Povero D, Yamashita H, Ren W, *et al.* Characterization and proteome of circulating extracellular vesicles as potential biomarkers for NASH. Hepatol Commun 2020; 4(9): 1263-78.
[http://dx.doi.org/10.1002/hep4.1556] [PMID: 32923831]

[54] Povero D, Eguchi A, Li H, *et al.* Circulating extracellular vesicles with specific proteome and liver microRNAs are potential biomarkers for liver injury in experimental fatty liver disease. PLoS One 2014; 9(12): e113651.
[http://dx.doi.org/10.1371/journal.pone.0113651] [PMID: 25470250]

[55] Newman LA, Useckaite Z, Johnson J, Sorich MJ, Hopkins AM, Rowland A. Selective isolation of liver-derived extracellular vesicles redefines performance of miRNA biomarkers for non-alcoholic fatty liver disease. Biomedicines 2022; 10(1): 195.
[http://dx.doi.org/10.3390/biomedicines10010195] [PMID: 35052873]

[56] Li W, Li C, Zhou T, *et al.* Role of exosomal proteins in cancer diagnosis. Mol Cancer 2017; 16(1): 145.
[http://dx.doi.org/10.1186/s12943-017-0706-8] [PMID: 28851367]

[57] Hubal MJ, Nadler EP, Ferrante SC, *et al.* Circulating adipocyte-derived exosomal MicroRNAs associated with decreased insulin resistance after gastric bypass. Obesity (Silver Spring) 2017; 25(1): 102-10.
[http://dx.doi.org/10.1002/oby.21709] [PMID: 27883272]

[58] Liu J, Yu X, Ting HJ, *et al.* Myeloperoxidase-sensitive T1 and T2 switchable MR imaging for diagnosis of nonalcoholic steatohepatitis. ACS Nano 2023; 17(4): 3324-33.
[http://dx.doi.org/10.1021/acsnano.2c06233] [PMID: 36773320]

[59] Nazeer SS, Saraswathy A, Nimi N, *et al.* Fluorescent carbon dots tailored iron oxide nano hybrid system for *in vivo* optical imaging of liver fibrosis. Methods Appl Fluoresc 2023; 11(2): 024002.
[http://dx.doi.org/10.1088/2050-6120/acc009] [PMID: 36854197]

[60] Misra SK, Kim B, Kolmodin NJ, Pan D. A dual strategy for sensing metals with a nano 'pincer'

scavenger for in vitro diagnostics and detection of liver diseases from blood samples. Colloids Surf B Biointerfaces 2015; 126: 444-51.
[http://dx.doi.org/10.1016/j.colsurfb.2014.12.048] [PMID: 25595484]

[61] Wang K, Margolis S, Cho JM, *et al.* Non-invasive detection of early-stage fatty liver disease via an on-skin impedance sensor and attention-based deep learning. Adv Sci (Weinh) 2024; 11(31): 2400596.
[http://dx.doi.org/10.1002/advs.202400596] [PMID: 38887178]

[62] Srilekha MK, Deepa SN, Shanker NR, Priya M. Human fatty liver volume measurement device using nano graphene polyvinyl sensor. IEEE Sens J 2023; 23(20): 25390-400.
[http://dx.doi.org/10.1109/JSEN.2023.3308769]

[63] Xiao G, Shi H, Zhang J, *et al.* Regulation of intestinal lipid metabolism by fusion-induced fatty liver based on graphene oxide nanopore DNA. Mater Express 2020; 10(6): 802-11.
[http://dx.doi.org/10.1166/mex.2020.1708]

[64] Kumar A, Purohit B, Mahato K, Mandal R, Srivastava A, Chandra P. Gold-iron bimetallic nanoparticles impregnated reduced graphene oxide based nanosensor for label-free detection of biomarker related to non-alcoholic fatty liver disease. Electroanalysis 2019; 31(12): 2417-28.
[http://dx.doi.org/10.1002/elan.201900337]

[65] Lee S, Tak E, Cho YJ, *et al.* Nano-biomarker-based surface-enhanced Raman spectroscopy for selective diagnosis of gallbladder and liver injury. Biochip J 2022; 16(1): 49-57.
[http://dx.doi.org/10.1007/s13206-022-00045-4]

[66] Muthukaruppankaruppiah S, Nagalingam SR, Murugasen P, Nandaamarnath R. Human fatty liver monitoring using nano sensor and IoMT. Intell Autom Soft Comput. 2023, 35(2), 2309-2323.
[http://dx.doi.org/10.32604/iasc.2023.029598]

[67] Cai S, Su Y, Shi M, Wang D, Chen DDY, Yan B. Simultaneous quantification of six proteins related to liver injury using nano liquid chromatography–tandem mass spectrometry. Rapid Commun Mass Spectrom 2024; 38(12): e9754.
[http://dx.doi.org/10.1002/rcm.9754] [PMID: 38605420]

[68] Zhao HY, Liu S, He J, *et al.* Synthesis and application of strawberry-like Fe_3O_4-Au nanoparticles as CT-MR dual-modality contrast agents in accurate detection of the progressive liver disease. Biomaterials 2015; 51: 194-207.
[http://dx.doi.org/10.1016/j.biomaterials.2015.02.019] [PMID: 25771010]

[69] Boll H, Figueiredo G, Fiebig T, *et al.* Comparison of Fenestra LC, ExiTron nano 6000, and ExiTron nano 12000 for micro-CT imaging of liver and spleen in mice. Acad Radiol 2013; 20(9): 1137-43.
[http://dx.doi.org/10.1016/j.acra.2013.06.002] [PMID: 23931428]

[70] Duan W, Liu G, Guo C, Qu Y. Preparation of nanomaterials Fe@Fe_3O_4 and its application in magnetic resonance imaging for liver functions. Sci Adv Mater 2021; 13(5): 906-16.
[http://dx.doi.org/10.1166/sam.2021.3994]

[71] Dong J, Han Y, Feng R, *et al.* Smart microenvironment-activatable silybin nano-prodrug for precise NIR-II fluorescence monitoring and on-demand therapy of acute liver injury. Biomaterials 2026; 326: 123673.
[http://dx.doi.org/10.1016/j.biomaterials.2025.123673] [PMID: 40907397]

[72] Wu Y, Sun LL, Han HH, He XP, Cao W, James TD. Selective FRET nano probe based on carbon dots and naphthalimide–isatin for the ratiometric detection of peroxynitrite in drug-induced liver injury. Chem Sci (Camb) 2024; 15(2): 757-64.
[http://dx.doi.org/10.1039/D3SC05010F] [PMID: 38179535]

[73] Li Y, Shang W, Liang X, *et al.* The diagnosis of hepatic fibrosis by magnetic resonance and near-infrared imaging using dual-modality nanoparticles. RSC Advances 2018; 8(12): 6699-708.
[http://dx.doi.org/10.1039/C7RA10847H] [PMID: 35540380]

[74] Balachandran YL, Wang W, Yang H, *et al.* Heterogeneous iron oxide/dysprosium oxide nanoparticles

target liver for precise magnetic resonance imaging of liver fibrosis. ACS Nano 2022; 16(4): 5647-59. [http://dx.doi.org/10.1021/acsnano.1c10618] [PMID: 35312295]

[75] Wu S, Meng X, Jiang X, *et al.* Harnessing X-ray energy-dependent attenuation of bismuth-based nanoprobes for accurate diagnosis of liver fibrosis. Adv Sci (Weinh) 2021; 8(11): 2002548. [http://dx.doi.org/10.1002/advs.202002548] [PMID: 34105274]

CHAPTER 10

Clinical Translation of Nanocarrier-based Drug Delivery Systems for the Treatment of Fatty Liver Disease

Pranav J Shah[1,*], **Priyanka Patil**[2], **Divya Gupta**[2], **Swati Gupta**[2], **Aarti Patel**[2] and **J.K Patel**[3]

[1] *Maliba Pharmacy College, UKA Tarsadia University, Surat, Gujarat, India*

[2] *Faculty of Pharmacy, Sigma University, Vadodara, Gujarat, India*

[3] *Viesain Pharma LLC, Atlanta, Georgia, USA*

Abstract: Fatty Liver Diseases (FLDs), including basic steatosis to Non-Alcoholic Steatohepatitis (NASH), are an increasing global health issue. Current therapeutic options for FLD are limited, highlighting the need for innovative approaches. Nano-medicines are revolutionising healthcare, with vaccines such as those from Pfizer/BioNTech and Moderna COVID-19 delivering billions of doses safely. This chapter highlights recent advances in nano-medicines for developing diagnostic and therapeutic tools for fatty liver disease without alcohol use, a growing global health challenge, paving the way for precision medicines. Nano carrier-based drug delivery systems (NDDS) offer a promising avenue for enhancing drug delivery to the liver, improving therapeutic efficacy, and minimising side effects. This chapter explores the potential of NDDS in FLD management, focusing on recent advancements in nanomaterial design, targeting strategies, and clinical translation, and discusses the challenges and opportunities associated with the development and clinical application of NDDS for FLD, including safety considerations, regulatory hurdles, and the need for well-designed clinical trials. Despite these challenges, NDDS has significant potential to improve the treatment of FLD and patient outcomes. The clinical trials investigating the efficacy of NDDS in FLD have shown promising results. Additionally, silibinin-loaded nanoparticles enhance mucosal penetration and oral absorption compared with conventional silibinin. Nanoparticulate approaches have shown promise in overcoming lipid metabolism disorders in preclinical trials, indicating potential effectiveness in humans.

Keywords: Non-alcoholic steatohepatitis, Novel drug delivery system, Nano-medicines, Nanocarrier, Nanomaterial design.

[*] **Corresponding author Pranav J Shah:** Maliba Pharmacy College, UKA Tarsaadia University, Surat, Gujarat, India; E-mail: pranav.shah@utu.ac.in

Anjali Sharma, Devkant Sharma, Ajmer Singh Grewal, Geeta Deswal & Ganga Reddy Velma (Eds.)

INTRODUCTION

The excessive accumulation of fat in the liver, known as fatty liver disease (FLD), is the leading cause of chronic liver disease, the main reason for liver transplants, and a significant contributor to the clinical and financial burdens worldwide. Clinically, the diagnosis is verified in patients without substantial alcohol use or other known causes of chronic liver disease using non-invasive imaging techniques or invasive procedures, such as a biopsy that shows 5% or more macro vesicular steatosis in hepatocytes [1]. The illness presents with several phenotypes, ranging from Non-Alcoholic Steatohepatitis (NASH) to mild steatosis or Non-Alcoholic Fatty Liver Disease (NAFLD). Hepatocellular carcinoma (HCC), cirrhosis, or liver fibrosis are more likely to develop in people with NASH. According to available data, there are several reversible cycles in the early phases before the disease progresses to fibrosis, indicating that the transition from NAFLD to NASH is a dynamic process. Both hepatocellular carcinoma (HCC) and NASH-related cirrhosis may occur as consequences of rapid fibrosis developing in approximately 10-20% of these cycles [2]. Besides the increased incidence of cardiovascular morbidity and mortality, NAFLD patients suffer from a significantly greater prevalence of atherosclerosis and other cardiovascular risk factors [3]. Fig. (**1**) illustrates the progression of Non-Alcoholic Fatty Liver Disease (NAFLD) from a healthy liver to cirrhosis, along with its underlying aetiology.

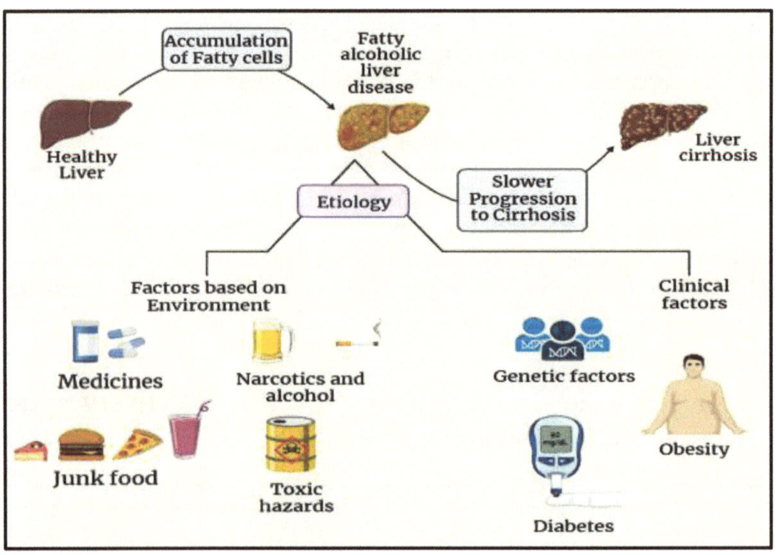

Fig. (1). Schematic diagram of Non-alcoholic Fatty Liver Disease (NAFLD) development from healthy liver to cirrhosis and its aetiology.

Patients with FLD often present with associated metabolic disorders, including insulin resistance, type 2 diabetes (T2D), hypertension, abdominal obesity, and dyslipidemia. Irrespective of other comorbidities, cardiovascular diseases are, by far, the commonest cause of death among FLD patients [4]. However, it is important to note that FLD can also develop in patients without metabolic syndrome. As highlighted in this chapter, FLD is a complex condition resulting from multiple interacting mechanisms and patient-specific pathways [5]. A diagnosis of FLD confirms the presence of hepatocellular steatosis, defined as an excess fat accumulation exceeding five percent of liver weight [6]. Steatosis has two types: macrovesicular and microvesicular. While macrovesicular steatosis is the most common type in patients with FLD, microvesicular steatosis is observed in roughly 10% of patients [7]. Prior studies have suggested FLD to be a benign condition. Compared to NASH, studies using paired or repeated liver biopsies suggested FLD has a much better overall prognosis, along with a lower risk of cirrhosis development. However, this idea was contested when more data became available, and FLD is now acknowledged as a progressive illness [8, 9]. The worldwide obesity and diabetes epidemics are the main causes of the rise in NAFLD as a health concern [10]. On the other hand, greater than 5% hepatic steatosis is a characteristic of metabolic-associated fatty liver disease (MAFLD), which does not rule out other liver disorders, including alcoholic liver disease [11]. Hepatic and systemic insulin resistance, gut dysbiosis, lipotoxicity, and hepatic immune dysfunction are all part of the pathogenesis, making this ailment a classic example of a systemic metabolic disease [12].

EPIDEMIOLOGY OF NAFLD

Non-Alcoholic Fatty Liver Disease (NAFLD), which presently affects an estimated 38% of the world's residents, has rapidly become the most common liver disease globally. Although only a small percentage of NAFLD patients progress to cirrhosis or hepatocellular carcinoma, the large overall prevalence of the disease means that a significant number of individuals remain at risk for these serious complications [13]. The global increase in metabolic syndrome, obesity, and diabetes has led to a considerable rise in the prevalence of NAFLD, which currently affects around 25% of the world's population [14]. Due to the increasing prevalence of non-communicable illnesses, major lifestyle changes over the past century have changed health priorities worldwide. The rising burden of NAFLD, which coincides with the global rise in obesity, is directly associated with the developing epidemic of chronic liver disease. It is now believed that 24% of people worldwide have NAFLD. While studies based on elevated liver enzymes have consistently overestimated the true prevalence, community surveys using proton NMR spectroscopy or ultrasonography have assessed the prevalence of

NAFLD in various countries. All continents are affected by NAFLD; however, South America and the Middle East have the greatest rates (31% and 32%, respectively), followed by Asia (27%), the USA (24%), and Europe (24%). Conversely, NAFLD is less prevalent in Africa, with a 14% prevalence [15]. In people with morbid obesity, the prevalence of NAFLD is estimated to be 75–92%, but in children, it varies from 13–14% [16]. Prevalence rates of NAFLD in the general populations of Bangladesh, India, Nepal, Pakistan, and Sri Lanka have been reported in 11 studies [17]. Following the formulation of consensus statements and recommendations by a diverse team of specialists, three rounds of assessment were conducted by a broader group of collaborators in this worldwide Delphi study until consensus was reached [18].

THE MOLECULAR PATHOGENESIS OF NAFLD

Steatosis: The first stage of NAFLD development is the build-up of triglycerides in hepatocytes. Steatosis, which is frequently linked to insulin resistance in both the liver and adipose tissue, is caused by an imbalance between fatty acid intake, de novo lipogenesis, and triglyceride utilization [19]. From a molecular standpoint, triglycerides stored in adipose tissue are excessively broken down into free fatty acids due to defective insulin signalling. CD36, FATP2, and FATP5 subsequently actively transport these free fatty acids into hepatocytes [20]. In particular, mice with liver-specific CD36 overexpression had increased hepatic steatosis, sufficient to replicate the liver effects of diet-induced obesity [21]. The notion that CD36 is a major player in the molecular pathophysiology of hepatic steatosis is further supported by the observation that CD36 expression in patients correlates with the severity of steatosis. Hepatic steatosis is associated with increased de novo lipogenesis and fatty acid absorption. At the molecular level, steatosis is influenced by the activation of the lysogenic master regulator SREBP1c and its target enzymes, such as acetyl-CoA carboxylase (ACC) and stearoyl-CoA desaturase (SCD1) [22]. Furthermore, increased signalling via the thyroid-stimulating hormone (TSH) and Thyroid Hormone Receptor β (THRβ) axis has been connected to hepatic triglyceride accumulation. This is believed to stimulate lipogenesis by activating SREBP1c [23]. However, patients with FLD have approximately 3 times higher lipogenesis levels [24]. The majority of hepatic lipids in obese NAFLD patients with fasting hypertriglyceridemia and hyperinsulinemia are absorbed from non-esterified fatty acids produced by adipose tissue lipolysis; diet and de novo lipogenesis contribute only 26% and 15%, respectively. Fructose is one dietary component that particularly promotes hepatic steatosis by lowering beta-oxidation and stimulating hepatic lipogenesis. It is interesting to note that animals that have both fructokinase A and C genetically deleted do not develop fatty liver from fructose, suggesting a clear link between fructose activation and triglyceride build-up [25]. Hepatic calcium regulation is also disrupted by hepatic steatosis. In particular, insulin-sensitive InsP3R channels are less activated in the presence of insulin resistance. Furthermore, steatosis alters the fluidity of the endoplasmic reticulum (ER) membrane and compromises the function of the ER calcium pump, SERCA, by disrupting the equilibrium between phosphatidylcholine and phosphatidylethanolamine. These molecular processes work together to lower calcium levels in the hepatocyte's ER, which in turn reduces the function of calcium-dependent chaperones and triggers a series of events, including ER stress, the unfolded protein response (UPR), and ER overload with misfolded proteins. However, it has been suggested that the unfolded protein response (UPR) reduces insulin sensitivity in several ways, including by first activating IRE1, which reduces insulin signaling by raising JNK activity, and then triggering TRB3, which directly blocks the insulin receptor [26]. As technology has advanced, more scientists have examined genetic predispositions and discovered several gene variants that can affect how the liver and other organs, including adipose tissue, metabolize sugar and lipids [27]. Lipotoxicity and hepatocellular stress can result from excessive absorption of saturated free fatty acids. Part of this damage arises from the stimulation of mitochondrial fatty acid β-oxidation, which increases the production of reactive oxygen species (ROS) beyond the cell's capacity to neutralize them. High ROS levels cause DNA damage, lipid peroxidation, and increased release of proinflammatory and profibrotic proteins by activating various stress signaling pathways, including TRAIL, JNK, and MLK3. Moreover, inflammation is associated with the liver's overexpression of CCR2/5, which encourages additional immune cell infiltration and exacerbates inflammation [28]. Another important source of hepatocellular ROS in FLD is gamma-oxidation in the ER, which is mediated by CYP2E1 and CYP4As, in addition to mitochondrial beta-oxidation of fatty acids. Hepatic CYP2E1 activity is higher in NASH patients than in those with benign steatosis, and its expression is localized in the steatotic regions of the liver [29, 30]. Fig. (**2**) describes the mechanistic pathways and causation of NAFLD, as well as its treatment alternatives.

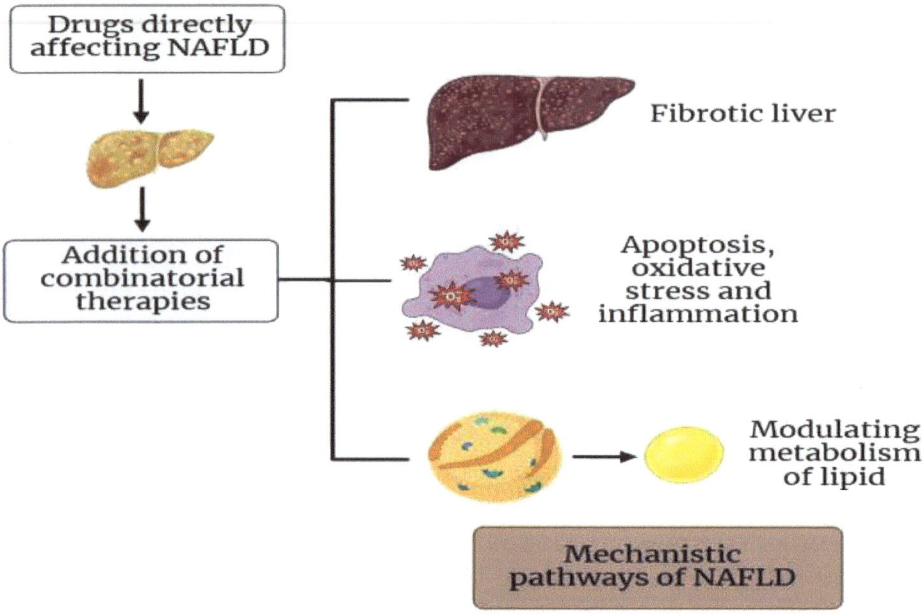

Fig. (2). Mechanistic pathways of NAFLD and the treatment alternatives.

CURRENT PHARMACOLOGIC THERAPIES

Therapeutic targets for Non-Alcoholic Fatty Liver Disease (NAFLD) have been categorized into four areas based on research: lipid toxicity and cell death; inflammation; extracellular matrix deposition for anti-fibrosis; and carbohydrate and lipid metabolism. Numerous medications can alleviate NASH by targeting distinct pathways [31]. Dietary guidelines, lifestyle modifications, weight loss, and management of underlying metabolic syndrome remain the cornerstone of treatment [32]. Amiodarone, tamoxifen, and steroids are examples of steatogenic medications that can cause liver fat infiltration as a side effect [33]. Fatty liver disease can be effectively managed through diet and lifestyle modifications; however, pharmacological intervention is necessary when these approaches prove insufficient [34].

Diet

Managing NAFLD involves identifying both modifiable factors, such as diet, exercise, and metabolic risk factors, and non-modifiable factors, including genetics, age, ethnicity, and sex, that contribute to disease progression. Most individuals with NAFLD have an unhealthy diet and insufficient physical activity. Therefore, the initial step in management is to target modifiable risk factors, aiming for a weight loss of 5–10% (or 3–5% for those without overweight or obesity). This weight reduction can decrease steatosis at the lower end of the range and help reverse fibrosis at the higher end [35].

Exercise

It has been shown that physical activity can reduce hepatic steatosis without dietary changes. Furthermore, it has been discovered to increase liver stiffness. Regular physical activity can improve the outcomes in NAFLD [36].

Vitamin E (alpha-tocopherol)

Oxidative stress results from an unbalanced synthesis of reactive oxygen species and the body's capacity to neutralize them. The transition from NAFLD to SH is accelerated by an excess of reactive oxygen species, which is driven by hepatic lipid accumulation. By boosting certain enzymes and regulating the inflammatory response, vitamin E has anti-fibrotic and antioxidant qualities [37].

(PPAR)-γ agonist

Pioglitazone, an agonist of the peroxisome proliferator-activated receptor (PPAR)-γ, aids in the reduction of insulin resistance in the liver, muscle, and adipose tissue. Pioglitazone treatment has shown significant improvement in NASH in individuals with and without diabetes, according to many prospective investigations [38].

Lipid-lowering drugs

NAFLD is closely associated with dyslipidemia and obesity. Statins, which are frequently used to treat dyslipidemia, function by blocking 3-hydroxy-3-methylglutaryl-coenzyme A (HMGCoA) reductase, which stops cholesterol synthesis. Statins are also thought to be a therapy option for NAFLD because of their possible anti-inflammatory properties [39].

Pentoxifylline

Pentoxifylline, a nonselective phosphodiesterase inhibitor and methylxanthine derivative, acts by preventing TNFα synthesis. Pentoxifylline has been investigated as a possible therapy for NAFLD/NASH, as TNFα is thought to be a major factor in the development of NAFLD [39].

Ursodeoxycholic Acid

A hydrophilic bile acid with cytoprotective and antiapoptotic qualities is ursodeoxycholic acid (UDCA). Therefore, research has been done on its possible impact on NAFLD/NASH [39].

Blockers of angiotensin receptors

The pathophysiology of NAFLD/NASH involves the renin-angiotensi--aldosterone system, which also affects insulin sensitivity. Thus, research has examined how angiotensin II type 1 blockers, such as telmisartan, valsartan, and losartan, affect NAFLD [39].

Probiotics and Synbiotics

Prebiotics are compounds that support the growth and/or activity of helpful microbes that support the host's well-being, whereas probiotics are microorganisms that provide health advantages when consumed. Synbiotics are dietary supplements that synergistically mix prebiotics and probiotics. Given that gut microbes contribute to the development of fibrosis, necroinflammation, hepatic steatosis, and insulin resistance, probiotics and synbiotics may be beneficial for NAFLD/NASH [39]. Probiotics and prebiotics, such as *Lactobacillus, Bifidobacterium spp.*, and *S. boulardii*, are used to treat NAFLD [39].

THR-b (thyroid hormone receptor b) Agonist

THR-β has been investigated as a therapeutic target for the development of novel therapeutics for NAFLD/NASH and is involved in several metabolic pathways, including cholesterol and glycolipid metabolism in the liver. A new THR-β agonist, Resmetirom (MGL-3196), targets the liver specifically [40].

Obeticholic Acid, or OCA, as an Agonist of the Farnesoid X Receptor (FXR)

Obeticholic acid (OCA) is a natural agonist of the Farnesoid X Receptor (FXR) and a semisynthetic derivative of chenodeoxycholic acid, the main bile acid in humans. FXR is a nuclear hormone receptor that controls the metabolism of fat and glucose. In NAFLD patients with type 2 diabetes mellitus, FXR improves insulin sensitivity when it is triggered by OCA [41].

Bariatric Surgery

Bariatric surgery greatly enhances glycemic control. Moreover, improvements in the inflammatory response and lipid metabolism are believed to reduce the severity of NAFLD [42].

CHALLENGES IN TREATING FATTY LIVER DISEASE

The primary drawbacks of conventional pharmaceutical therapies are their incapacity to provide the afflicted liver with a sufficient concentration of the therapeutic agent and their lack of focused medication delivery, which may cause unintended systemic side effects [43].

Liver-specific Targeting

It is challenging to deliver drugs to particular regions of the liver since it is a complex organ with a varied cell population [44].

Hepatotoxicity and Off-target Effects

Many drugs affect organs other than the liver, causing toxicity. Drugs may not effectively reach the liver in the desired concentrations when taken orally [45].

NANO CARRIER-BASED DRUG DELIVERY SYSTEMS

The pharmaceutical industry continuously advances its development strategies, focusing on two key factors: (i) designing medications to be highly selective for their target site in the body and (ii) ensuring a stable, reproducible drug concentration at the intended location, thereby reducing dosage frequency [46]. A new field, nanomedicine, has significant potential to develop highly effective, tailored treatments. Nanomedicines are composed of nanoparticles (NPs), which typically measure up to 100 nm in at least one dimension, although their overall diameter can extend to several hundred nanometres. There are two methods for producing these nanoparticles: bottom-up/self-assembly and top-down, which involves breaking larger structures into smaller ones using mechanical force.

Nanotechnology can enhance the delivery of macromolecules and poorly water-soluble medications, facilitate combination therapy, promote drug absorption across a range of epithelial and endothelial barriers, and enable tissue- or cell-specific drug delivery [47]. The idea of nanopharmaceuticals has been used by endowing already-existing active chemicals with new functions. These developments have made it easier to find materials at the molecular level and to evaluate compounds with special properties for biomedical applications due to nanotechnology [48]. By reducing renal excretion and hepatic clearance, nanomedicine can prolong the circulation time of the therapeutic payload, which sets them apart from traditional medications. 'Site-specific' medication administration is made possible, improving the therapeutic index and reducing toxicity. The idea of "the agnostic" combines therapeutic and diagnostic components, paving the way for next-generation nanoparticles that facilitate drug administration, controlled release, and non-invasive diagnostics. Nanomedicine is more than just a simple drug delivery device [47]. Nano medicines consist of nanomaterials or miniaturized devices with multifunctional components that are biocompatible, biodegradable, and highly viscoelastic, featuring an extended circulating half-life [49]. NDDSs containing various agents exhibit senescent cell clearance, ROS scavenging, local reduction in blood glucose levels, and anti-inflammatory effects [50]. Nanotechnology-based dietary supplements and pharmaceuticals developed by the food and pharmaceutical industries address challenges related to vitamin administration, including stability, absorption, and low bioavailability [51]. Nanostructures enable the controlled release of encapsulated medications at the prescribed dosage, as they remain in the bloodstream for a long time. Consequently, they limit plasma oscillations and lessen negative consequences [52]. Currently, more than 27 nanomedicines are approved for clinical use by the FDA or EMA. An enclosed payload, targeting or surface components, and a core material make up the organic, inorganic, or hybrid nanocarrier units employed in nanomedicine applications [53]. Major molecules, proteins, peptides, nucleic acids, and RNA oligonucleotides are just a few of the many payloads that may be loaded into these nanoparticles to facilitate both targeted and non-targeted distribution. Therapeutic and diagnostic substances have been delivered using a variety of nanostructure types to treat various illnesses [54]. Nanotechnology has enabled the advancement of biosensors for detecting pathogens and imaging techniques for diagnosing inflammatory diseases [55]. For drug delivery, a variety of nanocarriers have been developed, including micelles, nanoemulsions, nanospheres, nanocapsules, nanoshells, dendrimers, liposomes, solid lipid nanoparticles, polymersomes, polymer–drug conjugates, polymeric nanoparticles, peptide nanoparticles, gold nanoparticles, and carbon nanotubes [56]. Fig. (**3**) depicts the preparation of nanoparticles for the treatment of NAFLD.

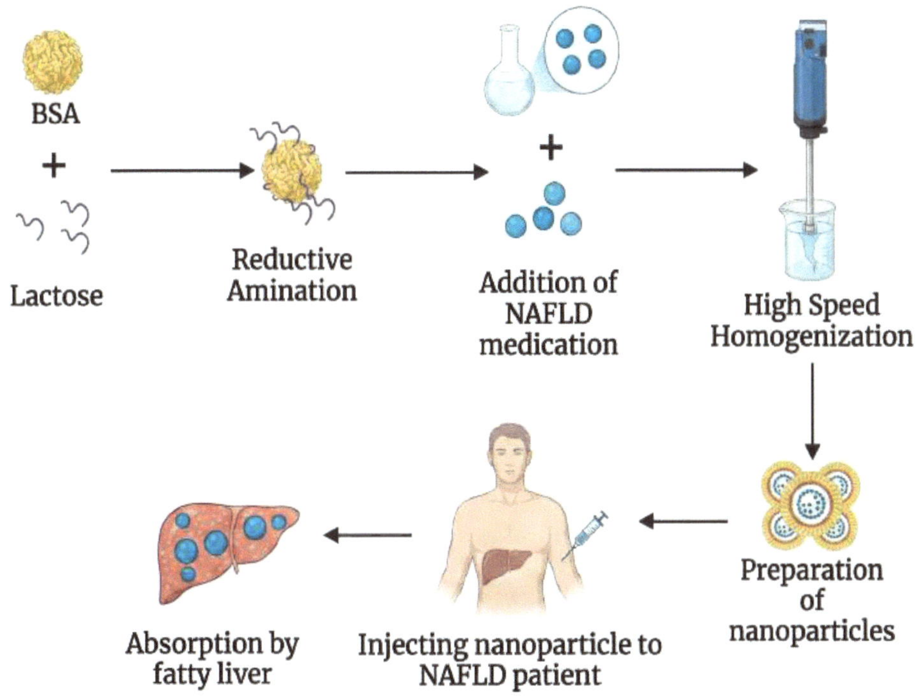

Fig. (3). Preparation of drug-loaded nanoparticles for the treatment of NAFLD.

Key types of nanocarriers include:

- **Nano crystals:** Used to increase the bioavailability of poorly soluble medications [57].
- **Solid lipid nanoparticles (SLNs):** Solid lipid nanoparticles that improve drug solubility and release profiles [57].
- **Polymeric nanoparticles:** These can include a range of medicinal substances, such as tiny molecules, proteins, or RNA [58]. Advanced drug delivery techniques use biodegradable and bioreducible polymers, and prospective future research applications are fuelling the field's advancement [59].
- **Liposomes:** Lipid bilayers are biocompatible and adaptable carriers that can transport both hydrophilic and hydrophobic medications [60]. Liposomes have a limited circulation time due to their rapid clearance from the bloodstream [61].

NANO MEDICINE FOR FLD THERAPEUTICS

The targeting mechanism of nanomaterials for fatty liver disease relies on their distinct properties and functions. Nanomaterials can deliver medications or other therapeutic agents to liver tissue or hepatocytes by selectively targeting their surfaces through surface modification and functionalization. There are two approaches to targeting nanomaterials: passive targeting and active targeting. Passive targeting occurs due to the intrinsic physical and chemical properties of nanomaterials, leading to their accumulation in liver tissue or on cell membranes. Passive targeting to liver cell membranes can occur through two mechanisms: static adsorption to the leukocyte surface or incorporation as a component of the cell membrane. The efficiency of nanomaterial targeting is also influenced by their size and shape. Smaller nanomaterials, due to their shape, exhibit high penetration capability, enabling them to traverse narrow blood vessels and gaps in vessel walls, thereby enhancing tissue diffusion [62]. In contrast, active targeting directs nanomaterials to liver tissue or hepatocytes via specific molecular-recognition mechanisms. For example, nanoparticles modified with surface ligands can enhance hepatic binding and actively target receptors on cells [63].

Passive Targeting

Passive targeting exploits the physical and chemical features of nanomaterials to facilitate their transport to liver tissue or hepatocytes. Nanomaterials serve various purposes toward passive targeting for the diagnosis and treatment of liver disease. For example, liposomes are characterized by a specific chemical composition and a phospholipid bilayer, which makes them more attractive to cell membranes, therefore increasing their targeting capability. Liposomes may also transport medicine directly to hepatocytes through endocytosis, thereby avoiding lysosomal degradation and ensuring drug potency and stability. The biological properties of liposomes, such as extended circulation, along with the specific physiological and pathological features of the diseased liver, account for their passive accumulation in regions that require treatment. The accumulation and release of liposomes in the diseased liver are aided by the hypoxic, acidic, and highly permeable microenvironment of the tissue [64]. Other factors noted to improve liposome targeting include changes in potential, local perfusion, microvascular permeability, and the influx of inflammatory cells [65]. The presence of negative charges can favorably increase liposome concentration in liver lesions. Surface charge, shape, and other biological characteristics are used by multifunctional nanoparticles to passively target hepatocytes.

Active Targeting

Active targeting of nanomaterials to liver tissue or hepatocytes is achieved through specific molecular-recognition mechanisms. Active targeting in nanotherapeutics is enabled by the high surface-area-to-volume ratio of nanomaterials, which allows a variety of functionalizations. Active targeting offers advantages over passive targeting by overcoming its limitations [66]. Liposomes, as an effective drug-delivery system, can target hepatocytes by binding to specific receptors on their surface. They can interact with hepatocyte membranes and internal molecules via specific signalling pathways, thereby promoting phagocytosis and drug degradation by hepatocytes. Altering liposome surface properties enables them to specifically target liver lesions [67]. Glycosylated liposomes can target overexpressed glycosylated receptors in the liver, such as glycosylated proteins on hepatocyte surfaces, to deliver drugs to diseased areas. During the inflammatory response in the liver, there is a change in the receptors on hepatocyte surfaces, creating a potential for targeting with liposomes. For example, the inflammatory response, by enhancing leukocyte accumulation, increases lipocyte expression of surface adhesion molecules in the liver, which can then bind to receptors on liposomes and thus provide a means for their targeted delivery. Several studies have demonstrated the ability of liver cells to recognize and internalize liposomes. This process is largely mediated by interactions with liver-specific receptors, such as the transferrin receptor (TfR) and the low-density lipoprotein receptor (LDLR), which facilitate targeted delivery to hepatic cells [68]. One well-known natural substance that is frequently utilized in clinical therapies for liver problems and has the potential to cure FLD is silibinin (Sil). However, because of its limited absorption and low bioavailability, its efficacy for treating FLD remains unknown. In addition to examining the mechanisms underlying Sil-Lip's activity, this study sought to design a Sil-loaded liposome (Sil-Lip) to overcome these drawbacks and enhance its therapeutic benefits in FLD. Using the well-established thin-film dispersion technique, Sil-Lip was developed, thoroughly described, and then assessed for therapeutic effectiveness [67]. Liver transcriptome analysis and 16S ribosomal RNA (16S rRNA) sequencing were conducted to explore the potential mechanisms of action of Sil-Lip. The results showed that Sil-Lip exhibited good stability in the gastrointestinal tract, effective penetration of the mucus layer, and enhanced oral absorption and bioavailability. In both *in vivo* and *in vitro* FLD models, Sil-Lip demonstrated superior effects on lipid metabolism disorders, insulin resistance, and inflammation compared with Sil alone [69]. Further analysis revealed that Sil-Lip's beneficial effects were mediated through modulation of intrahepatic insulin resistance-related and NF-κB signaling pathways, as well as the extrahepatic gut microbiota. The study concluded that Sil-Lip effectively enhanced the absorption and bioavailability of Sil, thereby amplifying its therapeutic effects on FLD by modulating intrahepatic insulin resistance-related pathways, NF-κB signaling, and the gut microbiota [69].

LIMITATIONS OF CURRENT APPROACHES AND CHALLENGES IN CLINICAL TRANSLATION

Despite the remarkable preclinical promise of nanocarrier-based drug delivery systems for fatty liver disease, their clinical translation remains hindered by several technological, biological, and regulatory challenges [70]. A major limitation is the lack of *in vivo* stability, as nanocarriers are often prone to aggregation, premature drug release, or rapid clearance by the reticuloendothelial system. These drawbacks compromise therapeutic efficacy and limit drug bioavailability in hepatic tissue [71, 72]. Furthermore, while nanocarrier-based systems have shown improved drug solubility and targeted delivery in animal models, translating these benefits to human applications is not straightforward due to the complexity of liver pathology and patient-to-patient variability.

Another significant challenge is immunogenicity, where nanocarriers may provoke unintended immune responses or long-term toxicological effects, especially when employing novel polymers, lipids, or surface modifications. For instance, although extracellular vesicles (EVs) are being investigated as natural nanocarriers due to their biocompatibility and low immunogenicity, issues, such as off-target effects, clearance mechanisms, and the risk of immune stimulation, remain unresolved [73, 74]. In addition, some nanocarrier systems fail to achieve efficient targeting of hepatocellular carcinoma (HCC) or specific liver cell populations, reducing their clinical value in complex conditions, such as non-alcoholic fatty liver disease (NAFLD) and non-alcoholic steatohepatitis (NASH). These targeting inefficiencies highlight the need for more precise ligand-recepto--mediated delivery strategies that can address the heterogeneity of liver disease progression [75].

Equally important are the challenges in scalability and regulatory approval. Large-scale manufacturing of nanocarriers while maintaining uniform particle size, surface properties, drug-loading capacity, and encapsulation efficiency is technically demanding and cost-intensive. Current good manufacturing practices (cGMP) for nanomedicines are still evolving, and the absence of standardized protocols further delays clinical adoption. Regulatory agencies also require extensive preclinical and clinical data on safety, biodistribution, and long-term toxicity, making the approval process particularly stringent. Thus, the future of nanocarrier-based therapies for fatty liver disease depends on developing robust, safe, and scalable systems that can withstand physiological conditions, minimize immune-related risks, and meet regulatory benchmarks for successful clinical translation [76].

FUTURE PROSPECTS

With rapid advances in nanotechnology and biomedicine, the use of targeted nanomaterials for treating liver diseases is increasingly promising. However, to maximize their success, challenges related to toxicity and stability must be addressed. Additionally, developing tailored, precise nanomaterials for specific liver diseases is crucial to improving treatment outcomes. In the future, approaches, such as bispecific or multispecific targeting methods for liver cancer cells, are expected to play a key role in advancing treatment strategies [77]. It is anticipated to lead to more precise targeting. In summary, targeted nanomaterials hold great promise as a novel therapeutic strategy for liver disease. Targeted nanomaterials are anticipated to become increasingly important in the treatment of liver disease as technology continues to advance and improve patient outcomes and quality of life.

CONCLUSION

Fatty liver disease is a widespread global health issue affecting millions of individuals. While several treatment options exist, their effectiveness is often limited, and many liver diseases remain untreatable. Recently, the development of targeted nanomaterials has emerged as a promising novel method of liver disease treatment. These nanomaterials may be customized with specific characteristics, such as size, shape, and surface charge, to target specific cells or tissues. They are intended to deliver medications or therapeutic agents directly to the afflicted liver cells. They can also be designed to release their therapeutic payloads in a controlled manner, thereby increasing effectiveness and reducing adverse effects. Targeted nanomaterials' capacity to overcome the drawbacks of conventional medication administration is one of their main advantages. In conclusion, targeted nanomaterials hold significant promise as a novel approach for treating liver diseases. While there are still challenges to overcome, the potential advantages of these nanoparticles are vast. As advancements in nanotechnology and biomedicine continue, targeted nanomaterials are likely to become an increasingly integral part of liver disease treatment, offering more effective and personalized solutions for patients.

LIST OF ABBREVIATIONS

ACC	Acetyl-CoA carboxylase
CYP2E1	Cytochrome P450 2E1
FLD	Fatty Liver Disease
FXR	Farnesoid X Receptor
HCC	Hepatocellular carcinoma

HMG-CoA	3-Hydroxy-3-methylglutaryl-coenzyme A
NDDS	Nanocarrier-based drug delivery systems
NAFLD	Non-Alcoholic Fatty Liver Disease
NASH	Non-Alcoholic Steatohepatitis
NPs	Nanoparticles
OCA	Obeticholic acid
PPAR-γ	Peroxisome proliferator-activated receptor-gamma
ROS	Reactive Oxygen Species
SCD1	Stearoyl-CoA desaturase
Sil	Silibinin
Sil-Lip	Silibinin-loaded liposome
SLNs	Solid lipid nanoparticles
SREBP1c	Sterol regulatory element-binding protein 1c
T2D	Type 2 diabetes
THR-β	Thyroid Hormone Receptor beta
UDCA	Ursodeoxycholic acid
UPR	Unfolded protein response

REFERENCES

[1] Bashir A, Duseja A, De A, Mehta M, Tiwari P. Non-alcoholic fatty liver disease development: A multifactorial pathogenic phenomena. Liver Res 2022; 6(2): 72-83.
[http://dx.doi.org/10.1016/j.livres.2022.05.002] [PMID: 39958625]

[2] Dhamija E, Paul SB, Kedia S. Non-alcoholic fatty liver disease associated with hepatocellular carcinoma. Indian J Med Res 2019; 149(1): 9-17.
[http://dx.doi.org/10.4103/ijmr.IJMR_1456_17] [PMID: 31115369]

[3] Vernon G, Baranova A, Younossi ZM. Systematic review: the epidemiology and natural history of non-alcoholic fatty liver disease and non-alcoholic steatohepatitis in adults. Aliment Pharmacol Ther 2011; 34(3): 274-85.
[http://dx.doi.org/10.1111/j.1365-2036.2011.04724.x] [PMID: 21623852]

[4] Sharma S, Sharma A, Gupta P, *et al.* The Green Path to Liver Health: Herbal Solutions for Non-alcoholic Steatohepatitis. Cardiovasc Hematol Disord Drug Targets 2025; 25(3): 168-92.
[http://dx.doi.org/10.2174/011871529X360903250211101856] [PMID: 40108906]

[5] Kemas AM, Youhanna S, Lauschke VM. Non-alcoholic fatty liver disease - opportunities for personalized treatment and drug development. Expert Rev Precis Med Drug Dev 2022; 7(1): 39-49.
[http://dx.doi.org/10.1080/23808993.2022.2053285]

[6] Han SK, Baik SK, Kim MY. Non-alcoholic fatty liver disease: Definition and subtypes. Clin Mol Hepatol 2023; 29 (Suppl.): S5-S16.
[http://dx.doi.org/10.3350/cmh.2022.0424] [PMID: 36577427]

[7] Tandra S, Yeh MM, Brunt EM, *et al.* Presence and significance of microvesicular steatosis in nonalcoholic fatty liver disease. J Hepatol 2011; 55(3): 654-9.
[http://dx.doi.org/10.1016/j.jhep.2010.11.021] [PMID: 21172393]

[8] Teli MR, James OFW, Burt AD, Bennett MK, Day CP. The natural history of nonalcoholic fatty liver: A follow-up study. Hepatology 1995; 22(6): 1714-9. [http://dx.doi.org/10.1002/hep.1840220616] [PMID: 7489979]

[9] Ekstedt M, Hagström H, Nasr P, *et al.* Fibrosis stage is the strongest predictor for disease-specific mortality in NAFLD after up to 33 years of follow-up. Hepatology 2015; 61(5): 1547-54. [http://dx.doi.org/10.1002/hep.27368] [PMID: 25125077]

[10] Pafili K, Roden M. Nonalcoholic fatty liver disease (NAFLD) from pathogenesis to treatment concepts in humans. Mol Metab 2021; 50: 101122. [http://dx.doi.org/10.1016/j.molmet.2020.101122] [PMID: 33220492]

[11] Habibullah M, Jemmieh K, Ouda A, Haider MZ, Malki MI, Elzouki AN. Metabolic-associated fatty liver disease: a selective review of pathogenesis, diagnostic approaches, and therapeutic strategies. Front Med (Lausanne) 2024; 11: 1291501. [http://dx.doi.org/10.3389/fmed.2024.1291501] [PMID: 38323033]

[12] Grander C, Grabherr F, Tilg H. Non-alcoholic fatty liver disease: pathophysiological concepts and treatment options. Cardiovasc Res 2023; 119(9): 1787-98. [http://dx.doi.org/10.1093/cvr/cvad095] [PMID: 37364164]

[13] Wong VWS, Ekstedt M, Wong GLH, Hagström H. Changing epidemiology, global trends and implications for outcomes of NAFLD. J Hepatol 2023; 79(3): 842-52. [http://dx.doi.org/10.1016/j.jhep.2023.04.036] [PMID: 37169151]

[14] Opioids er. Admission vital signs and laboratory charac-teristics as predictors of disposition status in a diverse cohort of hospitalized covid-19 patients in New Mexico. J Gen Intern Med 2023; 38(2): S81-S799.

[15] Younossi Z, Anstee QM, Marietti M, *et al.* Global burden of NAFLD and NASH: trends, predictions, risk factors and prevention. Nat Rev Gastroenterol Hepatol 2018; 15(1): 11-20. [http://dx.doi.org/10.1038/nrgastro.2017.109] [PMID: 28930295]

[16] Dyson JK, Anstee QM, McPherson S. Non-alcoholic fatty liver disease: a practical approach to diagnosis and staging. Frontline Gastroenterol 2014; 5(3): 211-8. [http://dx.doi.org/10.1136/flgastro-2013-100403] [PMID: 25018867]

[17] Dassanayake AS, Kasturiratne A, Rajindrajith S, *et al.* Prevalence and risk factors for non□alcoholic fatty liver disease among adults in an urban Sri Lankan population. J Gastroenterol Hepatol 2009; 24(7): 1284-8. [http://dx.doi.org/10.1111/j.1440-1746.2009.05831.x] [PMID: 19476560]

[18] Lazarus JV, Mark HE, Anstee QM, *et al.* Advancing the global public health agenda for NAFLD: a consensus statement. Nat Rev Gastroenterol Hepatol 2022; 19(1): 60-78. [http://dx.doi.org/10.1038/s41575-021-00523-4] [PMID: 34707258]

[19] Mavrogiannaki AN, Migdalis IN. Nonalcoholic Fatty liver disease, diabetes mellitus and cardiovascular disease: newer data. Int J Endocrinol 2013; 2013(1): 1-8. [http://dx.doi.org/10.1155/2013/450639] [PMID: 23653642]

[20] Glatz JFC, Luiken JJFP, Bonen A. Membrane fatty acid transporters as regulators of lipid metabolism: implications for metabolic disease. Physiol Rev 2010; 90(1): 367-417. [http://dx.doi.org/10.1152/physrev.00003.2009] [PMID: 20086080]

[21] Miquilena-Colina ME, Lima-Cabello E, Sánchez-Campos S, *et al.* Hepatic fatty acid translocase CD36 upregulation is associated with insulin resistance, hyperinsulinaemia and increased steatosis in non-alcoholic steatohepatitis and chronic hepatitis C. Gut 2011; 60(10): 1394-402. [http://dx.doi.org/10.1136/gut.2010.222844] [PMID: 21270117]

[22] Esler WP, Bence KK. Metabolic targets in nonalcoholic fatty liver disease. Cell Mol Gastroenterol Hepatol 2019; 8(2): 247-67. [http://dx.doi.org/10.1016/j.jcmgh.2019.04.007] [PMID: 31004828]

[23] Xiang L, Cao Y, Sun J, *et al.* Association between thyroid function and nonalcoholic fatty liver disease: a dose-response meta-analysis. Front Endocrinol (Lausanne) 2024; 15: 1399517. [http://dx.doi.org/10.3389/fendo.2024.1399517] [PMID: 38982990]

[24] Ishimoto T, Lanaspa MA, Rivard CJ, Roncal-Jimenez CA, Orlicky DJ, Cicerchi C, McMahan RH, Abdelmalek MF, Rosen HR, Jackman MR, MacLean PS, Diggle CP, Asipu A, Inaba S, Kosugi T, Sato W, Maruyama S, Sánchez-Lozada LG, Sautin YY, Hill JO, Bonthron DT, Johnson RJ. High-fat and high-sucrose (western) diet induces steatohepatitis that is dependent on fructokinase. Hepatology. 2013 Nov;58(5):1632-43.

[25] Ishimoto T, Lanaspa MA, Le MT, *et al.* Opposing effects of fructokinase C and A isoforms on fructose-induced metabolic syndrome in mice. Proc Natl Acad Sci USA 2012; 109(11): 4320-5. [http://dx.doi.org/10.1073/pnas.1119908109] [PMID: 22371574]

[26] Koh HJ, Toyoda T, Didesch MM, *et al.* Tribbles 3 mediates endoplasmic reticulum stress-induced insulin resistance in skeletal muscle. Nat Commun 2013; 4(1): 1871. [http://dx.doi.org/10.1038/ncomms2851] [PMID: 23695665]

[27] Hanson A, Wilhelmsen D, DiStefano JK. The role of long non-coding RNAs (lncRNAs) in the development and progression of fibrosis associated with nonalcoholic fatty liver disease (NAFLD). noncoding RNA. 2018 Aug 21;4(3):18.

[28] Emery MG, Fisher JM, Chien JY, Kharasch ED, Dellinger EP, Kowdley KV, Thummel KE. CYP2E1 activity before and after weight loss in morbidly obese subjects with nonalcoholic fatty liver disease. Hepatology. 2003 Aug;38(2):428-35.

[29] Weltman MD, Farrell GC, Hall P, Ingelman-Sundberg M, Liddle C. Hepatic cytochrome P450 2E1 is increased in patients with nonalcoholic steatohepatitis. Hepatology 1998; 27(1): 128-33. [http://dx.doi.org/10.1002/hep.510270121] [PMID: 9425928]

[30] Chalasani N, Gorski CJ, Asghar MS, *et al.* Hepatic cytochrome P450 2E1 activity in nondiabetic patients with nonalcoholic steatohepatitis. Hepatology 2003; 37(3): 544-50. [http://dx.doi.org/10.1053/jhep.2003.50095] [PMID: 12601351]

[31] Fu Y, Zhou Y, Shen L, *et al.* Diagnostic and therapeutic strategies for non-alcoholic fatty liver disease. Front Pharmacol 2022; 13: 973366. [http://dx.doi.org/10.3389/fphar.2022.973366] [PMID: 36408234]

[32] Pouwels S, Sakran N, Graham Y, *et al.* Non-alcoholic fatty liver disease (NAFLD): a review of pathophysiology, clinical management and effects of weight loss. BMC Endocr Disord 2022; 22(1): 63. [http://dx.doi.org/10.1186/s12902-022-00980-1] [PMID: 35287643]

[33] Guo X, Yin X, Liu Z, Wang J. Non-alcoholic fatty liver disease (NAFLD) pathogenesis and natural products for prevention and treatment. Int J Mol Sci 2022; 23(24): 15489. [http://dx.doi.org/10.3390/ijms232415489] [PMID: 36555127]

[34] Ray K. NAFLD—the next global epidemic. Nat Rev Gastroenterol Hepatol 2013; 10(11): 621-2. [http://dx.doi.org/10.1038/nrgastro.2013.197] [PMID: 24185985]

[35] Younossi ZM, Henry L. Understanding the burden of nonalcoholic fatty liver disease: time for action. Diabetes Spectr 2024; 37(1): 9-19. [http://dx.doi.org/10.2337/dsi23-0010] [PMID: 38385101]

[36] Shao Y, Chen S, Han L, Liu J. Pharmacotherapies of NAFLD: updated opportunities based on metabolic intervention. Nutr Metab (Lond) 2023; 20(1): 30. [http://dx.doi.org/10.1186/s12986-023-00748-x] [PMID: 37415199]

[37] Li S, Li H, Xu X, Saw PE, Zhang L. Nanocarrier-mediated antioxidant delivery for liver diseases. Theranostics 2020; 10(3): 1262-80. [http://dx.doi.org/10.7150/thno.38834] [PMID: 31938064]

[38] Trauner M, Fuchs CD. Novel therapeutic targets for cholestatic and fatty liver disease. Gut 2022; 71(1): 194-209.
[http://dx.doi.org/10.1136/gutjnl-2021-324305] [PMID: 34615727]

[39] Martín-Domínguez V, González-Casas R, Mendoza-Jiménez-Ridruejo J, García-Buey L, Moreno-Otero R. Pathogenesis, diagnosis and treatment of non-alcoholic fatty liver disease. Rev Esp Enferm Dig 2013; 105(7): 409-20.
[http://dx.doi.org/10.4321/S1130-01082013000700006] [PMID: 24206551]

[40] Rong L, Zou J, Ran W, *et al.* Advancements in the treatment of non-alcoholic fatty liver disease (NAFLD). Front Endocrinol (Lausanne) 2023; 13: 1087260.
[http://dx.doi.org/10.3389/fendo.2022.1087260] [PMID: 36726464]

[41] Mudaliar S, Henry RR, Sanyal AJ, *et al.* Efficacy and safety of the farnesoid X receptor agonist obeticholic acid in patients with type 2 diabetes and nonalcoholic fatty liver disease. Gastroenterology 2013; 145(3): 574-582.e1.
[http://dx.doi.org/10.1053/j.gastro.2013.05.042] [PMID: 23727264]

[42] Sahu P, Chhabra P, Mehendale AM. A comprehensive review on Non-alcoholic fatty liver disease. Cureus 2023; 15(12): e50159.
[http://dx.doi.org/10.7759/cureus.50159] [PMID: 38186528]

[43] Böttger R, Pauli G, Chao PH, AL Fayez N, Hohenwarter L, Li SD. Lipid-based nanoparticle technologies for liver targeting. Adv Drug Deliv Rev 2020; 154-155: 79-101.
[http://dx.doi.org/10.1016/j.addr.2020.06.017] [PMID: 32574575]

[44] Lee S, Zhang C, Liu Z, *et al.* Network analyses identify liver-specific targets for treating liver diseases. Mol Syst Biol 2017; 13(8): 938.
[http://dx.doi.org/10.15252/msb.20177703] [PMID: 28827398]

[45] Moosavian SA, Sathyapalan T, Jamialahmadi T, Sahebkar A. The emerging role of nanomedicine in the management of nonalcoholic fatty liver disease: A state-of-the-art review. Bioinorg Chem Appl 2021; 2021(1): 1-13.
[http://dx.doi.org/10.1155/2021/4041415] [PMID: 34659388]

[46] Mazdaei M, Asare-Addo K. A mini-review of nanocarriers in drug delivery systems. British Journal of Pharmacy 2022; 7(1): 1-3.
[http://dx.doi.org/10.5920/bjpharm.780]

[47] Athanasopoulou F, Manolakakis M, Vernia S, Kamaly N. Nanodrug delivery systems for metabolic chronic liver diseases: advances and perspectives. Nanomedicine (Lond) 2023; 18(1): 67-84.
[http://dx.doi.org/10.2217/nnm-2022-0261] [PMID: 36896958]

[48] Haripriyaa M, Suthindhiran K. Pharmacokinetics of nanoparticles: current knowledge, future directions and its implications in drug delivery. Future J Pharm Sci 2023; 9(1): 113.
[http://dx.doi.org/10.1186/s43094-023-00569-y]

[49] Ezike TC, Okpala US, Onoja UL, *et al.* Advances in drug delivery systems, challenges and future directions. Heliyon 2023; 9(6): e17488.
[http://dx.doi.org/10.1016/j.heliyon.2023.e17488] [PMID: 37416680]

[50] Liu M, Wei X, Zheng Z, *et al.* Recent advances in nano-drug delivery systems for the treatment of diabetic wound healing. Int J Nanomedicine 2023; 18: 1537-60.
[http://dx.doi.org/10.2147/IJN.S395438] [PMID: 37007988]

[51] Crintea A, Dutu AG, Sovrea A, *et al.* Nanocarriers for drug delivery: an overview with emphasis on vitamin D and K transportation. Nanomaterials (Basel) 2022; 12(8): 1376.
[http://dx.doi.org/10.3390/nano12081376] [PMID: 35458084]

[52] Patra JK, Das G, Fraceto LF, *et al.* Nano based drug delivery systems: recent developments and future prospects. J Nanobiotechnology 2018; 16(1): 71.
[http://dx.doi.org/10.1186/s12951-018-0392-8] [PMID: 30231877]

[53] Ross KA, Brenza TM, Binnebose AM, *et al.* Nano-enabled delivery of diverse payloads across complex biological barriers. J Control Release 2015; 219: 548-59.
[http://dx.doi.org/10.1016/j.jconrel.2015.08.039] [PMID: 26315817]

[54] Anselmo AC, Mitragotri S. Nanoparticles in the clinic: An update. Bioeng Transl Med 2019; 4(3): e10143.
[http://dx.doi.org/10.1002/btm2.10143] [PMID: 31572799]

[55] Huang Y, Guo X, Wu Y, *et al.* Nanotechnology's frontier in combatting infectious and inflammatory diseases: prevention and treatment. Signal Transduct Target Ther 2024; 9(1): 34.
[http://dx.doi.org/10.1038/s41392-024-01745-z] [PMID: 38378653]

[56] Alshawwa SZ, Kassem AA, Farid RM, Mostafa SK, Labib GS. Nanocarrier drug delivery systems: characterization, limitations, future perspectives and implementation of artificial intelligence. Pharmaceutics 2022; 14(4): 883.
[http://dx.doi.org/10.3390/pharmaceutics14040883] [PMID: 35456717]

[57] Mukherjee S, Ray S, Thakur RS. Solid lipid nanoparticles: A modern formulation approach in drug delivery system. Indian J Pharm Sci 2009; 71(4): 349-58.
[http://dx.doi.org/10.4103/0250-474X.57282] [PMID: 20502539]

[58] Lu H, Zhang S, Wang J, Chen Q. A review on polymer and lipid-based nanocarriers and its application to nano-pharmaceutical and food-based systems. Front Nutr 2021; 8: 783831.
[http://dx.doi.org/10.3389/fnut.2021.783831] [PMID: 34926557]

[59] Harun-Or-Rashid M, Aktar MN, Hossain MS, *et al.* Recent advances in micro-and nano-drug delivery systems based on natural and synthetic biomaterials. Polymers (Basel) 2023; 15(23): 4563.
[http://dx.doi.org/10.3390/polym15234563] [PMID: 38231996]

[60] Liu P, Chen G, Zhang J. A review of liposomes as a drug delivery system: current status of approved products, regulatory environments, and future perspectives. Molecules 2022; 27(4): 1372.
[http://dx.doi.org/10.3390/molecules27041372] [PMID: 35209162]

[61] Ulldemolins A, Seras-Franzoso J, Andrade F, *et al.* Perspectives of nano-carrier drug delivery systems to overcome cancer drug resistance in the clinics. Cancer Drug Resist 2021; 4(1): 44-68.
[http://dx.doi.org/10.20517/cdr.2020.59] [PMID: 35582007]

[62] Wu Y, Zhang J, He W, Li C, Wang Y. Nanomaterials for targeting liver disease: Research progress and future perspectives. Nano Biomed Eng 2023; 15(2): 199-224.
[http://dx.doi.org/10.26599/NBE.2023.9290024]

[63] Sun T, Kang Y, Liu J, *et al.* Nanomaterials and hepatic disease: toxicokinetics, disease types, intrinsic mechanisms, liver susceptibility, and influencing factors. J Nanobiotechnology 2021; 19(1): 108.
[http://dx.doi.org/10.1186/s12951-021-00843-2] [PMID: 33863340]

[64] Colino CI, Lanao JM, Gutierrez-Millan C. Targeting of hepatic macrophages by therapeutic nanoparticles. Front Immunol 2020; 11: 218.
[http://dx.doi.org/10.3389/fimmu.2020.00218] [PMID: 32194546]

[65] He S, Wang B, Zhang R, Zhou H, Yang Q. Preparation and evaluation of 2-methoxyestradiol-loaded pH-sensitive liposomes. Braz J Pharm Sci 2019; 55: e18204.
[http://dx.doi.org/10.1590/s2175-97902019000118204]

[66] Klein C, Brinkmann U, Reichert JM, Kontermann RE. The present and future of bispecific antibodies for cancer therapy. Nat Rev Drug Discov 2024; 23(4): 301-19.
[http://dx.doi.org/10.1038/s41573-024-00896-6] [PMID: 38448606]

[67] Ertas YN, Abedi Dorcheh K, Akbari A, Jabbari E. Nanoparticles for targeted drug delivery to cancer stem cells: a review of recent advances. Nanomaterials. 2021; 11: 1755 [Internet]. 2021.
[http://dx.doi.org/10.3390/nano11071755]

[68] Kim M, Jeong M, Hur S, *et al.* Engineered ionizable lipid nanoparticles for targeted delivery of RNA

therapeutics into different types of cells in the liver. Sci Adv 2021; 7(9): eabf4398.
[http://dx.doi.org/10.1126/sciadv.abf4398] [PMID: 33637537]

[69] Yan B, Zheng X, Wang Y, *et al.* Liposome-based silibinin for mitigating nonalcoholic fatty liver disease: Dual effects *via* parenteral and intestinal routes. ACS Pharmacol Transl Sci 2023; 6(12): 1909-23.
[http://dx.doi.org/10.1021/acsptsci.3c00210] [PMID: 38093834]

[70] Wang J, Zhang X, Xing J, Gao L, Lu H. Nanomedicines in diagnosis and treatment of prostate cancers: an updated review. Front Bioeng Biotechnol 2024; 12: 1444201.
[http://dx.doi.org/10.3389/fbioe.2024.1444201] [PMID: 39318666]

[71] AbouSamra MM. Liposomal nano-carriers mediated targeting of liver disorders: mechanisms and applications. J Liposome Res 2024; 34(4): 728-43.
[http://dx.doi.org/10.1080/08982104.2024.2377085] [PMID: 38988127]

[72] Alhalmi A, Beg S, Kohli K, Waris M, Singh T. Nanotechnology based approach for hepatocellular carcinoma targeting. Curr Drug Targets 2021; 22(7): 779-92.
[http://dx.doi.org/10.2174/18735592MTEycMjQp3] [PMID: 33302831]

[73] Takahashi Y, Sugimoto K, Inui H, Fukusato T. Current pharmacological therapies for nonalcoholic fatty liver disease/nonalcoholic steatohepatitis. World J Gastroenterol. 2015 Apr 7;21(13):3777-85.

[74] Liang J, Liu Y, Liu J, *et al.* Chitosan-functionalized lipid-polymer hybrid nanoparticles for oral delivery of silymarin and enhanced lipid-lowering effect in NAFLD. J Nanobiotechnology 2018; 16(1): 64.
[http://dx.doi.org/10.1186/s12951-018-0391-9] [PMID: 30176941]

[75] Khurana A, Hartmann P. Gut microbiome-specific nanoparticle-based therapeutics for liver diseases. World J Gastroenterol 2025; 31(27): 109105.
[http://dx.doi.org/10.3748/wjg.v31.i27.109105] [PMID: 40741099]

[76] Tan J. Extracellular vesicles as a next-generation therapeutic nanocarrier in disease treatments. In: Proceedings of SPIE, Vol. 12924, Third International Conference on Biological Engineering and Medical Science (ICBioMed2023); 2024. Article 129243V.
[http://dx.doi.org/10.1117/12.3013198]

[77] Huang R, Rao HY. [Fatty liver disease's renaming impacts on drug clinical trials]. Zhonghua Gan Zang Bing Za Zhi 2023; 31(8): 793-7.
[PMID: 37723059]

CHAPTER 11

Pharmacokinetics and Pharmacodynamics of Nanocarrier-based Therapeutics

Akashdeep Singh[1], **Sonu Kumar**[2], **Palak Sharma**[1], **Sanchit Dhankhar**[1], **Thakur Gurjeet Singh**[1] and **Samrat Chauhan**[1,*]

[1] *Chitkara College of Pharmacy, Chitkara University, Rajpura, Punjab, India*

[2] *Department of Pharmaceutical Sciences and Drug Research, Punjabi University, Patiyala, Punjab, India*

Abstract: Fatty liver disease, comprising non-alcoholic fatty liver disease (NAFLD) and its more acute form, non-alcoholic steatohepatitis (NASH), has emerged as a significant health challenge because of its intricate relationship with metabolic disorders worldwide. Despite several therapeutic developments, the effectiveness of traditional drug delivery methods is restricted due to their low bioavailability, fast degradation, and inadequate hepatic targeting. In contrast, nanocarrier-based therapeutics have emerged as viable strategies for enhancing the pharmacokinetics and pharmacodynamics of drugs. Pharmacokinetic studies revealed that nanocarrier delivery systems, including polymeric nanoparticles, liposomes, and lipid nanoparticles, can substantially enhance drug biodistribution and liver accumulation while reducing enzymatic degradation and premature clearance. In addition, they enable liver-targeted delivery via active targeting with surface ligands or passive accumulation via the increased permeability and retention effect, thereby minimizing systemic toxicity and improving therapeutic efficiency. Pharmacodynamic investigations demonstrated that nanocarrier-based systems effectively modulate key pathways, including inflammatory pathways, lipid metabolism, oxidative stress, and fibrosis inhibition, in the management of fatty liver disease. Furthermore, preclinical data reveal promising results with surface ligand nanocarriers, such as peptides and antibodies, which enhance cellular targeting via receptor-mediated drug uptake by hepatocytes and stellate cells. This chapter highlights the pharmacokinetics and pharmacodynamics of nanocarrier-based therapeutics for the management of fatty liver disease, discussing recent advancements, challenges, and potential future directions. By understanding these dynamics, highly effective, targeted treatments can be developed for the management of fatty liver disease, thereby addressing a significant, overlooked clinical need.

Keywords: Fatty liver disease, Liver-targeted drug delivery, Nanocarrier, Pharmacokinetics, Pharmacodynamics.

* **Corresponding author Samrat Chauhan:** Chitkara College of Pharmacy, Chitkara University, Patiyala, Punjab, India; E-mail: Chauhan.11@gmail.com

Anjali Sharma, Devkant Sharma, Ajmer Singh Grewal, Geeta Deswal & Ganga Reddy Velma (Eds.)

INTRODUCTION

Overview of Fatty Liver Disease (FLD)

Among liver pathologies, fatty liver disease (FLD) is the leading and most prevalent histological abnormality among liver disorders, which involves a pathological sequence starting from steatosis (simple fat accumulation in the liver), potentially evolving into steatohepatitis (inflammation), with or without perisinusoidal fibrosis, culminating in cirrhosis and liver cancer. Most recent data revealed that the mortality rate related to cirrhosis has increased by 65% annually, and a rising trend in liver cancer-related death has approximately doubled in the United States over the past three decades [1]. Furthermore, steatosis arises primarily from dysfunction of the lipid metabolic pathway, along with alterations in the body's energy regulation [2]. The FLDs are classified based on the underlying cause or etiological exposure involved in their progression. Initially, fatty liver disease (FLD) was classified as alcoholic liver disease (ALD) based on high alcohol intake, followed by non-alcoholic fatty liver disease (NAFLD), which is now also referred to as metabolic dysfunction–associated steatotic liver disease (MASLD) [3, 4]. Although NAFLD/MASLD is usually linked with metabolic disorders, such as diabetes and obesity, it is not restricted to individuals with these conditions [5]. Moreover, it is increasingly recognized that long-term exposure to workplace chemicals and environmental toxins may be associated with the development of FLD, which is termed toxicant-associated steatohepatitis (TASH) [6]. All these conditions could progress into more serious NAFLD/MASLD complications, like cirrhosis or hepatocellular carcinoma (HCC), liver fibrosis, metabolic dysfunction-associated steatohepatitis (MASH), or non-alcoholic steatohepatitis (NASH), which could be the reason for early morbidity and death in FLD patients globally. Therefore, the implementation of targeted treatment strategies and the adoption of healthier lifestyle changes are necessary to manage FLD [7, 8].

Non-Alcoholic Fatty Liver Disease (NAFLD)

MASH, an advanced form of NAFLD, is currently the leading cause of liver transplants in the U.S. and a critical reason for the development of HCC [9]. NAFLD, a term introduced by Schaffner in 1986, is characterized by steatosis (fat accumulation) in more than 5% of hepatocytes and is often associated with metabolic disorders, such as insulin resistance, primarily affecting individuals with type 2 diabetes (T2D), who consume little or no alcohol [10, 11]. It is estimated that NAFLD potentially affects up to one billion people globally and accounts for around 25% of the world's total population. A dynamic modeling study assessing the health burden of NAFLD and NASH in the US population projected that by 2030, NAFLD and NASH cases will increase by 21% and 63%, respectively, with liver-related deaths expected to rise substantially by 178%, reaching approximately 78,300 deaths [12]. In those affected by NAFLD, the leading cause of death is cardiovascular complications, trailed by cancer and then liver failure, representing the second cause of mortality worldwide [11]. Necroinflammation and hepatocellular damage, including hepatocyte ballooning, are characteristics of non-alcoholic steatohepatitis (NASH), which raises the risk for cirrhosis, fibrosis, and other liver-related issues [13, 14]. However, NAFLD may arise as a result of an interaction between the metabolism of lipids and the immune system-driven inflammatory response. The term metabolic dysfunction-associated fatty liver disease (MAFLD) was suggested in 2020 by a global panel of experts to highlight the role of cardiometabolic risk factors in both the onset and worsening of hepatic disorder, including patients with additional hepatic diseases [13].

Non-alcoholic Steatohepatitis *(NASH)*

The progressive form of NAFLD, called non-alcoholic steatohepatitis (NASH), is marked by liver inflammation and steatosis (accumulation of fat in the liver), primarily affecting obese women over 50 years of age, especially those suffering from type 2 diabetes mellitus [15]. Furthermore, the PNPLA3 gene, which is highly expressed in the liver, is recognized as a key genetic factor linked to the progression of NASH, cirrhosis, as well as HCC risk, especially in individuals who have metabolic issues like insulin resistance, obesity, hypertriglyceridemia, high blood pressure, and metabolic syndrome, along with additional environmental factors, particularly alcohol intake and smoking. However, the majority of studies confirmed that the actual contributing factor promoting NAFLD progression to NASH remains unknown and requires further study. It may be driven by a complex interaction of genetic and environmental factors [16]. Overall, the prevalence of NASH-associated comorbidities is high (approximately 15 to 94%) with the rise in cases of obese and NAFLD populations, indicating a wider NASH population burden, as one-third of patients with NAFLD progress to NASH. Although the prevalence of NASH is increasing, reliable non-invasive diagnostic methods remain unavailable [17]. Therefore, the primary objective is to understand the epidemiological profile and prevalence of NASH in the healthcare sector and highlight critical gaps in existing knowledge to provide accurate recommendations for early detection and successful interventions [18].

OBSTACLES IN CONVECTIONAL THERAPEUTIC STRATEGIES

Conventional therapeutic strategies for FLD, particularly non-alcoholic fatty liver disease (NAFLD), face multiple challenges:

New Drug Development

Although many therapeutic agents for the treatment of NAFLD-associated fibrosis are under investigation, no FDA-approved agents are available for clinical use. However, certain medications, such as insulin sensitizers and lipid-lowering drugs, have been used off-label to manage the condition, though their effectiveness in reversing liver injury remains limited. For example, metformin, glucagon-like peptide-1 receptor (GLP-1) agonists, and thiazolidinediones are being tested, but concerns about adverse effects and mixed results have inhibited their widespread adoption [19, 20].

Lifestyle Interventions

They are fundamental and, currently, the first-line treatments for NAFLD, given the absence of regulatory-approved drugs, and may include dietary and exercise adjustments. Most findings suggested the universal benefits of exercise and nutrition in controlling NAFLD progression, with 7-10% weight loss in obese patients and 3-5% in lean patients, leading to significant liver fat reduction [21]. However, if patients fail to embrace and adhere to necessary lifestyle modifications, treatment outcomes may be less effective [22].

Diagnostic Challenges

Based on several histopathological features of NAFLD and NASH according to staging and brunt grading (NASH Activity Score) system, accurate diagnosis of NAFLD and NASH can be challenging and often requires invasive liver biopsies. According to qualitative research conducted in the UK, general practitioners reported significant challenges in the diagnosis and treatment of NAFLD [23]. Although various non-invasive diagnostic techniques have been developed, such as imaging methods (FibroScan, also known as transient elastography) and serum biomarkers, many challenges remain in assessment, diagnosis, and risk stratification due to a lack of widespread clinical validation [20, 24]. Therefore, further research is required for clinical adoption and reliable disease monitoring [22].

Heterogeneity of NAFLD Progression

NAFLD is a wide range of conditions influenced by disease modifiers, such as sex, age, diet, smoking, hormonal status, gut microbiota, and concurrent disease, and it exhibits different rates of progression in every individual, ranging from mild steatosis to NASH, fibrosis, cirrhosis, and HCC. This heterogeneity of NAFLD complicates the development of standardized treatments, as therapies that work for one stage may not be suitable or effective for another [25, 26]. Hence, structural analysis of main pathogenic pathways and accurate classification of disease may lead to more accurate risk assessment and treatment outcomes.

Limited Targeted Therapies

Targeted treatment is difficult due to the complexity of the mediators and signaling molecules involved in the pathophysiology of NAFLD, including fibrotic, inflammatory, and metabolic pathways. The majority of novel interventions are still in the experimental stage and have not yet been established as safe and effective over the long term, which emphasises the need for further research and clinical validation [27].

ROLE OF ADVANCED DRUG DELIVERY SYSTEMS IN LIVER-TARGETED THERAPY

Current treatments available for liver diseases, such as NAFLD and its progressive form, NASH, are becoming more effective through the use of advanced drug delivery systems (ADDS). These innovative strategies are introduced to improve liver-specific drug targeting and reduce systemic adverse or off-target effects, thereby significantly increasing therapeutic efficacy in the treatment of NAFLD. The various advanced drug delivery systems used for liver-targeted therapy are summarized in Table **1**.

Table 1. Summary of various liver-targeted advanced drug delivery platforms, along with their description and examples.

Drug Delivery System	Description	Examples	Ref.
Nanoparticle-based Delivery Systems	Systemic toxicity has been reduced by engineered nanoparticles that enable targeted drug delivery to hepatocytes.	Gold nanoparticles for liver fibrosis, polymeric nanoparticles (PLGA, PEGylated nanoparticles).	[34, 35]

(Table 1) cont.....

Drug Delivery System	Description	Examples	Ref.
Lipid Nanoparticles (LNPs) for siRNA Delivery	Facilitates siRNA delivery into hepatocytes; lipid nanoparticles may silence genes linked to illness.	MC3-based LNPs for liver fibrosis and patisiran (FDA-approved for hereditary ATTR amyloidosis).	[36, 37]
Nano-Drug Delivery Systems (NDDS) in Metabolic Dysfunction-associated Steatohepatitis (MASH)	The absorption of drugs and the efficiency in metabolic dysfunction-associated steatohepatitis (MASH) are improved by nanoformulations.	DPP-4 inhibitors in lipid carriers and curcumin-loaded nanoparticles for hepatic inflammation.	[38]
Polysaccharide-based Delivery Systems	Hepatocellular carcinoma using chitosan nanoparticles and liver fibrosis with hyaluronic acid-drug conjugates.	Hyaluronic acid and chitosan are examples of natural polysaccharides that improve liver-targeted medication delivery.	[39, 40]
Hepatic Stellate Cell (HSC) Targeting	Targeted distribution to HSCs reduces off-target effects and supports the treatment of liver fibrosis.	HSC suppression using siRNA-loaded liposomes and vitamin A-conjugated nanoparticles.	[41, 42]

Nanoparticle-based Delivery Systems

It is a promising technique primarily used to deliver therapeutic agents to the liver [28]. The drug targeting hepatic cells can be encapsulated or linked to various carriers via nanoscale particle engineering. These techniques help to reduce off-target effects while increasing drug accumulation in the liver [29].

Lipid Nanoparticles (LNPs)-mediated siRNA Delivery

Lipid nanoparticles can effectively minimise NAFLD-associated fibrosis in preclinical models by delivering siRNA molecules that suppress genes implicated in liver disorders, thereby helping reduce hepatic fibrosis. Engineered lipid nanoparticles incorporating anisamide ligand for targeted RNA delivery target specific proteins implicated in liver fibrosis, resulting in downregulating the liver fibrotic tissue development and progression of the disease [29].

Advanced Drug Delivery Systems (ADDS) in MASH

ADDS have also been studied for their potential to improve MASH (Metabolic Dysfunction-Associated Steatohepatitis) management by optimizing the delivery and therapeutic effects of drug agents [28]. To minimise systemic exposure and achieve higher drug concentrations at the targeted site, the ADDS can be designed to target specific cellular components in the liver.

Hepatic Stellate Cell (HSC) Targeting

The pathophysiology of liver fibrosis is mainly dependent on hepatic stellate cells. Therapeutic agents used to treat liver fibrosis can be delivered to the specific site by targeting HSC with the help of ADDS [15]. Moreover, hyaluronic acid (HA)-coated polymeric micelles of olmesartan medoxomil (OLM), an anti-fibrotic agent, were evaluated for cellular uptake potential through in-vitro and in-vivo studies for liver fibrosis. The results suggested that targeted delivery to hepatic stellate cells (HSCs) resulted in a marked reduction in liver cirrhosis in a mouse model, confirming it as a potent drug delivery vehicle for the management of liver disorders [30].

Biomaterials as Drug Delivery Carrier

The literature findings highlighted that polysaccharides exhibit considerable therapeutic and protective potential against several hepatic disorders, such as NAFLD, fibrosis, drug-induced hepatic injury, hepatitis B, and HCC, through various biological pathways, as verified by both in-vitro and in-vivo studies [31]. Additionally, the presence of abundant functional groups (-COOH, -OH, and -NH2) in polysaccharides enables facile modification and makes them a controlled drug-delivery carrier for hepatoprotective agents, indicating their potential as biomaterials for liver diseases [32]. Moreover, several reviews have assessed the therapeutic potential of plant-derived polysaccharides for liver disorders by modulating cellular signaling pathways that regulate inflammation, oxidative stress, and apoptosis [33]. These systems aim to improve therapeutic efficacy while reducing adverse effects by enhancing drug delivery specificity, thereby resolving some of the primary issues with current treatment methodologies.

PHARMACOKINETIC AND PHARMACODYNAMIC OF NANO-CARRIER (NC)-BASED THERAPEUTICS

Nanocarrier (NC)-based therapeutics often exhibit distinct pharmacokinetic (PK) and pharmacodynamic (PD) profiles compared to their traditional formulations available on the market with the same active ingredient. A clear understanding of the PK and PD characteristics of NCs is essential for refining drug-delivery carrier systems, enhancing therapeutic outcomes, extending drug circulation time, and reducing systemic toxicity in targeted drug therapy, thereby representing a safer and more effective healthcare solution. Furthermore, the different routes of administration, such as oral, injectable, dermal, and pulmonary, present specific PK and PD characteristics that influence formulation optimization and the selection of delivery carriers. By understanding the PK/PD of NC-based therapeutics, researchers can predict dosage regimens or frequencies, estimate site-specific drug concentrations, and ensure controlled therapeutic action [43, 44]. NC's small size and large surface area enable the precise, targeted delivery of proteins, genes, small molecules, and imaging agents, which help diagnose and treat conditions, such as cancer, diabetes, liver disease, and brain diseases [44]. NCs provide better absorption, stability, regulated drug release, longer half-life, and fewer side effects than conventional techniques. Overall, the PK and PD evaluations are key for assessing the *in-vivo* behavior of NCs and to enhance the formulation design for better clinical translation, ultimately boosting regulatory filing, dosing strategies, and personalized medicinal approach [45].

Pharmacokinetics of Nanocarriers

Absorption and Bioavailability

The process of absorption refers to the movement of NCs and their encapsulated drugs from the site of administration to the bloodstream via several administration pathways, including oral, parenteral, inhalation, and transdermal. These pathways significantly affect the absorption of NCs, which, in turn, influence their biodistribution profile, pharmacokinetics, and the therapeutic efficacy of the therapeutic agent. Additionally, the extent of NCs' absorption is further affected by factors, such as the mucosal lining, NCs' stability, and the presence of a surface modifier. Among the various delivery routes, oral and intravenous (IV) delivery are the most commonly used and significant routes for NC-based therapeutics. The intravenous route helps avoid absorption barriers, allowing direct entry into the systemic circulation and thereby facilitating rapid and targeted drug delivery to specific tissues, such as the liver. For intravenous (IV) delivery, NCs smaller than 500 nm are ideal due to their longer circulation time, lower clearance rate, and greater accumulation in targeted pathological tissues via passive or active targeting [44, 46, 47].

Other non-invasive routes, such as oral, transdermal, and inhalation delivery, offer alternative options for NC absorption across biological barriers [48, 49]. These routes may initially allow NCs to accumulate in local lymph nodes before entering the bloodstream, thereby delaying drug absorption, prolonging residence time, and potentially reducing dosing frequency. Despite being convenient, the oral route is often hindered by limitations, such as enzyme-mediated breakdown, poor intestinal absorption, and a hepatic first-pass effect, which together can significantly lower drug bioavailability [50, 51]. Inhalation of NCs provides efficient drug absorption into the bloodstream via the lungs for local as well as systemic actions, by avoiding hepatic metabolism and promoting systemic distribution [52]. Upon inhalation, inhaled NCs are primarily taken up by macrophages and the lymphatic system and may be cleared by alveolar macrophages or accumulate in lymph nodes in the lungs [53]. Transdermal delivery helps avoid gastrointestinal barriers and directly delivers therapeutic agents through the skin, with a controlled-release profile [54]. The primary challenge associated with the transdermal route is the skin barrier, which is composed of three layers: epidermis, dermis, and subcutaneous tissue. NCs must cross all skin layers, including the cuticle, which is a major entry barrier, for absorption into the bloodstream. Therefore, it is essential to understand how NCs are absorbed and distributed in biological system in order to improve their therapeutic effectiveness and reduce off-target responses [47, 55].

Mechanisms of Nanocarrier Absorption into the Bloodstream

The ability of NCs to be absorbed into the bloodstream is influenced by various factors, including their physicochemical characteristics, chosen route of administration, and their capacity to interact with physiological barriers [56]. After oral administration, NCs cross the enzymatic and chemical barriers to enter the gastrointestinal (GI) system. They can be absorbed via various mechanisms, including carrier-mediated transcytosis, M cell absorption, paracellular transport through tight junctions, and passive diffusion across cell membranes. After absorption by the intestinal epithelium, they can enter the bloodstream via the intestinal lymphatic system or the hepatic portal vein [57]. In-vivo absorption of nanoparticles is typically energy-dependent, with absorption efficiency varying based on nanoparticle properties [58]. The literature suggests that nanocomposites whose surfaces were modified with ethylene glycol-chitosan or pH-sensitive Eudragit® L100–55 tend to be internalized through clathrin-mediated endocytosis and paracellular transport, while polymeric nanoparticles of carboxylated chitosan are predominantly absorbed through M cell-mediated paracellular transport [59].

For inhaled NCs, absorption occurs through macrophage uptake and lymphatic transport. Some particles are rapidly cleared from the lungs by alveolar macrophages, while others accumulate or are localized in regional lymph nodes within the lungs' microenvironment, contributing to their systemic distribution [60]. In case of transdermal delivery, NCs must penetrate the skin's natural barrier, which includes the dermis, epidermis, and subcutaneous tissue. NCs mainly enter the bloodstream via two primary routes: the transepidermal route (across the stratum corneum) and the transappendageal route (through hair follicles and sweat glands). Although the transepidermal pathway is the main route, the transappendageal route also allows the penetration of macromolecules and nanoparticles; however, very few of them are able to pass through the stratum corneum [61]. Hence, the stratum corneum presents a significant challenge to NCs' absorption. Conversely, when delivered by intramuscular or subcutaneous route, NCs can travel across connective tissues and enter the bloodstream via capillary or lymphatic endothelium, where they are predominantly taken up by macrophages and lymphocytes. It is essential to understand these absorption mechanisms to minimize off-target effects, enhance NCs' bioavailability, and optimize drug delivery [62]. The mechanism of NCs' absorption into the bloodstream via different routes of administration is shown in Fig. (**1**).

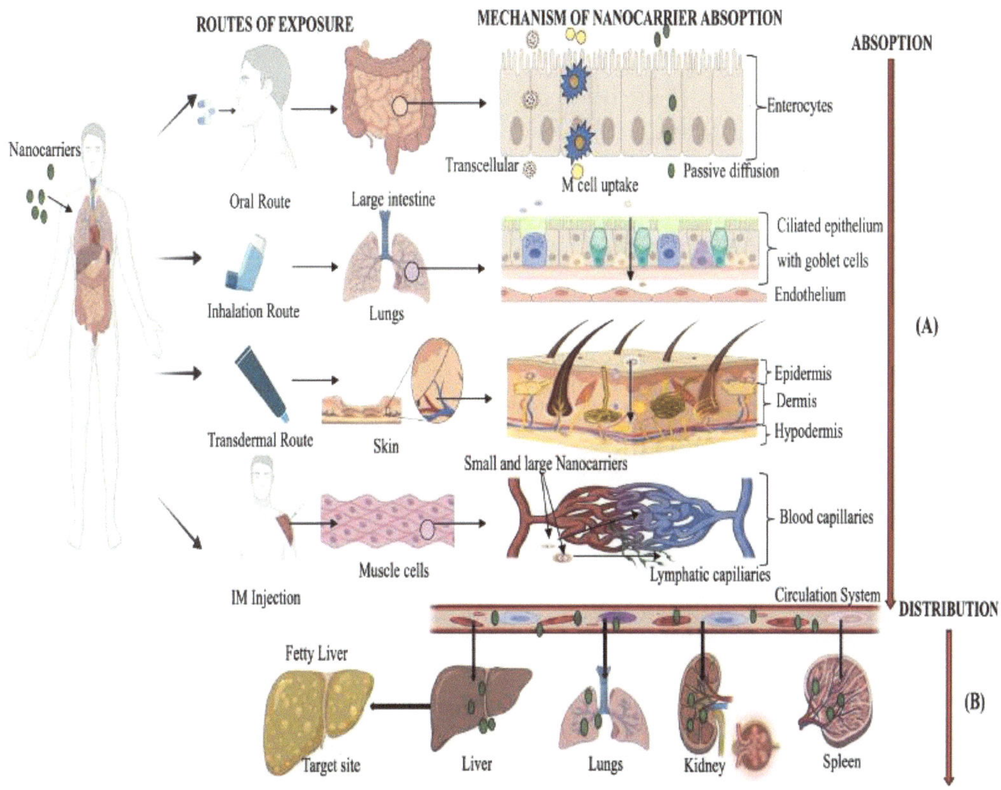

Fig. (1). Diagrammatic illustration of A) Mechanisms of nanocarrier absorption into the bloodstream, and B) Distribution profile of nanocarriers to various organs.

Distribution to the Liver

The process by which nanocarriers (NCs) deliver drugs from the bloodstream to tissues, intercellular fluid, and cells is known as distribution. Blood flow, vascular permeability, plasma protein interactions, the mononuclear phagocytic system (MPS), the complement system, and NC interactions with tissue cells are among the variables that affect the distribution of NCs once they are absorbed and move through the body via the blood [47]. The liver significantly contributes to NCs' distribution and clearance mechanism due to its highly fenestrated endothelial structure, rich blood supply, and role in the mononuclear phagocytic system (MPS). The fenestrations of sinusoidal endothelial capillaries, which range in size from 50 to 100 nm, facilitate the uptake of NCs, and their retention is influenced by local macrophages (Kupffer cells), which affects the pharmacokinetic behaviour and therapeutic performance of drugs [63].

LIVER-SPECIFIC TARGETING MECHANISMS

The liver plays a vital role in both metabolism and detoxification, making it a primary target for the treatment of liver-associated diseases, including NAFLD, hepatitis, liver fibrosis, cirrhosis, and HCC. NCs are mainly delivered to the liver via two primary mechanisms: active targeting and passive targeting. Table **2** lists nanocarrier-based formulations delivered to the liver *via* active and passive targeting mechanisms.

Table 2. List of nanocarrier-based formulations delivered to the liver through active targeting and passive targeting mechanisms.

Active Targeting Mechanisms				
Nanocarrier	**Size**	**Use**	**Description**	**Ref.**
Galactose-Functionalized Nanoparticles	100-200 nm	Targeted drug delivery to hepatocytes in liver diseases	Designed to bind to the Asialoglycoprotein receptor (ASGPR) on hepatocytes, enhancing cellular uptake.	[66]
Galactose-Functionalized Liposomes	~100 nm	Targeted delivery to hepatocytes in liver diseases	Galactose moieties on liposomes bind to Asialoglycoprotein receptors on hepatocytes.	[69]
Folate-Conjugated Nanoparticles	100-200 nm	Treatment of hepatocellular carcinoma	Folate ligands target folate receptors overexpressed on liver cancer cells, improving drug accumulation.	[64]
Lipid-Based Nanoparticles (LNPs)	Varies	Delivery of genetic material for liver diseases	LNPs facilitate the delivery of nucleic acids to hepatocytes, enhancing gene therapy approaches for liver conditions.	[70]

(Table 2) cont.....

Active Targeting Mechanisms				
Nanocarrier	**Size**	**Use**	**Description**	**Ref.**
Passive Targeting Mechanisms				
Lipid-Based Nanoparticles (LNPs)	20-200 nm	Potential treatment for nonalcoholic fatty liver disease (NAFLD)	LNPs exploit the liver's fenestrated endothelium and lack of basal lamina, facilitating passive accumulation in hepatic tissues.	[69]
Polymeric Nanoparticles	20-200 nm	Investigational use for liver diseases	These nanoparticles passively accumulate in the liver due to their size and the organ's unique vasculature, enhancing drug delivery to hepatic cells.	[66]
Polymeric Nanoparticles	20-200 nm	Delivery of chemotherapeutic agents for liver cancer	These nanoparticles passively accumulate in liver tumors through the EPR effect, enhancing drug delivery to malignant cells while minimizing systemic toxicity.	[69]

Passive Targeting (Permeability and Retention Effect)

The strategy of passive targeting, also known as the enhanced permeability and retention (EPR) effect, is widely used in NC-based drug delivery, particularly for treating various tumors and liver diseases. This mechanism improves drug deposition at the disease site without the need for specific ligand-receptor interactions. The liver's sinusoidal endothelium lacks a basement membrane and contains fenestrations, making it highly permeable to NCs. This allows passive accumulation of NCs in hepatic tissues, aiding in site-specific drug delivery for the management of various liver disorders. The EPR effect promotes drug retention at the tumor site by allowing NCs to accumulate in tumors due to their poor lymphatic drainage and leaky vasculature [63].

Active Targeting *via* Surface Ligands

The process of active liver targeting involves modifying the surface of NCs with specialized exogenous ligands, such as carbohydrates, antibodies, peptides, or proteins, that identify and bind to specific receptors on liver cells. The liver is composed of both non-parenchymal cells, including sinusoidal endothelial cells (SECs), hepatic stellate cells (HSCs), and Kupffer cells (KCs), and parenchymal cells, mainly hepatocytes, which control important liver functions. These cells contribute to liver metabolism, detoxification, immunological response, and general hepatic homeostasis. They have unique morphologies, pathoanatomical traits, and physiological functions. Therefore, the targeted active strategies minimize off-target effects and increase treatment efficacy by increasing drug delivery to hepatic cells [64, 65].

Active targeting using surface ligands improves selectivity and ensures accurate drug delivery, but passive targeting via the enhanced permeability and retention (EPR) effect may result in non-specific accumulation [66, 67]. Active targeting delivers active substances to specific liver cell types to maximise therapeutic efficacy and minimise side effects. Firstly, the surface-modified NCs undergo passive absorption, which further triggers the endocytosis process, leading to targeting NCs to specific liver cell receptors. Various liver cells express different receptors, such as asialoglycoprotein (ASGPR) receptor, transferrin (Tf) receptor, glycyrrhizin/glycyrrhetinic acid receptor, hyaluronan receptor for endocytosis (HARE), low-density lipoprotein (LDL) receptor, high-density lipoprotein (HDL) receptor, and immunoglobulin A binding protein. Among all, the ASGPR receptor is a key target for hepatocyte-specific ligand drug delivery to enhance cellular uptake and therapeutic precision [65, 68].

ROLE OF NANOCARRIER IN LIVER-TARGETED DRUG DELIVERY

The uptake and retention of NCs in liver cells are influenced by multiple factors, including surface charge, size, and ligand properties. Passive targeting of NCs to specialized liver cells is primarily governed by the size of hepatic sinusoidal fenestrae, which selectively allow NPs smaller than 100 nm to reach hepatocytes and hepatic stellate cells (HSCs) [69 - 70]. In contrast, larger NPs (>100 nm) are more likely to be engulfed by SECs and KCs present in the liver. The size-dependent interactions serve a vital function in regulating NPs distribution and optimizing targeted drug delivery within the liver [71, 72]. The various NCs, such as solid lipid nanoparticles (SLNs), liposomes, polymers, and targeted moieties, with a size range of 100-200 nm, offer promising strategies for delivering drugs, siRNA, and antibodies for liver-targeted therapy and imaging. Furthermore, the conjugation of NCs with specific ligands enables their applications in drug delivery, radiology imaging, and diagnostics [73]. Currently, liposomes are being evaluated in clinical trials for the treatment of liver fibrosis and HCC due to their ability to encapsulate both water-soluble and lipid-soluble drugs, thereby enhancing therapeutic efficacy. Surface-modified human serum albumin-based liposomes serve as effective carriers for targeting activated HSCs *via* specific protein-binding pathways, making them a potential treatment option for liver diseases [65].

Metabolism and Elimination

Metabolic Pathways Involved in the Breakdown of Nanocarriers

The metabolism of NCs encompasses a series of biochemical processes that facilitate their transformation, degradation, and subsequent elimination from the body. These processes involve the breakdown of NC components, combined with the controlled release of the active drug, ensuring therapeutic effectiveness while reducing the risk of systemic toxicity. Upon administration from various routes, NCs interact with biological systems, and their fate is primarily dictated by their physicochemical properties, such as particle size, shape, and surface characteristics [74, 75]. The liver, with its hepatocytes, Kupffer cells, and hepatic macrophages, serves as the primary organ for NC biotransformation and clearance. Hepatocytes are equipped with abundant transporters, phase I and phase II metabolic enzymes, and a well-developed biliary excretion system, facilitating the metabolism and elimination of NCs. Enzymatic degradation in the liver (first-pass metabolism), primarily mediated by cytochrome P450 (CYP) enzymes, governs the metabolic fate of NCs, influencing their pharmacokinetics and biodistribution [76, 77] (Fig. **2**). Additionally, extrahepatic metabolism of NCs occurs in the gastrointestinal (GI) tract epithelium, lungs, kidneys, skin, and placenta. The lungs, due to their extensive vascular network, and other organs, such as the kidneys, skin, and placenta, which have xenobiotic-metabolizing capabilities, contribute to NCs metabolism to varying extents [77]. Studies indicate that 30-90% of conventional NCs, particularly those lacking surface modifications, accumulate in the liver, making it a key site for NCs metabolism and clearance [78]. The biodegradability of NCs significantly impacts their clearance pathways. In contrast, nonbiodegradable NCs exhibit slower metabolism, leading to prolonged retention and potential bioaccumulation in the liver, which raises concerns regarding long-term toxicity [79].

Routes of Elimination

The liver and kidneys serve as the primary excretory organs, ensuring effective clearance of NCs from the body (Fig. **2**). The elimination of NCs determines their therapeutic effectiveness, circulation duration, and potential side effects [56, 80]. Renal excretion plays a significant role in clearing NCs, and studies indicate that particles with a hydrodynamic diameter (HD) greater than 15 nm are unable to undergo renal clearance, whereas those with an HD of 5.5 nm or less are efficiently eliminated through urine.

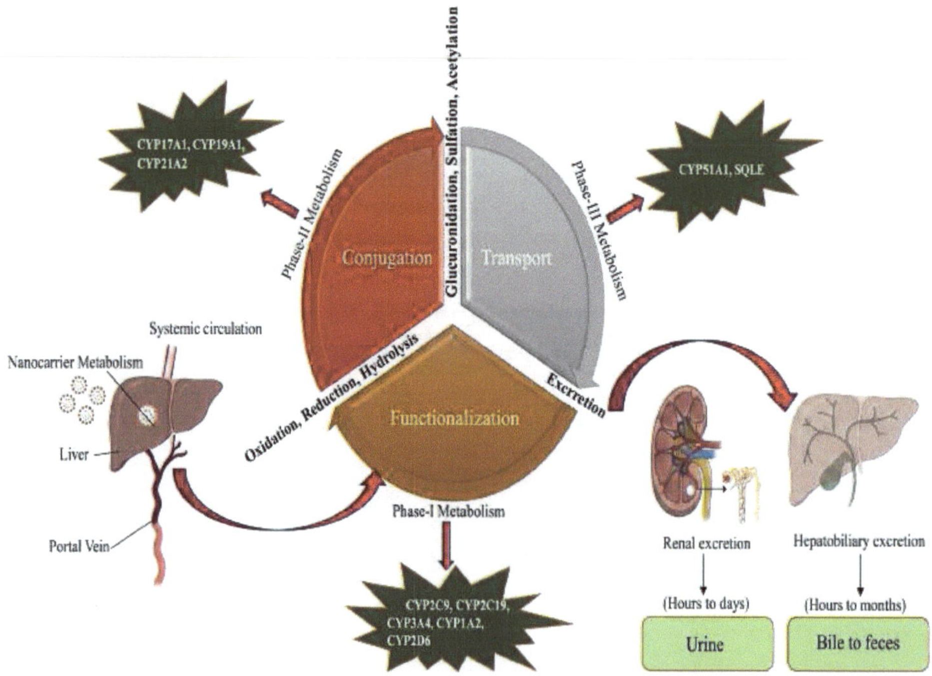

Fig. (2). Routes of elimination and the importance of CYP in nanocarrier metabolism.

Nanoparticles larger than 8 nm may interact electrostatically with the negatively charged glomerular capillary wall, leading to partial reabsorption by renal tubules into the blood circulation after passing into Bowman's cavity, while others are excreted in urine [81]. Certain biodegradable nanomaterials degrade into smaller, low-molecular-weight substances in the liver, facilitating renal excretion; however, these metabolites may accumulate in the kidneys and contribute to renal dysfunction, as observed with compounds, such as cyclodextrin analogues and poloxamers [82]. In addition to renal clearance, the hepatobiliary route plays a crucial role in eliminating NCs from the body. Kupffer cells degrade NCs without facilitating bile excretion, whereas hepatocytes process NCs for biliary removal [83]. Hepatobiliary clearance is slower than renal clearance, taking hours to months. In cases where NCs are resistant to macrophage degradation or renal elimination, surface ligand modifications can enhance hepatocyte uptake, thereby promoting effective hepatobiliary excretion. The liver effectively captures and removes NCs with a hydrodynamic diameter of 10-20 nm, making particle size a crucial parameter influencing hepatobiliary excretion [78].

Physicochemical Properties of Nanocarriers and their Impact on Pharmacokinetics

The key properties of NCs, such as particle size, morphology, and surface attributes, significantly influence their interactions with biological systems and pharmacokinetics, ultimately affecting drug disposition, efficacy, and safety within the body. These properties collectively determine NCs' absorption, circulation time, biodistribution, and accumulation at target tissues. The in-vivo ADME (absorption, distribution, metabolism, and excretion) profile of NCs can be regulated by a number of mechanisms, including surface conditioning, mononuclear phagocyte system (MPS) uptake, enhanced permeability and retention (EPR) effect, blood circulation dynamics, and lymphatic transport. Additionally, all of these mechanisms do not function independently; instead, they interact synergistically to dictate the ultimate fate of NCs [77, 84, 85]. The effects of the physicochemical properties of NCs on pharmacokinetics and biodistribution are thoroughly discussed below and depicted in Fig. (**3**).

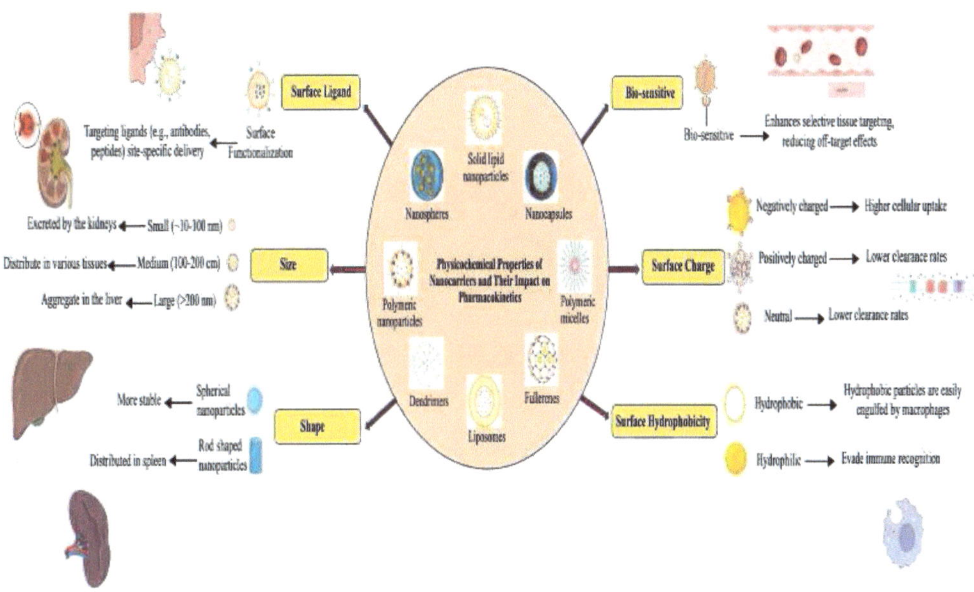

Fig. (3). Physicochemical properties of nanocarriers and their impact on pharmacokinetics.

Size

The size or dimension of the NCs plays a significant role in the internalization process, such as endocytosis, which affects transmembrane transport capacity and rate. For example, intestinal cells absorb small nanoparticles, whereas M cells mainly absorb larger nanoparticles [86, 87]. NCs' size also significantly affects their in-vivo distribution, ability to reach target sites like tumors, and helps to achieve sustained drug release [88]. NCs larger than 10 nm can bypass renal elimination and penetrate deeper tissues, while those between 10 and 20 nm can distribute widely due to tight endothelial connections but are rapidly excreted through the glomerulus. Furthermore, smaller NCs with highly curved surfaces exhibit reduced complement activation and diminished macrophage uptake, leading to prolonged circulation times. Conversely, larger NCs (>200 nm) are rapidly engulfed by the mononuclear phagocyte system (MPS), leading to preferential accumulation in the spleen and liver and reducing their systemic availability [89, 90].

Shape

The morphology of NCs plays a vital role in their biological interactions and pharmacokinetics. The literature suggests that rod- and disk-shaped NPs exhibit higher transport efficiency in intestinal cells than spherical NPs after oral administration [91]. Furthermore, macrophage phagocytosis of NCs and subsequent internalization, affecting their circulation time and therapeutic efficacy, is related to the shape of NCs [92].

NCs, particularly non-spherical NCs (*e.g.*, rods, ellipses, and stars), significantly influence vascular transport and biodistribution. Discoid and elongated NCs demonstrated improved tumor targeting by minimizing interactions with the mononuclear phagocyte system (MPS) and enhancing vascular marginalization [93]. Additionally, gold nanoballs exhibit higher liver accumulation than gold nanorods, highlighting the role of shape in optimizing NCs design for targeted therapies [94]. Spherical and star-shaped gold nanoparticles (GNPs) exhibit similar in vivo accumulation, whereas nanorods show lower penetration and faster excretion. Despite their similarities, spherical and star GNPs differ in liver localization, with only star-shaped GNPs accumulating in the lungs, highlighting shape-dependent biodistribution patterns [95]. Furthermore, mesoporous silica nanoparticles (MSNs) suggested that short-rod MSNs predominantly accumulate inside the liver and exhibit a faster clearance rate, whereas long-rod MSNs tend to localize in the spleen [96].

Surface Charge

Surface charge significantly influences NCs' interactions, affecting opsonin adsorption, macrophage recognition, phagocytosis, and overall biodistribution. NCs with a positive surface charge tend to adhere strongly to negatively charged phospholipid bilayers, enhancing cell penetration and displaying selective binding to negatively charged tumor cell surfaces. Compared to anionic and PEGylated liposomes, cationic liposomes exhibit superior absorption and transport efficiency in intestinal cells, making them more effective for targeted drug delivery and intracellular uptake [97]. However, positively charged nanoparticles often disrupt cell membranes, leading to cytotoxicity and immune responses, which can limit their clinical application. Additionally, strong nonspecific interactions between cationic NCs and serum constituents enhance phagocytosis, leading to their rapid clearance from the bloodstream [98]. The positively charged NCs tend to localize in the glomerulus region, while neutral ones are primarily found in the renal arteries, indicating differences in kidney filtration. In spleen tissue, both positively and negatively charged NCs predominantly concentrate within the red pulp, while neutral NCs tend to localize in the white pulp and along the spleen's outer edge. Additionally, cationic nanoparticles accumulate significantly in liver cells, whereas uncharged nanoparticles are associated with Kupffer cells of the liver, and anionic nanoparticles are more widely distributed throughout the liver [99, 100].

Surface Hydrophobicity

Nanoparticles with hydrophilic polymer coatings, such as PEG, PVA, and PAA, enhance mucus penetration and improve oral absorption but may lower intestinal membrane permeability. In contrast, hydrophobic nanoparticles facilitate intestinal absorption by modifying membrane fluidity. Hydrophobic nanoparticles are more susceptible to immune system recognition and rapid clearance by the reticuloendothelial system (RES), limiting their effectiveness in tumor targeting. However, hydrophilic coatings such as PEG, poloxamer, and dextran help prolong circulation time by reducing immune recognition and macrophage uptake. Hence, adjustment of surface hydrophobicity, particularly through PEG modification, is a promising approach to reducing RES clearance and enhancing drug delivery efficiency [77].

Target Ligand

Surface modification with targeting ligands significantly improves NCs' absorption and accumulation while reducing their clearance from the body. Although passive targeting primarily influences nanoparticle accumulation at target sites, ligand density on the NCs' surface significantly alters their *in-vivo* behavior [101]. The PEGylated NCs, which lack targeted specificity but display anti-EGFR ligands on the surface, exhibit a shortened circulation half-life, which further decreases with increasing ligand density [102, 93]. This effect may be due to increased nonspecific protein adsorption as ligand density rises. However, despite shorter blood retention, higher ligand density enhances nanoparticle accumulation in tumors. Studies indicate that an optimal ligand density maximizes cell-targeting efficiency, regardless of NC's size or surface targeting ligand. Interestingly, smaller EGFR-targeted NCs transition from the spleen towards the liver, likely due to EGFR overexpression in liver tissue, whereas this phenomenon is not observed in larger nanoparticles [103].

Bio-sensitive NCs

Surface modification of NCs not only enhances their absorption and retention but also enables bio-sensitive nanocarriers (NCs) to be triggered by internal environmental factors, such as pH or enzymatic changes, to facilitate drug release at target sites. Since tumor tissues have a lower pH (4.0-5.0) than normal extracellular fluid or blood (7.2-7.4), pH-responsive NC systems can be designed for targeted delivery of therapeutic agents. Additionally, pH-sensitive carboxymethyl chitosan nanoparticles were prepared, and their surfaces were subsequently modified with perfluorobutyric anhydride to develop fluorinated nanoparticles. The results suggested that these nanoparticles exhibited greater stability at normal pH (7–9) but swelled in mildly acidic environments, accelerating drug release over a more extended period and increasing blood absorption, resulting in superior *in vivo* antitumor activity [104].

PHARMACODYNAMICS OF NANOCARRIERS IN FLD

Nanocarrier-mediated Drug Release Within Liver Cells

The interaction of NCs with liver cells plays a vital role in determining their fate within the body. However, the exact physicochemical properties that govern liver sequestration and cellular interactions remain unclear. Despite hepatocytes being the dominant liver cell type, most NCs are primarily absorbed by non-parenchymal cells [78]. NCs typically enter liver cells via endocytic pathways, though some may passively penetrate the plasma membrane. Post-endocytosis, NCs are encapsulated in early endocytic vesicles rather than being delivered directly into the cytoplasm. Conversely, NCs that enter via membrane penetration bypass this process and reach the cytoplasm immediately, making this approach particularly beneficial for targeted drug delivery [105].

Kupffer cells, located in liver sinusoids, act as the body's first line of innate immunity by engulfing pathogens, foreign substances, and apoptotic cells. These resident macrophages identify nanoparticles as foreign agents and internalize them via multiple scavenger receptors, including clathrin-dependent and caveolin-dependent endocytosis and macropinocytosis [76]. The liver sinusoidal endothelial cells, which line hepatic sinusoids, actively clear NCs from the bloodstream via scavenger receptors [106]. The NCs' uptake depends on their physicochemical properties, particularly hydrodynamic size. NCs larger than 100 nm or aggregated sub-100 nm particles tend to interact more with Kupffer cells, while LSECs more readily absorb smaller monodisperse NCs. The adsorption of specific serum proteins onto nanoparticles also influences their distribution within liver cells [107].

The study on poly-aconitylated human serum albumin (Aco-HSA) liposomes has provided insights into strategies for targeting LSECs [108]. Furthermore, hepatic stellate cell (HSC)-targeting NCs show promise for the treatment of liver fibrosis [109]. However, delivering NCs to HSCs poses challenges because they are located within the Disse space, adjacent to endothelial cells. Most NCs are likely to be taken up by Kupffer cells and LSECs before they can interact with stellate cells. To enhance targeting, NCs can be engineered to bind selectively to surface receptors, including the mannose 6-phosphate (M6P) receptor, the insulin-like growth factor-II (IGF-II) receptor, retinol-binding protein (RBP), collagen type VI, and integrin. Although HSCs account for less than 10% of liver cells, effective targeting could improve therapeutic outcomes for liver-related diseases [78].

Cellular Uptake Mechanism of Nanocarriers

Liver cells utilize various mechanisms for NCs uptake, with endocytosis being the primary pathway for nanocarrier internalization [76]. Endocytosis is broadly classified into pinocytosis (cell drinking) and phagocytosis (cell eating). While pinocytosis is responsible for the uptake of fluids and dissolved substances via small vesicles, phagocytosis is a process that enables specialized cells, such as monocytes, dendritic cells, and neutrophils, to engulf large particles into intracellular phagosomes. These two processes can be distinguished by the size of their vesicles: phagocytosis involves the uptake of large particles via vesicles approximately 250 nm in diameter, while pinocytosis facilitates fluid uptake through vesicles ranging from a few nanometers to hundreds of nanometers in diameter. Furthermore, pinocytosis is categorized into five main types: clathrin-dependent endocytosis, caveolin-dependent endocytosis, clathrin/caveolin-independent endocytosis, macropinocytosis, and passive uptake [110]. NCs enter cells through various endocytic pathways, as illustrated in Fig. (**4**).

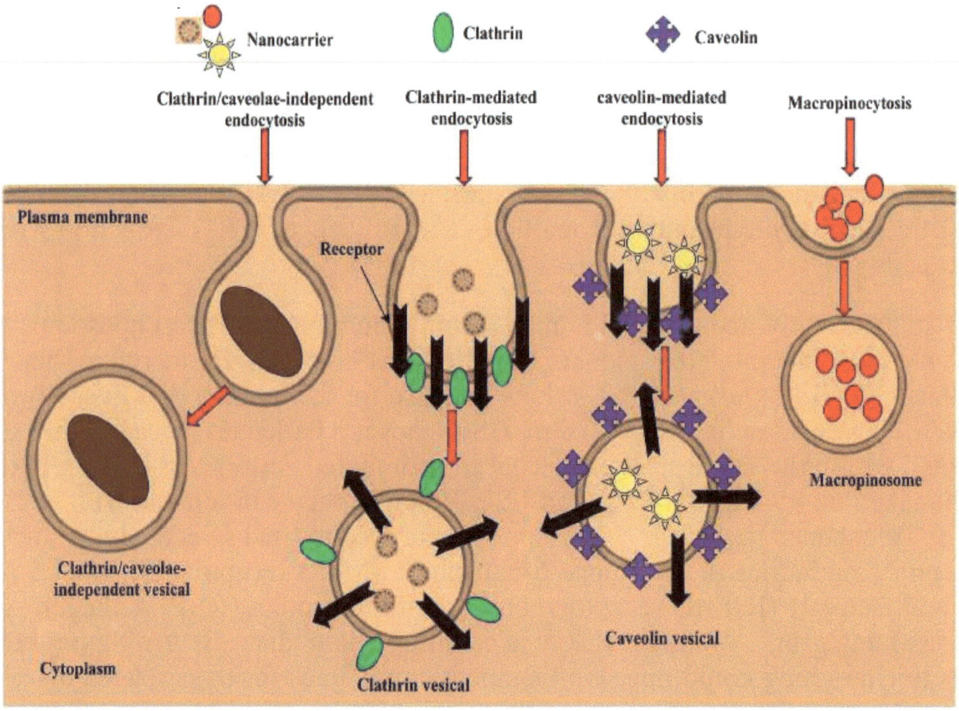

Fig. (4). Cellular uptake mechanism of nanocarriers *via* different endocytotic pathways.

Clathrin-dependent Endocytosis

Clathrin-dependent endocytosis is a key cellular mechanism for the selective internalization of NCs into the cells. The essential nutrients and components of the plasma membrane required by cells are absorbed through this pathway, including iron via transferrin receptors and cholesterol via low-density lipoprotein (LDL) receptors [111]. In this process, some specific ligands found in the extracellular fluid attach themselves to cell membrane receptors to create ligand-receptor complexes. Clathrin-coated vesicles are prepared to target certain clathrin-rich areas of the membrane, where they are easily swallowed [105]. The clathrin coat is removed once the vesicles enter the cell and fuse with early endosomes. The endo-lysosomal route subsequently transports drugs from endosomes to lysosomes for further processing [112, 113].

Caveolin-dependent Endocytosis

Caveolin-dependent endocytosis is a cellular uptake process that involves the invasion of flask-shaped membranes called caveolae, which are present in muscle, fibroblast, adipocyte, endothelial, and epithelial cells. The characteristic shape of these structures, which are usually 50-80 nm in size, is due to the presence of the membrane protein caveolin-1 [105]. The regulation of lipids, fatty acids, membrane proteins, and cell signalling depends on this mechanism. Unlike other endocytic routes, caveolae avoid lysosomal uptake by fusing with caveosomes, which maintain a neutral pH and protect internalized drugs from lysosomal breakdown. Due to this protective mechanism, viruses and bacteria often exploit this entry route to evade destruction. This mechanism is used in nanomedicine for drug delivery because it enables NCs to avoid lysosomal breakdown [110, 114].

Clathrin/Caveolin-independent Endocytosis

In addition to the above-mentioned endocytosis mechanisms, NCs, cellular fluids, hormones, and toxins may also enter cells via independent clathrin/caveolin-independent pathways. This allows for a variety of intracellular trafficking and cellular absorption methods [105].

Macropinocytosis

Macropinocytosis is a specialized form of pinocytosis in which cells internalize substantial amounts of extracellular fluid into large vesicles, known as macropinosomes, ranging from 0.5 to 10 µm in size. This cellular mechanism contributes significantly to the internalization of apoptotic and necrotic cells, bacteria, viruses, and the presentation of antigens [115]. Unlike other endocytic mechanisms, macropinocytosis enables the uptake of micron-sized nanoparticles, making it an essential route for the internalization of large nanoparticles. It occurs in most cell types, except for brain microvessel endothelial cells. Due to its ability to engulf large particles, this pathway is widely utilized in NCs-based drug delivery systems [105, 116].

Passive Uptake

The primary mechanisms for NCs uptake include various endocytic pathways. However, other processes, such as passive diffusion via van der Waals forces, steric interactions (adhesive interactions), and pore formation, may also contribute to nanoparticle internalization across the cell membrane [105]. Once NCs enter a cell, drug release proceeds via various mechanisms depending on nanoparticle composition, cellular uptake pathway, and intracellular environment. The main drug release mechanisms are: endosomal escape, lysosomal degradation, diffusion-controlled release, stimuli-responsive release, and carrier degradation, etc [117].

Impact of Nanocarriers on Cellular Uptake

Improve Cellular Uptake

The absorption of lipophilic medicines can be improved by engineering NCs to interact with liver cells. Conjugated linoleic acid (CLA)-loaded tocopherol nanostructured lipid carriers (NLCs) were prepared, and their anti-adipogenic activity was investigated in an in-vitro model and an in-vivo obese rat model fed a high-fat diet, and compared with free α-tocopherol and CLA. The results suggested that the prepared NLCs with a smaller size achieved superior adipocyte uptake and showed better inhibition of adipocyte differentiation than the large particles, thereby enhancing CLA delivery into adipocytes by 5.5-fold compared to the free form [118].

Targeted Delivery to the Liver

NCs can deposit effectively in the liver due to its distinct vasculature and sinusoidal endothelial cells. Delivering lipophilic medications to hepatic tissues is easier because of this property, which results in higher local drug concentrations and lower systemic exposure [36].

Overcoming Physiological Obstacles

Drug distribution is hampered by various biological barriers, and NCs are designed to overcome these by improving solubility, delaying early breakdown, and increasing the bioavailability and cellular uptake of lipophilic drugs, encapsulated within lipid-based structures. This results in prolonged drug circulation throughout the body and more successful therapeutic outcomes [119].

Delivery of siRNA

Small interfering RNA (siRNA) delivery by NCs, especially lipid-based nanoparticles, has been shown to be beneficial for targeting hepatocytes [120]. The inclusion of cationic lipids in these nanoparticles enhances the binding of negatively charged siRNA, promotes efficient cellular uptake, and facilitates gene silencing [121]. This approach has shown potential to alter the expression of genes associated with FLD pathophysiology.

Targeted Therapeutic Effects in Hepatocytes and other Liver Cells

Immune Modulation

There are opportunities to develop NCs that will deliver immunomodulatory medications to Kupffer cells and other hepatic immune cells [122]. The pro-inflammatory milieu associated with FLD can be altered by modulating the function of these cells with NCs, thereby decelerating the progression of the disease.

Anti-Inflammatory Actions

FLD development and progression are significantly impacted by oxidative stress. In this case, NCs can be used to deliver antioxidants effectively to hepatocytes, helping lower reactive oxygen species (ROS) levels and preventing cellular injury and inflammation [123]. Targeted delivery increases the bioavailability of antioxidants at the pathologic site and provides a tactical advantage over systemic delivery. The pharmacodynamics of nanocarriers for FLD is presented in Table **3**.

Table 3. Pharmacodynamics of Nanocarriers for FLD.

Topic	Description	Examples	Ref.
Nanocarrier-Mediated Drug Release Within Liver Cells	Nanocarriers facilitate the controlled release of therapeutic agents within hepatocytes, thereby enhancing drug efficacy and reducing systemic side effects.	Lipid-based nanocarriers are utilized for encapsulating drugs, protecting them from degradation, and allowing gradual release within liver cells.	[124]
Impact of Nanocarriers on Cellular Uptake			
Lipophilic Drugs	The liver's unique architecture, featuring fenestrations lined by sinusoidal endothelial cells, promotes enhanced nanoparticle uptake, making it an ideal target for nanocarrier-delivery of lipophilic drugs.	Polymeric nanocarriers promote bioavailability and therapeutic efficacy of hydrophobic drugs by increasing their solubility and stability.	[125]
siRNA Delivery	Nanocarriers, particularly lipid-based nanoparticles, have been advantageous in delivering small interfering RNA (siRNA), promoting efficient cellular uptake and gene silencing in liver cells.	DNAsome nanocarriers are designed for efficient hepatocyte-specific siRNA delivery, enhancing insulin sensitization through TSC22D4 knockdown.	[126]
Targeted Therapeutic Effects in Hepatocytes and Other Liver Cells			

(Table 3) cont.....

Topic	Description	Examples	Ref.
Immune Modulation	Nanocarriers can be developed and functionalized to deliver immunomodulatory agents specifically to liver-resident immune cells, such as Kupffer cells, changing the inflammatory environment associated with FLD.	Functionalized nanocarriers are utilized for targeted drug delivery in cancer therapy, which can be adapted for immune modulation in liver diseases.	[127]
Anti-Inflammatory Actions	Oxidative stress plays a significant role in FLD progression. Nanocarrier-mediated delivery of antioxidants directly to hepatocytes can effectively minimize reactive oxygen species (ROS) levels, mitigating inflammation and cellular damage.	Redox-manipulating nanocarriers are designed to exploit redox imbalances, achieving precise drug release and enhancing therapeutic efficacy.	[128]

CONCLUSION

This chapter discusses the pharmacokinetics (ADME) and pharmacodynamics of NCs formulations, along with the impact of physicochemical properties of nanocarriers (NCs) on various routes of administration and in-vivo processes. NCs-based therapeutics have shown significant improvement in treating fatty liver diseases, including NAFLD and its progressive form, NASH. This could be attributed to increased drug bioavailability and controlled release, which facilitate effective liver targeting by enhancing drug absorption. By altering distribution profiles, NCs also help to minimize systemic toxicity and ensure site-specific drug delivery. Furthermore, the composition of NCs enhances drug stability, extends circulation time, and prevents therapeutic molecules from enzymatic breakdown during metabolism. NCs also affect the elimination of drugs by increasing hepatic retention and reducing renal clearance. To further enhance liver targeting, techniques such as ligand modifications are employed, facilitating drug delivery to hepatic stellate cells and hepatocytes via endocytosis and receptor-mediated cellular uptake. Therefore, this targeted approach improves the selective uptake of drugs by diseased liver cells, increasing therapeutic potential and reducing off-target effects.

LIST OF ABBREVIATIONS

FLD Fatty Liver Disease

NAFLD Non-Alcoholic Fatty Liver Disease

NASH Non-Alcoholic Steatohepatitis

MASLD Metabolic Dysfunction-Associated Steatotic Liver Disease

MASH Metabolic Dysfunction-Associated Steatohepatitis

ALD	Alcoholic Liver Disease
TASH	Toxicant-Associated Steatohepatitis
HCC	Hepatocellular Carcinoma
FDA	Food and Drug Administration
GLP-1	Glucagon-Like Peptide-1
PK/PD	Pharmacokinetics / Pharmacodynamics
PBPK	Physiologically Based Pharmacokinetics
ADME	Absorption, Distribution, Metabolism, Excretion
NCs	Nanocarriers
ROS	Reactive Oxygen Species
siRNA	Small Interfering RNA
LDL	Low-Density Lipoprotein
ER	Endoplasmic Reticulum
UPR	Unfolded Protein Response
PERK	Protein Kinase R-like Endoplasmic Reticulum Kinase
eIF2α	Eukaryotic Initiation Factor 2 Alpha
CHOP	C/EBP Homologous Protein

REFERENCES

[1] Tapper EB, Parikh ND. Mortality due to cirrhosis and liver cancer in the United States, 1999–2016: observational study. BMJ 2018; 362: k2817.
[http://dx.doi.org/10.1136/bmj.k2817]

[2] Fabbrini E, Magkos FJN. Hepatic steatosis as a marker of metabolic dysfunction. Nutrients 2015; 7(6): 4995-5019.
[http://dx.doi.org/10.3390/nu7064995]

[3] Rinella ME, Sookoian S. From NAFLD to MASLD: updated naming and diagnosis criteria for fatty liver disease. J Lipid Res 2024; 65: 100485.
[http://dx.doi.org/10.1016/j.jlr.2023.100485]

[4] Wahlang B, Jin J, Beier JI, *et al.* Mechanisms of environmental contributions to fatty liver disease. Curr Environ Health Rep 2019; 6(3): 80-94.
[http://dx.doi.org/10.1007/s40572-019-00232-w]

[5] Younossi ZM, Koenig AB, Abdelatif D, Fazel Y, Henry L, Wymer M. Global epidemiology of nonalcoholic fatty liver disease: meta-analytic assessment of prevalence, incidence, and outcomes. Hepatology 2016; 64(1): 73-84.
[http://dx.doi.org/10.1002/hep.28431]

[6] Cave M, Falkner KC, Ray M, *et al.* Toxicant-associated steatohepatitis in vinyl chloride workers. Hepatology 2010; 51(2): 474-81.
[http://dx.doi.org/10.1002/hep.2]

[7] Chan W-K, Chuah K-H, Rajaram RB, Lim LL, Ratnasingam J, Vethakkan SR. Metabolic dysfunction-associated steatotic liver disease (MASLD): a state-of-the-art review 2023; 32(3): 197-213.

[8] Ahmadizar F, Younossi ZMJJoCG. Exploring Biomarkers in Nonalcoholic Fatty Liver Disease

Among Individuals With Type 2 Diabetes Mellitus. 2025; 59(1): 36-46

[9] Younossi ZM, Yilmaz Y, Yu M-L, *et al.* Clinical and patient-reported outcomes from patients with nonalcoholic fatty liver disease across the world: data from the global non-alcoholic steatohepatitis (NASH)/non-alcoholic fatty liver disease (NAFLD) registry. Clin Gastroenterol Hepatol. 2021.

[10] Han SK, Baik SK, Kim MY. Non-alcoholic fatty liver disease: Definition and subtypes. Clin Mol Hepatol 2022; 29(suppl): S5-S16.

[11] Loomba R, Friedman SL, Shulman GI. Mechanisms and disease consequences of nonalcoholic fatty liver disease. Cell 2021; 184(10): 2537-64.
[http://dx.doi.org/10.1016/j.cell.2021.04.008]

[12] Estes C, Razavi H, Loomba R, Younossi Z, Sanyal AJ. Modeling the epidemic of nonalcoholic fatty liver disease demonstrates an exponential increase in burden of disease. Hepatology 2018; 67(1): 123-33.
[http://dx.doi.org/10.1002/hep.29466]

[13] Powell E, Wong VW-S, Rinella M. Non-alcoholic fatty liver disease. Lancet 2021; 397(10290): 2212-24.
[http://dx.doi.org/10.1016/S0140-6736(20)32511-3]

[14] Pafili K, Roden MJMM. Nonalcoholic fatty liver disease (NAFLD) from pathogenesis to treatment concepts in humans. 2021;50:101122.
[http://dx.doi.org/10.1016/j.molmet.2020.101122]

[15] Pouwels S, Sakran N, Graham Y, *et al.* Non-alcoholic fatty liver disease (NAFLD): a review of pathophysiology, clinical management and effects of weight loss. BMC Endocr Disord 2022; 22(1): 63.

[16] Szczerbinska A, Rolinski J, Surdacka A, Cichoz-Lach H. Diagnostic and Prognostic Potential of CXCL9 and CXCL10 Chemokines in Alcohol-Associated Liver Disease. Int J Mol Sci 2025; 26(23): 11717.
[http://dx.doi.org/10.3390/ijms262311717] [PMID: 41373861]

[17] Filozof C, Goldstein BJ, Williams RN, Sanyal A. Non-alcoholic steatohepatitis: limited available treatment options but promising drugs in development and recent progress towards a regulatory approval pathway. Drugs 2015; 75(12): 1373-92.
[http://dx.doi.org/10.1007/s40265-015-0437-3]

[18] Povsic M, Wong OY, Perry R. A structured literature review of the epidemiology and disease burden of non-alcoholic steatohepatitis (NASH). 2019;36:1574-94

[19] Rafiq N, Younossi ZM. Nonalcoholic fatty liver disease: a practical approach to evaluation and management. 2009;13(2):249-66

[20] Chen JYS, Chua D, Lim CO, Ho WX, Tan NS. Lessons on drug development: a literature review of challenges faced in nonalcoholic fatty liver disease (NAFLD) clinical trials. 2022;24(1):158

[21] Wong VWS, Wong GLH, Chan RSM, *et al.* Beneficial effects of lifestyle intervention in non-obese patients with non-alcoholic fatty liver disease. J Hepatol 2018; 69(6): 1349-56.
[http://dx.doi.org/10.1016/j.jhep.2018.08.011]

[22] Petroni ML, Brodosi L, Bugianesi E, Marchesini G. Management of non-alcoholic fatty liver disease. BMJ 2021; 372: m4747.
[http://dx.doi.org/10.1136/bmj.m4747]

[23] Forlano R, Sigon G, Mullish BH, Yee M, Manousou PJM. Screening for NAFLD-current knowledge and challenges. Metabolites. 2023 Apr 9;13(4):536
[http://dx.doi.org/10.3390/metabo13040536]

[24] Dinani AM, Kowdley KV, Noureddin M. Application of artificial intelligence for diagnosis and risk stratification in NAFLD and NASH: The state of the art. Hepatology. 2021 ;74(4):2233-2240.

[http://dx.doi.org/10.1002/hep.31869]

[25] Cotter TG, Rinella M. Nonalcoholic fatty liver disease 2020: The state of the disease. Gastroenterology. 2020 ;158(7):1851-1864.
[http://dx.doi.org/10.1053/j.gastro.2020.01.052]

[26] Tacke F, Weiskirchen R. Non-alcoholic fatty liver disease (NAFLD)/non-alcoholic steatohepatitis (NASH)-related liver fibrosis: mechanisms, treatment and prevention. Ann Transl Med. 2021 ;9(8):729
[http://dx.doi.org/10.21037/atm-20-4354]

[27] Liang C, Li J, Tian B, *et al.* Foresight regarding drug candidates acting on the succinate–GPR91 signalling pathway for non-alcoholic steatohepatitis (NASH) treatment. Biomedicine & Pharmacotherapy 2017 Dec 1; 144: 112298.

[28] Athanasopoulou F, Manolakakis M, Vernia S, Kamaly N. Nanodrug delivery systems for metabolic chronic liver diseases: advances and perspectives. Nanomedicine. 2023;18(1):67–84.
[http://dx.doi.org/10.2217/nnm-2022-0261]

[29] Han X, Gong N, Xue L, *et al.* Ligand-tethered lipid nanoparticles for targeted RNA delivery to treat liver fibrosis. Nat Commun. 2023; 14:75
[http://dx.doi.org/10.1038/s41467-022-35637-z]

[30] Yoshizaki Y, Yamasaki M, Nagata T, *et al.* Drug delivery with hyaluronic acid-coated polymeric micelles in liver fibrosis herapy. ACS Biomater Sci Eng. 2023;9(6).
[http://dx.doi.org/10.1021/acsbiomaterials.3c00327]

[31] Yuan Y, Che L, Qi C, Meng Z. Protective effects of polysaccharides on hepatic injury: A review. Int J Biol Macromol 2019; 141: 822-30.
[http://dx.doi.org/10.1016/j.ijbiomac.2019.09.002]

[32] Wang J, Wang H, Yang X, Wang K, Zhang Y. Recent advances in the role of polysaccharides in liver diseases: a review. Front Pharmacol. 2025;16:1535717.
[http://dx.doi.org/10.3389/fphar.2025.1535717]

[33] Wei X, Luo D, Li H, *et al.* The roles and potential mechanisms of plant polysaccharides in liver diseases: a review. Front Pharmacol. 2024; 15: 1400958.
[http://dx.doi.org/10.3389/fphar.2024.1400958]

[34] Ezhilarasan D. Advantages and challenges in nanomedicines for chronic liver diseases: A hepatologist's perspectives. Eur J Pharmacol. 2021; 893: 173832
[http://dx.doi.org/10.1016/j.ejphar.2020.173832]

[35] Liu Z, Li Y, Li W, *et al.* Multifunctional nanohybrid based on porous silicon nanoparticles, gold nanoparticles, and acetalated dextran for liver regeneration and acute liver failure theranostics. Adv Mater. 2018 ;30 (24): e1703393.
[http://dx.doi.org/10.1002/adma.201703393]

[36] Chu R, Wang Y, Kong J, Pan T, Yang Y, He JJ. Lipid nanoparticles as the drug carrier for targeted therapy of hepatic disorders. J Mater Chem B 2024; 12: 4759-4784.

[37] Kulkarni J, Witzigmann D, Chen S, Cullis P, van der Meel R. Lipid nanoparticle technology for clinical translation of siRNA therapeutics. Acc Chem Res 2019; 52(9)

[38] Kerry RG, Mahapatra GP, Maurya GK, *et al.* Molecular prospect of type-2 diabetes: nanotechnology-based diagnostics and therapeutic intervention. Rev Endocr Metab Disord. 2020; 22(2): 421-451.
[http://dx.doi.org/10.1007/s11154-020-09606-0]

[39] Gao F, Feng X, Li X. Recent advances in polymeric nanoparticles for the treatment of hepatic diseases Front Pharmacol 2025; 16: 1528752
[http://dx.doi.org/10.3389/fphar.2025.1528752]

[40] Speciale A, Muscarà C, Molonia MS, Cristani M, Cimino F, Saija A. Recent advances in

glycyrrhetinic acid-functionalized biomaterials for liver cancer-targeting therapy. Molecules. 2022; 27(6): 1775
[http://dx.doi.org/10.3390/molecules27061775]

[41] Bakrania A, Mo Y, Zheng G, Bhat M. 2023. RNA nanomedicine in liver diseases. Hepatology. 2025 ;81(6):1847-1877
[http://dx.doi.org/10.1097/HEP.0000000000000606]

[42] Ezhilararasan D, Lakshmi T, Raut B. Novel nano-based drug delivery systems targeting hepatic stellate cells in the fibrotic liver. J Nanomater 2021; 2021: 4674046.

[43] Liu E, Zhang M, Huang Y. Pharmacokinetics and pharmacodynamics (PK/PD) of bionanomaterials. In: Grumezescu AM, editor. Biomedical nanomaterials. Weinheim: Wiley-VCH; 2016. p. 1-60.
[http://dx.doi.org/10.1002/9783527694396.ch1]

[44] Gharat SA, Momin MM, Khan T. Pharmacokinetics and pharmacodynamics of novel drug delivery systems: from basic concepts to applications: a machine-generated literature overview. Cham: Springer Nature; 2024

[45] Glassman PM. Muzykantov VR. Pharmacokinetic and pharmacodynamic properties of drug delivery systems. J Pharmacol Exp Ther. 2019 ;370(3):570-80.

[46] Couvreur P. Nanoparticles in drug delivery: past, present and future. Adv Drug Deliv Rev. 2013 ;65(1):21-3.
[http://dx.doi.org/10.1016/j.addr.2012.04.010]

[47] Zhang A, Meng K, Liu Y, Pan Y, Qu W, Chen D, *et al.* Absorption, distribution, metabolism, and excretion of nanocarriers in vivo and their influences. Adv Colloid Interface Sci. 2020; 284: 102261.
[http://dx.doi.org/10.1016/j.cis.2020.102261]

[48] Sillu D, Sudhakara Reddy M, Agnihotri S. Nanocarriers for drug delivery: general characteristics. In: Nanomaterials for Drug Delivery and Neurological Diseases Management. Springer Nature; 2024. p. 3–20
[http://dx.doi.org/10.1007/978-981-97-0308-1_1]

[49] Wu L, Liu M, Shan W, Zhu X, Li L, Zhang Z. Lipid-based nanocarriers for oral drug delivery. J Control Release. 2017;252:1–15
[http://dx.doi.org/10.1016/j.jconrel.2017.02.019.]

[50] Maurya R, Vikal A, Patel P, Narang RK, Kurmi BD. "Enhancing Oral Drug Absorption: Overcoming Physiological and Pharmaceutical Barriers for Improved Bioavailability". AAPS PharmSciTech 2024; 25(7): 228.
[http://dx.doi.org/10.1208/s12249-024-02940-5] [PMID: 39354282]

[51] Li M, Zou P, Tyner K, Lee S. Physiologically based pharmacokinetic (PBPK) modeling of pharmaceutical nanoparticles AAPS J 2017; 19(1): 26-42
[http://dx.doi.org/10.1208/s12248-016-0010-3]

[52] Pramanik S, Mohanto S, Manne R, *et al.* Nanoparticle-based drug delivery system: the magic bullet for the treatment of chronic pulmonary diseases. Mol Pharm. 2021; 18(10): 3655–3681.
[http://dx.doi.org/10.1021/acs.molpharmaceut.1c00353]

[53] Yuan D, He H, Wu Y, Fan J, Cao Y. Physiologically based pharmacokinetic modeling of nanoparticles. J Pharm Sci. 2019; 108(1): 58-72

[54] Kurmi BD, Tekchandani P, Paliwal R, Paliwal S. Transdermal drug delivery: opportunities and challenges for controlled delivery of therapeutic agents using nanocarriers. Curr Drug Metab. 2017; 18(5): 481–495
[http://dx.doi.org/10.2174/1389200218666170222150555]

[55] Peng X, Wang J, Zhou F, Liu Q, Zhang Z. Nanoparticle-based approaches to target the lymphatic system for antitumor treatment. Cell Mol Life Sci. 2021; 78(12): 5139-5161.
[http://dx.doi.org/10.1007/s00018-021-03842-6]

[56] Gharat SA, Momin MM, Khan T. Absorption, distribution, metabolism and excretion of novel drug delivery systems. In: Pharmacokinetics and Pharmacodynamics of Novel Drug Delivery Systems: From Basic Concepts to Applications. Springer; 2024. p. 19–79

[57] Wang Y, Mo Y, Sun Y. Intestinal nanoparticle delivery and cellular response: a review of the bidirectional nanoparticle–cell interplay in mucosa based on physicochemical properties. J Nanobiotechnology. 2024; 22(1): 669
[http://dx.doi.org/10.1186/s12951-024-02345-0]

[58] Ishii M, Fukuoka Y, Deguchi S, Otake H, Tanino T, Nagai N. Energy-dependent endocytosis is involved in the absorption of indomethacin nanoparticles in the small intestine. Int J Mol Sci. 2019; 20(3): 476
[http://dx.doi.org/10.3390/ijms20030476]

[59] Lee SH, Song JG, Han HK. Development of pH-responsive organic–inorganic hybrid nanocomposites as an effective oral delivery system of protein drugs. J Control Release. 2019; 311: 74–84
[http://dx.doi.org/10.1016/j.jconrel.2019.08.010]

[60] Jin Z, Gao Q, Wu K, Ouyang J, Guo W, Liang X-J. Harnessing inhaled nanoparticles to overcome the pulmonary barrier for respiratory disease therapy. Adv Drug Deliv Rev. 2023; 198: 115111.

[61] Lane ME, Rahma A. Non-deformable nanoparticles and transdermal penetration. Fundamentals of Pharmaceutical Nanoscience. Springer Nature 2024; pp. 295-311.
[http://dx.doi.org/10.1007/978-3-031-59478-6_12]

[62] Stack T, Liu Y, Frey M, Bobbala S, Vincent M, Scott EA. Enhancing subcutaneous injection and target tissue accumulation of nanoparticles via co-administration with macropinocytosis inhibitory nanoparticles (MiNP). Nat Nanotechnol. 2021; 6(5): 393–400

[63] Onzi G, Guterres SS, Pohlmann AR, Frank LA. Passive targeting and the enhanced permeability and retention (EPR) effect. In: Advances in Pharmacokinetics and Pharmacodynamics. 2021: 1–13

[64] Jain A, Mishra AK, Hurkat P, Shilpi S, Mody N, Jain SK. Navigating liver cancer: precision targeting for enhanced treatment outcomes. Drug Deliv Transl Res. 2025:1–27

[65] Jacob S, Nair A, Boddu S, Abuhijjleh R, Selvaraju K, Babu T, *et al.* The emerging role of lipid nanosystems and nanomicelles in liver diseases. Int J Pharm. 2023; 27(18).

[66] Luo F, Yu Y, Li M, *et al.* Polymeric nanomedicines for the treatment of hepatic diseases. J Nanomedicine. 2022; 20(1): 488

[67] Upponi J, Torchilin V. Passive *vs* active targeting: an update of the EPR role in drug delivery to tumors. 2014

[68] Ramírez-Cortés F, Ménová P. Hepatocyte targeting via the asialoglycoprotein receptor. RSC Med Chem. 2025; 16: 525-544
[http://dx.doi.org/10.1039/D4MD00652F]

[69] Dilliard SA, Siegwart DJ. Passive, active and endogenous organ-targeted lipid and polymer nanoparticles for delivery of genetic drugs. Nat Rev Mater. 2023; 8: 282-300
[http://dx.doi.org/10.1038/s41578-022-00529-7]

[70] Mahmoud K, Swidan S, El-Nabarawi M, Teaima M. Lipid-based nanoparticles as a novel treatment modality for hepatocellular carcinoma: a comprehensive review on targeting and recent advances. J Nanobiotechnol. 2022; 20(1): 109

[71] Böttger R, Pauli G, Chao P-H, Fayez NA, Hohenwarter L, Li SD. Lipid-based nanoparticle technologies for liver targeting. Adv Drug Deliv Rev. 2020; 154: 79-101
[http://dx.doi.org/10.1016/j.addr.2020.06.004]

[72] Thacharodi A, Singh P, Meenatchi R. Revolutionizing healthcare and medicine: The impact of modern technologies for a healthier future-A comprehensive review. Health Care Sci. 2024; 3(5): 329-349
[http://dx.doi.org/10.1002/hcs2.115]

[73] Cheng Z, Huang H, Yin M, Liu H. Applications of liposomes and lipid nanoparticles in cancer therapy: current advances and prospects. Exp Hematol Oncol. 2025; 14(1): 11

[74] Shah N. editor. Nanocarriers: Drug Delivery System. Singapore: Springer Singapore; 2021. [http://dx.doi.org/10.1007/978-981-33-4497-6]

[75] Cai X, Jin M, Yao L, He B, Ahmed S, Safdar W, *et al.* Physicochemical properties, pharmacokinetics, toxicology and application of nanocarriers J Mater Chem B 2023; 11(4): 716-733 [http://dx.doi.org/10.1039/D2TB02001G]

[76] Colino CI, Lanao JM, Gutierrez-Millan C. Targeting of hepatic macrophages by therapeutic nanoparticles. Front Immunol. 2020; 11: 218. [http://dx.doi.org/10.3389/fimmu.2020.00218]

[77] Haripriyaa M, Suthindhiran K. Pharmacokinetics of nanoparticles: current knowledge, future directions and its implications in drug delivery. J Pharm Sci. 2023; 9(1): 113 [http://dx.doi.org/10.1016/j.jphs.2023.113]

[78] Zhang YN, Poon W, Tavares AJ, McGilvray ID, Chan WCW. Nanoparticle–liver interactions: Cellular uptake and hepatobiliary elimination. J Control Release. 2016; 240: 332-348 [http://dx.doi.org/10.1016/j.jconrel.2016.03.017]

[79] Li X, Wang B, Zhou S, *et al.* Surface chemistry governs the sub-organ transfer, clearance and toxicity of functional gold nanoparticles in the liver and kidney. J Nanobiotechnol. 2020; 18:45 [http://dx.doi.org/10.1186/s12951-020-00599-1]

[80] Soares DCF, Ferreira TH, de Aguiar Ferreira C, Cardoso VN, de Sousa EMB. Boron nitride nanotubes radiolabeled with 99mTc: Preparation, physicochemical characterization, biodistribution study, and scintigraphic imaging in Swiss mice. Int J Pharm. 2012; 423(2): 489-495 [http://dx.doi.org/10.1016/j.ijpharm.2011.11.031]

[81] Poon W, Zhang Y-N, Ouyang B. Elimination pathways of nanoparticles. ACS Nano. 2019; 13(5): 5785-5798 [http://dx.doi.org/10.1021/acsnano.9b01383] [PMID: 30990673]

[82] Emanuele M, Balasubramaniam B. Differential effects of commercial-grade and purified poloxamer 188 on renal function. Drug-Induced Renal Inj. 2014; 14: 73-83 [http://dx.doi.org/10.1016/j.drir.2014.02.002]

[83] Dalla Costa T, Carreño F, Haas SE. Pharmaceutical Nanocarriers: Disposition. In: Talevi A, editor. The ADME Encyclopedia. Cham: Springer; 2022 [http://dx.doi.org/10.1007/978-3-030-84860-6_112]

[84] Parmar K, Patel J, Pathak Y. Factors affecting the clearance and biodistribution of polymeric nanoparticles. In: Patel JK, Pathak YV, editors. Pharmacokinetics and Pharmacodynamics of Nanoparticulate Drug Delivery Systems. Cham: Springer; 2022 [http://dx.doi.org/10.1007/978-3-030-83395-4_14]

[85] Saker R, Regdon G, Sovány T. Pharmacokinetics and toxicity of inorganic nanoparticles and the physicochemical properties/factors affecting them. J Drug Deliv Sci Technol. 2024; 99: 105979 [http://dx.doi.org/10.1016/j.jddst.2024.105979]

[86] Cheng X, Tian X, Wu A, *et al.* Protein corona influences cellular uptake of gold nanoparticles by phagocytic and nonphagocytic cells in a size-dependent manner. ACS Appl Mater Interfaces. 2015; 7(37): 20568-20575 [http://dx.doi.org/10.1021/acsami.5b04290]

[87] Malhaire H, Gimel J-C, Roger E, Benoît J-P, Lagarce F. How to design the surface of peptide-loaded nanoparticles for efficient oral bioavailability? Adv Drug Deliv Rev. 2016; 106(Pt B): 320–336 [http://dx.doi.org/10.1016/j.addr.2016.03.011]

[88] Lee JH, Sahu A, Jang C, Tae G. The effect of ligand density on in vivo tumor targeting of

nanographene oxide. J Control Release. 2015; 209: 219-228 [http://dx.doi.org/10.1016/j.jconrel.2015.04.035]

[89] Parmar K, Patel JK. Surface modification of nanoparticles to oppose uptake by the mononuclear phagocyte system. Surface modification of nanoparticles for targeted drug delivery. Springer 2019; pp. 221-36.

[90] Zhao Z, Ukidve A, Krishnan V, Mitragotri S. Effect of physicochemical and surface properties on in vivo fate of drug nanocarriers. Adv Drug Deliv Rev. 2019; 143: 3-21 [http://dx.doi.org/10.1016/j.addr.2019.01.002]

[91] Banerjee A, Qi J, Gogoi R, Wong J, Mitragotri S. Role of nanoparticle size, shape and surface chemistry in oral drug delivery. J Control Release. 2016; 238: 176-185 [http://dx.doi.org/10.1016/j.jconrel.2016.07.051]

[92] Sharma G, Valenta DT, Altman Y, Harvey S, Xie H, Mitragotri S. Polymer particle shape independently influences binding and internalization by macrophages. J Control Release. 2010; 147(3): 408-412 [http://dx.doi.org/10.1016/j.jconrel.2010.07.116]

[93] Reuter KG, Perry JL, Kim D, Luft JC, Liu R, DeSimone JM. Targeted PRINT hydrogels: The role of nanoparticle size and ligand density on cell association, biodistribution, and tumor accumulation. Nano Lett. 2015; 15(10): 6371-6378 [http://dx.doi.org/10.1021/acs.nanolett.5b01362]

[94] Alarcon JF, Soliman M, Lüdtke TU, Clemente E, Dobricic M, Violatto MB, *et al.* Long-term retention of gold nanoparticles in the liver is not affected by their physicochemical characteristics. ACS Nano. 2023; 15(19): 8740-8753. [http://dx.doi.org/10.1021/acsnano.3c04683]

[95] Wang J, Xie Y, Wang L, *et al.* In vivo pharmacokinetic features and biodistribution of star and rod shaped gold nanoparticles by multispectral optoacoustic tomography. Sci Rep. 2015; 5:7529 [http://dx.doi.org/10.1038/srep07529]

[96] Huang X, Li L, Liu T, *et al.* The shape effect of mesoporous silica nanoparticles on biodistribution, clearance, and biocompatibility in vivo. ACS Nano. 2011; 5(7): 5390-5399 [http://dx.doi.org/10.1021/nn200185u]

[97] Efimova A, Abramova T. Complexes of anionic and cationic liposomes for encapsulation of bioactive substances. Russ J Gen Chem 2024; 94(11): 3126-32. [http://dx.doi.org/10.1134/S1070363224110148]

[98] Saha K, Rahimi M, Yazdani M, *et al.* Regulation of macrophage recognition through the interplay of nanoparticle surface functionality and protein corona. ACS Nano 2016; 10(4): 4421-30. [http://dx.doi.org/10.1021/acsnano.5b08177]

[99] Du B, Yu M, Zheng J. Transport and interactions of nanoparticles in the kidneys. Nat Rev Mater 2018; 3(10): 358-74. [http://dx.doi.org/10.1038/s41578-018-0046-9]

[100] Arnida M, Ray A, Peterson C, Ghandehari H. Geometry and surface characteristics of gold nanoparticles influence their biodistribution and uptake by macrophages. Eur J Pharm Biopharm. 2011; 77(3): 417-423 [http://dx.doi.org/10.1016/j.ejpb.2010.12.011]

[101] Wu L, Liu M, Shan W, Cui Y, Zhang Z, Huang Y. Lipid nanovehicles with adjustable surface properties for overcoming multiple barriers simultaneously in oral administration. Int J Pharm 2017; 520(1-2): 216-27.

[102] Ma X, Hui H, Jin Y, *et al.* Enhanced immunotherapy of SM5-1 in hepatocellular carcinoma by conjugating with gold nanoparticles and its in vivo bioluminescence tomographic evaluation. Biomaterials. 2016; 87: 46-56.

[http://dx.doi.org/10.1016/j.biomaterials.2016.02.007]

[103] Jun H, Jang E, Kim H, *et al.* TRAIL & EGFR affibody dual-display on a protein nanoparticle synergistically suppresses tumor growth. Biomaterials. 2022; 349: 367-378

[104] Cheng X, Zeng X, Zheng Y, Wang X, Tang R. Surface-fluorinated and pH-sensitive carboxymethyl chitosan nanoparticles to overcome biological barriers for improved drug delivery in vivo. Colloids Surf B Biointerfaces. 2019; 208: 59-69

[105] de Almeida MS, Susnik E, Drasler B, Taladriz-Blanco P, Petri-Fink A, Rothen-Rutishauser B. Understanding nanoparticle endocytosis to improve targeting strategies in nanomedicine. Chem Soc Rev. 2021; 50(9): 5397-5434

[106] Bhandari S, Larsen AK, McCourt P, Smedsrød B, Sørensen KK. The scavenger function of liver sinusoidal endothelial cells in health and disease. Front Immunol. 2021; 12: 757469 [http://dx.doi.org/10.3389/fimmu.2021.757469]

[107] He Y, Wang Y, Wang L, Jiang W, Wilhelm S. Understanding nanoparticle-liver interactions in nanomedicine. Expert Opin Drug Deliv. 2024; 21(6): 829-843

[108] Kamps JA, Morselt HW, Swart PJ, Meijer DKF, Scherphof GL. Massive targeting of liposomes, surface-modified with anionized albumins, to hepatic endothelial cells. Proc Natl Acad Sci USA. 1997; 94(21): 11681-11685 [http://dx.doi.org/10.1073/pnas.94.21.11681]

[109] Chen Z, Jain A, Liu H, Zhao Z, Cheng K. Targeted drug delivery to hepatic stellate cells for the treatment of liver fibrosis. J Pharmacol Exp Ther. 2019; 370(3): 695-702 [http://dx.doi.org/10.1124/jpet.118.254014]

[110] Foroozandeh P, Aziz AA. Insight into cellular uptake and intracellular trafficking of nanoparticles. Nanoscale Res Lett. 2018; 13(1): 339. [http://dx.doi.org/10.1186/s11671-018-2728-5]

[111] Ferguson JP, Huber SD, Willy NM, *et al.* Mechanoregulation of clathrin-mediated endocytosis. J Cell Sci. 2017; 130(21): 3631-3636 [http://dx.doi.org/10.1242/jcs.205877]

[112] Cocucci E, Aguet F, Boulant S, Kirchhausen T. The first five seconds in the life of a clathrin-coated pit. Cell. 2012; 150(3): 495-507 [http://dx.doi.org/10.1016/j.cell.2012.06.054]

[113] Baschieri F, Porshneva K, Montagnac G. Frustrated clathrin-mediated endocytosis—causes and possible functions. J Cell Sci. 2020; 133(11): jcs240861 [http://dx.doi.org/10.1242/jcs.240861]

[114] Kiss AL, Botos E. Caveolae and the regulation of endocytosis. Cell Signal. 2012; 24(1): 14-28 [http://dx.doi.org/10.1016/j.cellsig.2011.09.014]

[115] Lin XP, Mintern JD, Gleeson PA. Macropinocytosis in different cell types: similarities and differences. Membranes (Basel). 2020; 10(8): 177. [http://dx.doi.org/10.3390/membranes10080177]

[116] Kuhn DA, Vanhecke D, Michen B, *et al.* Different endocytotic uptake mechanisms for nanoparticles in epithelial cells and macrophages. J Nanobiotechnology. 2014; 12:16 [http://dx.doi.org/10.1186/1477-3155-12-16]

[117] Desai N, Rana D, Salave S, Benival D, Khunt D, Prajapati BG. Achieving endo/lysosomal escape using smart nanosystems for efficient cellular delivery. Molecules. 2024; 29(13): 3131 [http://dx.doi.org/10.3390/molecules29133131]

[118] Hsu CY, Liao CC, Lin ZC, *et al.* Facile adipocyte uptake and liver/adipose tissue delivery of conjugated linoleic acid-loaded tocol nanocarriers for a synergistic anti-adipogenesis effect. J Nanobiotechnology. 2024; 22(1): 50

[http://dx.doi.org/10.1186/s12951-024-00845-7]

[119] Suhag D, Kaushik S, Taxak VB. Drug delivery *via* lipid-based nanocarriers. In: Handbook of Biomaterials for Medical Applications, Volume 1: Fundamentals. Springer; 2024. p.297-328

[120] Nguyen L, Nguyen TT, Kim JY, Jeong JH. Advanced siRNA delivery in combating hepatitis B virus: mechanistic insights and recent updates. J Nanobiotechnology. 2024; 22(1): 745

[121] Sato Y, Matsui H, Sato R, Harashima H. Neutralization of negative charges of siRNA results in improved safety and efficient gene silencing activity of lipid nanoparticles loaded with high levels of siRNA. J Control Release. 2018; 284: 179-187.
[http://dx.doi.org/10.1016/j.jconrel.2018.06.011]

[122] Kaps L, Limeres MJ, Schneider P, *et al.* Liver cell type-specific targeting by nanoformulations for therapeutic applications. ACS Nano. 2023; 24(14): 11869-11884
[http://dx.doi.org/10.1021/acsnano.3c02076]

[123] Liu J, Han X, Zhang T, Tian K, Li Z, Luo F. Reactive oxygen species (ROS) scavenging biomaterials for anti-inflammatory diseases: from mechanism to therapy. J Hematol Oncol. 2023; 16(1): 116.
[http://dx.doi.org/10.1186/s13046-023-02761-9]

[124] Perrigue PM, Murray RA, Mielcarek A, Henschke A, Moya SE. Degradation of drug delivery nanocarriers and payload release: a review of physical methods for tracing nanocarrier biological fate. Pharmaceutics. 2021; 13(6): 770
[http://dx.doi.org/10.3390/pharmaceutics13060770]

[125] Bhalani DV, Nutan B, Kumar A, Singh Chandel AK. Bioavailability enhancement techniques for poorly aqueous soluble drugs and therapeutics. Biomedicines. 2022; 10: 2055
[http://dx.doi.org/10.3390/biomedicines10092055]

[126] Mohammadi A, Ebrahimnejad P, Kenari SA, Kashi Z, Gill P. Nanomolecular silencing of TSC22D4 mRNA via a DNAsome-siRNA for enhancing insulin sensitization in hepatocytes. Iran J Basic Med Sci. 2025; 28(3): 385-392
[http://dx.doi.org/10.22038/ijbms.2024.81998.17744] [PMID: 39906612]

[127] Xia W, Tao Z, Zhu B, *et al.* Targeted delivery of drugs and genes using polymer nanocarriers for cancer therapy. Int J Mol Sci. 2021; 22(17): 9118
[http://dx.doi.org/10.3390/ijms22179118]

[128] Meng X, Shen Y, Zhao H, Lu X, Wang Z, Zhao Y. Redox-manipulating nanocarriers for anticancer drug delivery: a systematic review. J Nanobiotechnol. 2024; 22(1): 587
[http://dx.doi.org/10.1186/s12951-024-02859-w]

CHAPTER 12

Safety and Toxicity Considerations of Nanocarrier-based Therapeutics

Himanshu Sharma[1], **Akashdeep Singh**[1], **Vishnu Mittal**[2] and **Pooja Mittal**[3,*]

[1] *Chitkara College of Pharmacy, Chitkara University, Rajpura, Punjab, India*

[2] *Department of Pharmaceutics, Adesh Institute of Pharmacy and Biomedical Sciences, Adesh University, Bathinda, Punjab, India*

[3] *GITAM School of Pharmacy, GITAM (Deemed to be University), Sangareddy, Telangana, India*

Abstract: A novel strategy in pharmaceuticals, nano-formulations increase therapeutic effectiveness, decrease side effects, and enhance medication dispersion. In this study, the laws, safety, and ethics related to nano-formulations are covered in great detail. Regulatory obstacles, such as the need for particular legislation designed for medications using nanotechnology, are a significant issue. A thorough analysis of characterisation methods, stability evaluations, and the development of standardised production and quality control procedures are all necessary to address these issues. To ensure effectiveness and safety while accelerating the transition of research into clinical applications, regulatory authorities worldwide must create flexible frameworks to streamline approval processes. Risk-benefit analyses, informed consent, and fair access to technical innovations are the main ethical factors in nano-formulations. Making moral decisions requires weighing potential advantages against potential disadvantages and maintaining open communication with all stakeholders. Furthermore, healthcare systems worldwide face moral conundrums about the fair distribution and cost of these cutting-edge treatments. Important safety issues include knowing how nanoparticles interact with the biological environment, their potential toxicity, and their long-term impacts. Thorough safety evaluations, including in vitro and in vivo studies, are necessary to assess biocompatibility and mitigate unanticipated risks associated with nanocarriers. Ongoing safety evaluations are also conducted through post-marketing surveillance and continuous monitoring. Regulatory authorities, researchers, physicians, and ethicists must work together to fully use these formulations while maintaining patient safety, moral behaviour, and legal obligations.

Keywords: Bio-compatibility, Nanocarrier, Safety, Therapeutics, Toxicity.

* **Corresponding author Pooja Mittal:** GITAM School of Pharmacy, GITAM (Deemed to be) University, Sangareddy, Telangana, India; E-mail: poojamittal2009@gmail.com

Anjali Sharma, Devkant Sharma, Ajmer Singh Grewal, Geeta Deswal & Ganga Reddy Velma (Eds.)

INTRODUCTION

Although still in its infancy, nanomedicine, the application of nanotechnology in medicine, has the potential to drastically transform the healthcare industry [1]. The rapidly expanding area of nanomedical research is being actively supported by government funding and legislation. As nanomedicines advance, they might provide many advantages over traditional therapies, including improved targeting, safety, effectiveness, bioavailability, dose response, and personalization [2]. Perhaps the most exciting concept in nanomedical research is the creation and manufacture of multifunctional nanoparticle (NP) complexes that simultaneously deliver therapeutic and diagnostic drugs to specific sites. These abilities might greatly enhance the monitoring, diagnosis, and treatment of patients. Despite these possible advantages, little is known about the pharmacokinetics, pharmacodynamics, and toxicity of certain nanomaterials.

Rising Interest Due to Enhanced Drug Delivery, Targeting, and Bioavailability

Nanotechnology has applications across the pharmaceutical, cosmetic, electronic, food, and numerous other industries. According to the Woodrow Wilson International Center for Scholars' Project on Emerging Nanotechnologies, approximately 800 products currently incorporate nanotechnology [3]. It has been employed in digital cameras, cell phones, computers, water filtration systems, and cosmetics. Research is also underway to enhance the solubility of food ingredients and develop packaging that can detect and prevent spoilage. In the medical field, nanotechnology has advanced various products and procedures, including medications, antimicrobial materials, medical imaging, sunscreens, burn and wound dressings, dental bonding agents, protective coatings for eyeglasses, and skin care products. Moreover, nanotechnology has improved drug targeting and absorption, increased the sensitivity of biomarker detection, enhanced therapeutic delivery, and advanced diagnostic imaging [4].

Importance of Safety and Toxicity Evaluation in Clinical Translation

The merging of nanotechnology with medicine gives rise to the interdisciplinary domain of nanomedicine [5]. Advances in genetics, proteomics, molecular and cellular biology, materials science, and bioengineering have supported this growing discipline, which focuses on physiological processes at the nanoscale. Most cellular internal operations naturally occur at the nanoscale, since various physiologically significant components, such as water, glucose, proteins, enzymes, receptors, haemoglobin, and antibodies, already have sizes within the nanoscale range. Many researchers are currently employing nanotechnology to enhance medical processes, equipment, and gadgets in terms of sensitivity, safety, efficacy, and customisation. Nanotherapeutics may deliver benefits, including enhanced solubility, greater dose responsiveness, reduced toxicity, and improved absorption, compared with standard drugs [6]. Another major area of scientific interest is the production of magnetic nanoparticles (NPs) for the targeted delivery of diverse pharmacological or diagnostic chemicals.

The potential for detecting magnetic nanoparticles (NPs) via MRI and correlating the results with post-therapy histology has generated significant interest in magnetic NP targeting applications. Polymer/SPIO composites are the most commonly employed NPs for theranostics (diagnostics). The backbone of a polymer/IO conjugate may incorporate a number of anticancer drugs. The drugs may combine to perhaps boost efficacy by releasing at the tumour location. As SPIO NPs emit heat when exposed to an alternating magnetic field, external electromagnetic fields can also be used to remotely activate them for thermal ablation therapy [7].

TYPES OF NANOCARRIERS

Liposomes

In recent years, a lot of studies have focused on liposomes for the controlled delivery of medications. Liposomes are frequently stable owing to their biodegradable nature [8]. The inner core of the liposome holds the medicines. Liposomes may be used in a range of therapeutic applications due to their low toxicity, biodegradability, biocompatibility, and ability to encapsulate both hydrophilic and hydrophobic drugs. Liposomes were engineered to carry CD147 antibodies, a polyclonal antibody highly expressed in liver cancer cell lines and HCC tissues. Using CD147 as the target, a novel liposome-based carrier was developed to deliver doxorubicin. The results demonstrated that this nanocarrier exhibited enhanced cytotoxic effects in the HCC3736 model, as well as in Huh-7 and HepG2 cells [9].

The anticancer potential of hepatoblastoma (HB) against HepG2 cells was investigated using butyric acid (BA)-loaded chitosan-coated and uncoated liposomes. It was observed that the cytotoxic impact of chitosan-coated liposomes loaded with BA was greater than that of both free BA and uncoated liposomes. The experimental data indicated that sorafenib-loaded liposomes enhanced biocompatibility, reduced biotoxicity, and increased anti-tumour activity compared with free sorafenib. The study suggests that liposomes offer a novel, acceptable therapeutic approach as nanocarriers to extend the duration of HCC therapy.

Polymer Nanoparticles

The drug-loading efficiency, bioavailability, and targeted delivery of polymeric nanoparticles are inferior to those of traditional delivery vectors [10]. However, the gap between what state-of-the-art laboratories can synthesize and what can be produced cost-effectively remains the primary reason polymeric nanoparticles have not been widely adopted in clinical practice. Despite this, their remarkable functional versatility, adaptability, and ability to deliver a broad range of therapeutics make polymeric nanoparticles one of the most promising non-lipi--based drug delivery platforms [11].

Solid Lipid Nanoparticles

Scientists are developing SLNs as an alternative, spherical colloidal carrier for drug delivery and release. SLNs have an average size of 150–300 nm and are composed of around 0.1–30 (% w/w) solid fat; but, depending on the surfactant used in synthesis, they may be larger than 1000 nm [12]. The size and solid-t--liquid fat ratio of SLNs affect their drug-loading capacity, long-term stability, and drug-release characteristics. A substantial drug load capacity, the ability to load hydrophilic or lipophilic therapeutic medications, and little to no adverse effects on healthy tissue are just a few of the many desirable properties that SLNs provide, as was previously mentioned. Furthermore, they are easy to produce in large numbers. Oral administration of medication is the most common use of SLNs as nanocarriers.

Dendrimers

Dendrimers are hyper-branched, nanoscale polymeric structures with a pronounced tree-like form. They have a lot of promise for medication administration because of their internal canals and high degree of surface functioning, but their toxicity has been a major concern [13]. The toxicity of dendrimers is strongly influenced by their size, synthesis, and surface charge. Cationic dendrimers, particularly those with amine-terminal groups, such as polyamidoamine (PAMAM), are known to be cytotoxic due to their interactions with cell membranes, leading to membrane rupture, oxidative stress, and mitochondrial damage [14]. Hemolysis and immunogenicity have also been reported. Their toxicity may be reduced and their biocompatibility increased by surface modification with neutral or anionic moieties, such as acetylation or PEGylation.

Carbon-based Nanocarriers (*e.g.*, Carbon Nanotubes, Graphene Oxide)

Due to their high surface area, mechanical robustness, and ease of functionalization, carbon-based nanocarriers, such as graphene oxide (GO) and carbon nanotubes (CNTs), are increasingly used in nanomedicine [15]. However, there are still concerns about their safety. The toxicity of CNTs is influenced by their size, length, surface chemistry, and degree of aggregation. It has been shown that pristine CNTs, particularly when inhaled, induce inflammation, oxidative stress, and granuloma formation. Graphene oxide's reactive oxygen species (ROS) have the potential to damage DNA and induce apoptosis. Functionalization may reduce some of the adverse effects of these nanomaterials; however, environmental impacts and long-term accumulation remain concerns. Inconsistent results from *in vivo* studies highlight the need for comprehensive toxicological evaluations prior to clinical translation.

Metallic Nanoparticles (*e.g.*, Gold, Silver)

Metallic nanoparticles are metallic entities measuring 1–100 nm in length, breadth, and thickness. They may be used in medical and biotechnology applications, as well as for delivering medications and genes [16]. These metallic nanoparticles may readily associate with peptides, antibodies, and DNA/RNA to target specific cells. By conjugating with biocompatible polymers, such as polyethylene glycol, they may also be enlarged *in vivo* for medical and gene-delivery applications. Furthermore, their ability to convert light into heat enables the thermal ablation of specific cancer cells. The different types of nanocarriers are shown in Fig. (**1**).

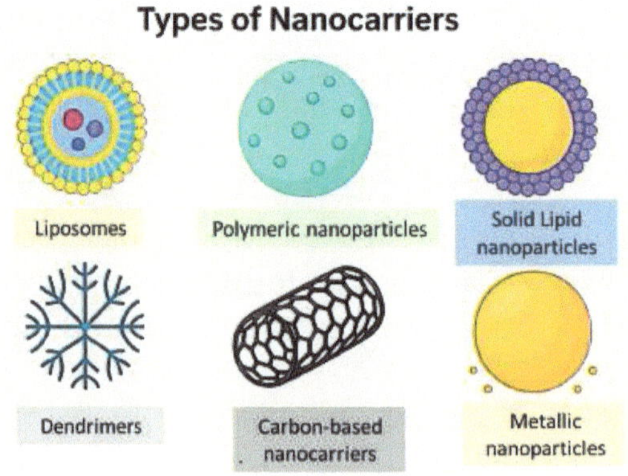

Fig. (1). Types of nanocarriers.

MECHANISMS OF NANOCARRIER TOXICITY

The toxicity of nanocarriers arises from a variety of interrelated mechanisms that are influenced by their physicochemical properties, biological interactions, and exposure routes. The generation of reactive oxygen species (ROS), which results in oxidative stress, inflammation, cellular damage, and even necrosis or apoptosis, is one of the primary pathways [17, 18]. Nanocarriers, especially metallic nanoparticles and carbon-based chemicals, may disrupt mitochondrial function, impede cellular respiration, and cause oxidative stress that damages DNA. Another crucial technique is membrane disruption, particularly by cationic nanoparticles like dendrimers. Through electrostatic interactions, these particles can disrupt cell membranes, increase permeability, cause ion imbalance, and eventually lead to cell lysis. Furthermore, because some nanoparticles can induce immunotoxic effects by activating the complement system or releasing cytokines, immunological activation is a significant concern. Low biodegradability and bioaccumulation may lead to chronic toxicity, as some nanocarriers can have long-term detrimental effects and accumulate in organs, including the liver, spleen, and lungs. The surface charge, size, and hydrophobicity of nanoparticles largely dictate their toxicity profiles; these factors also affect how the body absorbs, distributes, metabolizes, and excretes them [19].

IN VITRO AND *IN VIVO* TOXICITY EVALUATION

Studies on blood interactions and hemocompatibility assess the effects of nanomaterials on blood, while *in vitro* experiments evaluate cell viability (Table **1**). Animal models are employed to measure acute and chronic toxicity. Additional research focuses on biodistribution, clearance, and histopathology to determine the safety, accumulation, elimination, and tissue-level effects of nanoparticles.

Table 1. Comprehensive toxicity evaluation method.

Toxicity Evaluation	Method	Details	Ref.
***In Vitro* Cytotoxicity Assays**	MTT, LDH, Trypan Blue	Used to measure cell viability and membrane integrity in response to nanoparticle exposure.	[20]
Hemocompatibility Studies	Hemolysis, Coagulation (PT, aPTT), Platelet Aggregation	Assesses impact on red blood cells, coagulation cascade, and platelet function.	[21]

(Table 1) cont.....

Toxicity Evaluation	Method	Details	Ref.
Blood Interaction Studies	Complement Activation (CH50, C3a, SC5b-9)	Detects potential immune response through activation of complement proteins.	[22]
Animal Models: Acute Toxicity	Single high-dose exposure	Observes short-term toxicological effects and organ responses.	[23]
Animal Models: Chronic Toxicity	Repeated low-dose exposure over time	Evaluates long-term safety, systemic accumulation, and delayed effects.	[24]
Biodistribution Studies	Radiolabeling, Fluorescent Tracking, ICP-MS	Tracks nanoparticle distribution and clearance in major organs.	[25]
Clearance Studies	Renal (urine) *vs* Hepatic (bile, feces) Elimination	Determines excretion routes and elimination half-life of nanoparticles.	[26]
Histopathological Analysis	Tissue staining and microscopic examination	Identifies microscopic tissue damage or inflammation post-exposure.	[27]

IMPACT OF SURFACE ON NANOPARTICLE PROPERTIES

The surface features of nanoparticles have a substantial influence on their physicochemical and biological behaviour, as well as on their effectiveness in drug delivery applications [28]. The physicochemical features of nanoparticles, such as particle size, surface charge, hydrophobicity, and the presence of functional groups, may influence their stability, solubility, dispersibility, drug release rate, and toxicity.

Particle Size and Surface Charge

The size and surface charge of nanoparticles significantly influence their physicochemical and biological properties. Among the essential properties affected by particle size are stability, biodistribution, and cellular uptake of nanoparticles [29]. The capacity of tiny nanoparticles, generally in the 10–100 nm range, to enter tissues more effectively and to be less likely to be recognized and destroyed by the reticuloendothelial system (RES) may allow for longer circulation times and greater accumulation in target areas. However, due to their rapid renal clearance, tiny nanoparticles (<10 nm) may not be very effective. However, the manner in which nanoparticles interact with proteins and biological membranes is dictated by their surface charge. Positively charged nanoparticles often exhibit greater cellular uptake due to electrostatic attraction to negatively charged cell membranes; however, opsonisation and RES uptake may also render them dangerous and rapidly eliminated from the circulation. Neutral or negatively charged nanoparticles may exhibit longer circulation times but reduced cellular uptake, as they generally have lower clearance rates and decreased protein adsorption.

Hydrophobicity

Hydrophobic surfaces tend to aggregate in aqueous environments to minimize contact with water molecules, whereas hydrophilic surfaces generally exhibit greater dispersion [30]. This aggregation can result in poor dispersion and reduced stability in biological fluids, potentially hindering circulation and delivery to target sites. Hydrophobicity is a key factor influencing nanoparticle interactions with biological membranes and proteins. Hydrophobic surfaces may enhance plasma protein adsorption, leading to opsonization and subsequent clearance by the reticuloendothelial system (RES), thereby reducing therapeutic efficacy and shortening circulation time [31]. However, hydrophobic nanoparticles are also well-suited for encapsulating and delivering hydrophobic drugs.

Regulatory and Ethical Considerations

Throughout research and implementation, the safety and ethical concerns raised by nano-based drug delivery systems should be closely considered.

• ***Implications for Ethics***

Concerns over unknown risks and potential effects on human health and the environment are heightened by the growing use of nanotechnology in drug delivery [32]. Strict regulatory oversight is necessary to assess risks and benefits, strike a balance between safety and creativity, and address ethical quandaries. Ethical issues pertaining to accessibility and cost arise when ensuring that all socioeconomic groups have equal access to nanomedicines.

• ***Safety Concerns***

In-depth safety evaluations are essential because different nanoparticles may exhibit different toxicological characteristics. Reducing harmful effects requires an understanding of how nanoparticles bioaccumulate and spread throughout the body [33]. Nanomaterials' immunogenic potential must be assessed, as they may elicit allergic or immunological responses.

• ***Effect on the Environment***

Concerns with ecological safety arise from the potential impact on the environment and the disposal of items based on nanotechnology [34]. Formulations based on nanocarriers must be well researched, risk-managed, and manufactured responsibly in order to reduce potential risks and ensure their safety.

• ***Analysing and Assessing Risks***

There is a need to conduct thorough *in vitro* and *in vivo* toxicity studies to identify the likely disadvantages of nanomaterials [35] and to examine the fate of nanocarriers to determine how they spread and most likely accumulate in the body.

• ***Optimisations of Formulation and Materials***

To reduce the risk of negative consequences, it is necessary to prioritize the use of harmless, biocompatible nanomaterials. Additionally, nanocarrier surfaces may be altered to decrease immunogenicity and improve biocompatibility [36]. For a thorough evaluation and approval of nanotechnology-based formulations, regulatory laws and regulations must be adhered to. Risk management plans should be created to address any identified risks and dangers.

• ***Social and Moral Factors***

Encouraging open discussion of the benefits, drawbacks, and unknowns of formulations based on nanotechnology is essential [37]. Stakeholders, such as the general public, legislators, and medical experts, should be involved in discussions on the safety and implications of nanotechnology.

STRATEGIES TO IMPROVE SAFETY

Lipid-based nanocarriers, which securely transport drugs and break down after delivering their payload, are used to reduce systemic toxicity. Combining lipids and polymers may create mixed systems that improve the safety, security, and delivery of pharmaceuticals [38]. Surface coatings, such as polyethylene glycol (PEGylation) or biodegradable polymers, confer nanocarriers a "stealth" effect that enhances immunological detection and prolongs their half-life in circulation [39]. Specialised ligands or biomimetic coatings, such as cell membranes, may be added to functionalised surfaces to improve targeting and further restrict the immune response. To boost drug accumulation in disease regions and limit exposure to healthy organs, targeting components (peptides, antibodies) can be added to nanocarriers and directed to specific cells or tissues. It has been established that this tailored strategy decreases adverse effects while allowing higher, more effective drug dosages.

CASE STUDIES AND CLINICAL TRANSLATION

Although nanocarrier-based treatments significantly enhance the delivery of customised medications, a thorough assessment of the risks and safety issues is necessary before their use in humans [36]. The toxicity of several nanocarrier systems, including carbon-based materials, quantum dots, liposomes, polymeric nanoparticles, dendrimers, and metallic nanoparticles, is determined by their physicochemical properties, structure, and biological interactions. Despite being widely used because they pose no risks, liposomes may cause haemolysis, activate the immune system, or accumulate in the liver. To lessen these effects, the right PEGylation and fat-reduction strategies must be identified. As PLGA and other biodegradable polymer-based polymeric nanoparticles may leak hazardous liquids or monomers, special cleaning techniques are necessary. Adding PEG or neutral groups to the surface of dendrimers may significantly reduce the risks, even if their charge remains dangerous, particularly if it is cationic. Functionalisation improves their safety and spreadability when compared to other carbon-based carriers, such as graphene and carbon nanotubes. The need for surface coverage and dosage control is highlighted by the potential for dose-dependent damage and the production of reactive oxygen species (ROS) from metallic nanoparticles, such as gold and silver [40]. However, mesoporous silica nanoparticles, in particular, have the potential to cause lung inflammation. If their biodegradability is thoroughly studied, they may show promise. Table **2** summarizes various nanocarrier types, their potential toxicities, and the strategies employed to mitigate these effects.

Table 2. Nanocarrier types, associated toxicities, and key safety considerations.

Nanocarrier Type	Potential Toxicity	Safety Considerations	Ref.
Liposomes	Hemolysis, complement activation, liver accumulation	Use of PEGylation to reduce immune response; optimize lipid composition	[41]
Polymeric nanoparticles	Cytotoxicity from residual monomers or solvents	Purification techniques; use biocompatible polymers like PLGA	[42]
Dendrimers	Charge-dependent toxicity (especially cationic types)	Surface modification with PEG or neutral groups to reduce cytotoxicity	[43]
Carbon-based nanocarriers (*e.g.*, CNTs, graphene)	Oxidative stress, inflammation, genotoxicity	Functionalization to improve dispersion and reduce toxicity	[44]
Metallic nanoparticles (*e.g.*, Au, Ag, Fe)	Dose-dependent cytotoxicity, ROS generation	Surface coating, dose optimization, and long-term clearance studies	[45]
Silica nanoparticles	Lung inflammation, oxidative damage	Use of mesoporous silica; thorough evaluation of biodegradability	[46]
Quantum dots	Heavy metal toxicity	Use of non-toxic core materials, encapsulation strategies	[47]

FUTURE DIRECTIONS AND CHALLENGES

Developing nanocarrier-based formulations for clinical translation requires addressing issues, such as toxicity, scalability, and regulatory constraints [36]. Formulation processes are streamlined, scalable manufacturing techniques are used, and repeatability is maintained without compromising nanocarrier quality and characteristics to address scaling issues. Before clinical translation, comprehensive toxicity evaluations are conducted to ensure safety profiles using surface changes, biocompatible materials, and *in vitro* and *in vivo* models [48]. The European Medicines Agency (EMA) and the Food and Drug Administration (FDA) have established regulatory standards that must be adhered to in order to meet regulatory criteria for consistent manufacturing and the completion of toxicological studies [49]. To address immune response issues, nanocarriers are designed to be less immunogenic and biocompatible, and to undergo rigorous preclinical testing to ensure safety and effectiveness. Since nanocarriers are designed to remain stable over an extended period, stability testing under various conditions is conducted to determine shelf life and ensure consistent performance. To ensure the safe and effective transition of nanocarrier-based formulations from bench to bedside, a multidisciplinary approach integrating material research, pharmaceutical development, and regulatory compliance is required. Nanocarrier-based formulations have great promise for novel discoveries across many medical specialties. By delivering medications in a targeted manner, nanocarriers reduce systemic toxicity and enhance therapeutic efficacy in the fight against cancer [50].

CONCLUSION

Formulations based on nanocarriers hold tremendous potential for more specialised and efficient therapeutic interventions in a number of medical sectors. However, if their clinical translation and financial sustainability are to succeed, numerous issues must be solved. Scalability, stability, biocompatibility, reduced toxicity, regulatory considerations, and addressing safety and ethical issues are among the key hurdles. A multidisciplinary approach involving materials research, drug development, and regulatory compliance is required to address these challenges. Future methodologies offer opportunities for discoveries by highlighting the projected advantages of nanocarrier-based formulations for ocular pharmaceutical delivery, neurological diseases, infectious illnesses, regenerative medicine, diagnostic imaging, and cancer treatment. Notable breakthroughs in clinical trials and the regulatory approval of some nanobased medications, such as liposomal doxorubicin and albumin-bound paclitaxel, imply that these technologies may find usage beyond the laboratory. It is vital to conduct detailed risk assessments, optimise materials, adhere to regulations, examine ethical considerations, monitor continuously, and pursue breakthrough research to reduce potential hazards and ensure the safe and ethical development of nanocarrier-based formulations. The successful translation and application of nanocarrier-based formulations in clinical settings will depend on overcoming obstacles and implementing practical measures, such as interdisciplinary collaborations, regulatory standardisation, personalised medicine approaches, and technological advancements.

LIST OF ABBREVIATIONS

- **NPs** Nanoparticles
- **NP** Nanoparticle
- **ROS** Reactive Oxygen Species
- **MRI** Magnetic Resonance Imaging
- **SPIO** Superparamagnetic Iron Oxide
- **IO** Iron Oxide
- **HB** Hepatoblastoma
- **BA** Butyric Acid
- **HCC** Hepatocellular Carcinoma
- **PEG** Polyethylene Glycol
- **PEGylation** Surface modification with Polyethylene Glycol
- **PAMAM** Polyamidoamine
- **GO** Graphene Oxide
- **CNTs** Carbon Nanotubes
- **Au** Gold
- **Ag** Silver
- **Fe** Iron
- **PLGA** Poly(lactic-co-glycolic acid)
- **RES** Reticuloendothelial System
- **ICP-MS** Inductively Coupled Plasma Mass Spectrometry
- **PT** Prothrombin Time
- **aPTT** Activated Partial Thromboplastin Time
- **CH50** Total Complement Hemolytic Activity
- **C3a** Complement Component 3a
- **SC5b-9** Soluble Membrane Attack Complex

REFERENCES

[1] Boisseau P, Loubaton B. Nanomedicine, nanotechnology in medicine. C R Phys 2011; 12(7): 620-36. [http://dx.doi.org/10.1016/j.crhy.2011.06.001]

[2] Fornaguera C, García-Celma M. Personalized nanomedicine: a revolution at the nanoscale. J Pers Med 2017; 7(4): 12.
[http://dx.doi.org/10.3390/jpm7040012] [PMID: 29023366]

[3] Davies JC. Nanotechnology oversight. Washington, DC: Project on Emerging Nanotechnologies 2008.

[4] Alrushaid N, Khan FA, Al-Suhaimi EA, Elaissari A. Nanotechnology in cancer diagnosis and treatment. Pharmaceutics 2023; 15(3): 1025.
[http://dx.doi.org/10.3390/pharmaceutics15031025] [PMID: 36986885]

[5] Oberdörster G. Safety assessment for nanotechnology and nanomedicine: concepts of nanotoxicology. J Intern Med 2010; 267(1): 89-105.
[http://dx.doi.org/10.1111/j.1365-2796.2009.02187.x] [PMID: 20059646]

[6] Malik S, Muhammad K, Waheed Y. Emerging applications of nanotechnology in healthcare and medicine. Molecules 2023; 28(18): 6624.
[http://dx.doi.org/10.3390/molecules28186624] [PMID: 37764400]

[7] Ashikbayeva Z, Tosi D, Balmassov D, Schena E, Saccomandi P, Inglezakis V. Application of nanoparticles and nanomaterials in thermal ablation therapy of cancer. Nanomaterials (Basel) 2019; 9(9): 1195.
[http://dx.doi.org/10.3390/nano9091195] [PMID: 31450616]

[8] Torchilin VP. Recent advances with liposomes as pharmaceutical carriers. Nat Rev Drug Discov 2005; 4(2): 145-60.
[http://dx.doi.org/10.1038/nrd1632] [PMID: 15688077]

[9] Kiranmayi P, Soumya V, Malla RR. Theranostics application of nanocarriers in hepatocellular carcinoma Theranostics and Precision Medicine for the Management of Hepatocellular Carcinoma. Elsevier 2022; Vol. 3: pp. 15-27.
[http://dx.doi.org/10.1016/B978-0-323-99283-1.00017-3]

[10] Castro KC, Costa JM, Campos MGN. Drug-loaded polymeric nanoparticles: a review. Int J Polym Mater 2022; 71(1): 1-13.
[http://dx.doi.org/10.1080/00914037.2020.1798436]

[11] Sork H. Profiling and exploiting lipid-based nanoparticles *in vitro* and *in vivo*. Stockholm: Karolinska Institutet 2018. Available from: https://hdl.handle.net/10616/46369

[12] Hernández-Esquivel R-A, Navarro-Tovar G, Zárate-Hernández E, Aguirre-Bañuelos P. Solid lipid nanoparticles (SLN). In: Nanocomposite materials for biomedical and energy storage applications. London: IntechOpen; 2022.

[13] Irfan M, Saeed A, Akram S, Yameen S. Dendrimers chemistry and applications: a short review. Frontiers in Chemical Sciences 2020; 1(1): 29-40.
[http://dx.doi.org/10.52700/fcs.v1i1.6]

[14] Janaszewska A, Lazniewska J, Trzepiński P, Marcinkowska M, Klajnert-Maculewicz B. Cytotoxicity of dendrimers. Biomolecules 2019; 9: 330.
[http://dx.doi.org/10.3390/biom9080330] [PMID: 31374911]

[15] Patel KD, Singh RK, Kim HW. Carbon-based nanomaterials as an emerging platform for theranostics. Mater Horiz 2019; 6(3): 434-69.
[http://dx.doi.org/10.1039/C8MH00966J]

[16] Kumar H, Venkatesh N, Bhowmik H, Kuila A. Metallic nanoparticle: a review. Biomed J Sci Tech Res 2018; 4(2): 3765-75.

[17] Egbuna C, Parmar VK, Jeevanandam J, *et al.* Toxicity of nanoparticles in biomedical application: nanotoxicology. J Toxicol 2021; 2021(1): 1-21.
[http://dx.doi.org/10.1155/2021/9954443] [PMID: 34422042]

[18] Vega-Villa KR, Takemoto JK, Yáñez JA, Remsberg CM, Forrest ML, Davies NM. Clinical toxicities

of nanocarrier systems. Adv Drug Deliv Rev 2008; 60(8): 929-38.
[http://dx.doi.org/10.1016/j.addr.2007.11.007] [PMID: 18313790]

[19] Saker R, Regdon G Jr, Sovány T. Pharmacokinetics and toxicity of inorganic nanoparticles and the physicochemical properties/factors affecting them. J Drug Deliv Sci Technol 2024; 99: 105979.
[http://dx.doi.org/10.1016/j.jddst.2024.105979]

[20] Mani S, Swargiary G. *In vitro* cytotoxicity analysis: MTT/XTT, trypan blue exclusion. Animal Cell Culture: Principles and Practice Techniques in Life Science and Biomedicine for the Non-Expert. Cham: Springer 2023; pp. 267-84.
[http://dx.doi.org/10.1007/978-3-031-19485-6_18]

[21] Bhatt A, Nair RP, Rashmi R, Raju R, Geeverghese R, Lekshmi P. Product evaluation: blood compatibility studies. Biomedical Product and Materials Evaluation: Standards and Ethics. Cambridge: Woodhead Publishing 2022; pp. 435-59.
[http://dx.doi.org/10.1016/B978-0-12-823966-7.00022-0]

[22] Harboe M, Thorgersen EB, Mollnes TE. Advances in assay of complement function and activation. Adv Drug Deliv Rev 2011; 63(12): 976-87.
[http://dx.doi.org/10.1016/j.addr.2011.05.010] [PMID: 21664392]

[23] Keller KA, Banks C. Multidose general toxicology studies. Toxicological Testing Handbook: Principles, Applications, and Data Interpretation. Informa Healthcare 2006.

[24] Rhomberg LR, Baetcke K, Blancato J, *et al.* Issues in the design and interpretation of chronic toxicity and carcinogenicity studies in rodents: approaches to dose selection. Crit Rev Toxicol 2007; 37(9): 729-837.
[http://dx.doi.org/10.1080/10408440701524949] [PMID: 17957539]

[25] Skotland T, Iversen TG, Llorente A, Sandvig K. Biodistribution, pharmacokinetics and excretion studies of intravenously injected nanoparticles and extracellular vesicles: Possibilities and challenges. Adv Drug Deliv Rev 2022; 186: 114326.
[http://dx.doi.org/10.1016/j.addr.2022.114326] [PMID: 35588953]

[26] Zhao Y, Sultan D, Liu Y. Biodistribution, excretion, and toxicity of nanoparticles. Theranostic Bionanomaterials. Cambridge: Elsevier 2019; pp. 27-53.
[http://dx.doi.org/10.1016/B978-0-12-815341-3.00002-X]

[27] Poole JA, Gaurav R, Schwab A, *et al.* Post-endotoxin exposure-induced lung inflammation and resolution consequences beneficially impacted by lung-delivered IL-10 therapy. Sci Rep 2022; 12(1): 17338.
[http://dx.doi.org/10.1038/s41598-022-22346-2] [PMID: 36243830]

[28] Yusuf A, Almotairy ARZ, Henidi H, Alshehri OY, Aldughaim MS. Nanoparticles as drug delivery systems: a review of the implication of nanoparticles' physicochemical properties on responses in biological systems. Polymers (Basel) 2023; 15(7): 1596.
[http://dx.doi.org/10.3390/polym15071596] [PMID: 37050210]

[29] He C, Hu Y, Yin L, Tang C, Yin C. Effects of particle size and surface charge on cellular uptake and biodistribution of polymeric nanoparticles. Biomaterials 2010; 31(13): 3657-66.
[http://dx.doi.org/10.1016/j.biomaterials.2010.01.065] [PMID: 20138662]

[30] van Oss CJ. Hydrophobicity and hydrophilicity of biosurfaces. Curr Opin Colloid Interface Sci 1997; 2(5): 503-12.
[http://dx.doi.org/10.1016/S1359-0294(97)80099-4]

[31] Karmali PP, Simberg D. Interactions of nanoparticles with plasma proteins: implication on clearance and toxicity of drug delivery systems. Expert Opin Drug Deliv 2011; 8(3): 343-57.
[http://dx.doi.org/10.1517/17425247.2011.554818] [PMID: 21291354]

[32] Allhoff F, Lin P. Nanotechnology & society: Current and emerging ethical issues. Springer 2009.
[http://dx.doi.org/10.1007/978-1-4020-6209-4]

[33] Subhan MA, Subhan T, Choudhury KP, Neogi N. Safety measures, regulations, ethical, and legal issues for nanomaterials Handbook of Nanomaterials. Elsevier 2024; Vol. 2: pp. 791-828.

[34] Inbathamizh L, Harsha Varthan M, Kumar RR, Rohinth M, Tawfeeq Ahmed Z. Nanotechnology: ethical impacts, health issues, and safety issues. Modern Nanotechnology: Volume 2: Green Synthesis Sustainable Energy and Impacts. Cham: Springer 2023; pp. 455-77.

[35] Park MVDZ, Lankveld DPK, van Loveren H, de Jong WH. The status of in vitro toxicity studies in the risk assessment of nanomaterials. Nanomedicine (Lond) 2009; 4(6): 669-85. [http://dx.doi.org/10.2217/nnm.09.40] [PMID: 19663595]

[36] Kardani SL. Nanocarrier-based formulations: Regulatory Challenges, Ethical and Safety Considerations in Pharmaceuticals. Asian J Pharm 2024; 18(2) [http://dx.doi.org/10.22377/ajp.v18i02.5444]

[37] Verma V, Gupta P, Singh P, Pandey NK. Considerations in the development and deployment of nanotechnology. Nanotechnology in Societal Development. Cham: Springer 2024; pp. 505-40. [http://dx.doi.org/10.1007/978-981-97-6184-5_15]

[38] Lim SB, Banerjee A, Önyüksel H. Improvement of drug safety by the use of lipid-based nanocarriers. J Control Release 2012; 163(1): 34-45. [http://dx.doi.org/10.1016/j.jconrel.2012.06.002] [PMID: 22698939]

[39] Fam SY, Chee CF, Yong CY, Ho KL, Mariatulqabtiah AR, Tan WS. Stealth coating of nanoparticles in drug-delivery systems. Nanomaterials (Basel) 2020; 10(4): 787. [http://dx.doi.org/10.3390/nano10040787] [PMID: 32325941]

[40] Ur Rahim H, Qaswar M, Uddin M, Giannini C, Herrera ML, Rea G. Nano-enable materials promoting sustainability and resilience in modern agriculture. Nanomaterials (Basel) 2021; 11(8): 2068. [http://dx.doi.org/10.3390/nano11082068] [PMID: 34443899]

[41] Mohamed M, Alaaeldin E, Hussein A, Sarhan HA. Liposomes and PEGylated liposomes as drug delivery system. J Adv Biomed Pharm Sci 2020; 3(2): 80-8.

[42] Sharma S, Parmar A, Kori S, Sandhir R. PLGA-based nanoparticles: A new paradigm in biomedical applications. Trends Analyt Chem 2016; 80: 30-40. [http://dx.doi.org/10.1016/j.trac.2015.06.014]

[43] Zeng Y, Kurokawa Y, Win-Shwe TT, *et al.* Effects of PAMAM dendrimers with various surface functional groups and multiple generations on cytotoxicity and neuronal differentiation using human neural progenitor cells. J Toxicol Sci 2016; 41(3): 351-70. [http://dx.doi.org/10.2131/jts.41.351] [PMID: 27193728]

[44] Díez-Pascual AM. Carbon-based nanomaterials. Int J Mol Sci 2021; 22: 7726. [http://dx.doi.org/10.3390/ijms22147726]

[45] Lin Z, Monteiro-Riviere NA, Riviere JE. Pharmacokinetics of metallic nanoparticles. Wiley Interdiscip Rev Nanomed Nanobiotechnol 2015; 7(2): 189-217. [http://dx.doi.org/10.1002/wnan.1304] [PMID: 25316649]

[46] Sahu D, Vijayaraghavan R, Kannan GM. Silica nanoparticle induces oxidative stress and provokes inflammation in human lung cells. J Exp Nanosci 2015; 10(13): 983-1000. [http://dx.doi.org/10.1080/17458080.2014.951409]

[47] Zhu C, Chen Z, Gao S, *et al.* Recent advances in non-toxic quantum dots and their biomedical applications. Prog Nat Sci 2019; 29(6): 628-40. [http://dx.doi.org/10.1016/j.pnsc.2019.11.007]

[48] Dobrovolskaia MA. Pre-clinical immunotoxicity studies of nanotechnology-formulated drugs: Challenges, considerations and strategy. J Control Release 2015; 220(Pt B): 571-83. [http://dx.doi.org/10.1016/j.jconrel.2015.08.056] [PMID: 26348388]

[49] Bode G. Regulatory guidance: ICH, EMA, FDA. In: Drug Discovery and Evaluation: Methods in

Clinical Pharmacology. 2nd ed. Berlin: Springer; 2020. p. 1085□1138.

[50] Sohail M, Guo W, Li Z, *et al.* Nanocarrier-based drug delivery system for cancer therapeutics: a review of the last decade. Curr Med Chem 2021; 28(19): 3753-72. [http://dx.doi.org/10.2174/1875533XMTEwbNDMs2] [PMID: 33019919]

CHAPTER 13

Case Studies: Nanocarriers Based Drug Delivery in Fatty Liver Disease

Rakesh Sindhu[1,*], **Gagandeep Kaur**[2] **Parul Sood**[2], **Soumya Banerjee**[2], **Nitin Jangra**[2] and **Aanandita Thakur**[2]

[1] *School of Pharmacy, Sharda University, Noida, Uttar Pradesh, India*

[2] *School of Pharmacy, Chitkara University, Solan, Himachal Pradesh, India*

Abstract: Non-alcoholic fatty liver disease (NAFLD) has become a global health concern due to its rising prevalence and its correlation with metabolic syndrome, diabetes, and cardiovascular disorders. Efficient drug delivery to the liver is a considerable challenge in managing fatty liver diseases due to the modified microenvironment and compromised liver function. Nanotechnology offers a viable approach for targeted medication delivery to the liver, which possesses distinct anatomical and physiological characteristics that make it an optimal target for nanomedicine. Various categories of nanomaterials, including inorganic nanomaterials, polymer nanomaterials, and multifunctional nanoparticles (NPs), have been investigated as potential agents for targeting this organ in the context of liver illnesses. Nanomedicine enhances internalization and penetration, thereby facilitating targeted drug delivery, combination therapy, and theranostics. Recent advancements in nanomedicine have led to efforts to integrate nanomaterials, including liposomes, polymer nanoparticles, micelles, and cocrystals, into pharmacotherapy for liver diseases. This integration significantly enhances drug solubility and targeting, thereby improving therapeutic efficacy and minimizing toxic side effects. This chapter explores a wide range of nanotechnology-based systems as potential innovative approaches for treating liver diseases, focusing on the different categories of nanocarriers, their advantages, and the challenges they pose.

Keywords: Non-alcoholic fatty liver, Nanocarriers, Nano-formulations, Nanotechnology.

INTRODUCTION

Non-alcoholic fatty liver disease (NAFLD) is more common than alcoholic fatty liver disease. It is characterized by deposition of excessive fat in the liver without

* **Corresponding author Pooja Mittal:** School of Pharmacy, Sharda University, Noida, Uttar Pradesh, India; E-mail: drrakeshsindhu@gmail.com

Anjali Sharma, Devkant Sharma, Ajmer Singh Grewal, Geeta Deswal & Ganga Reddy Velma (Eds.)

or with little consumption of alcohol by patients [1]. It is a multi-factorial progressive liver disease encompassing a range of multiple liver disease conditions, ranging from benign simple hepatic steatosis (grade 1) to non-alcoholic steatohepatitis with lobular inflammation (grade 2), having substantial potential to progress to liver fibrosis (grade 3) to liver cirrhosis, followed by liver carcinoma and finally liver failure [2]. Epidemiological studies have documented a 38% prevalence of NAFLD globally in 2019, which has been increasing rapidly [3, 4]. NAFLD is also referred to as metabolic dysfunction-associated steatosis liver disease (MDASLD), as it has been found to be associated with several metabolic disorders, including type-2 diabetes, insulin resistance, obesity, dyslipidemia, hypertension, and cardiovascular disorders [5 - 7]. The growing prevalence of NAFLD has led to a rise in hepatic-related mortality and the need for hepatic transplantation; therefore, there is an urgent demand for an effective and therapeutic strategy to manage this disease or prevent disease progression. Currently, management of NAFLD primarily involves liver modifications, insulin-sensitizing agents, lipid-lowering medications, and dietary interventions. However, many promising drugs have failed to demonstrate therapeutic efficacy in late-stage clinical trials due to limited liver concentrations [8]. In this chapter, we review recent case studies on nanocarrier-based drug delivery systems aimed at hepatocytes, Kupffer cells, hepatic stellate cells, and liver sinusoidal endothelial cells for the treatment of NAFLD. The development of several novel drug carriers, such as liposomes, nanoparticles, nanoemulsions, and micelles, for poorly water-soluble pharmaceuticals, intended to improve bioavailability and reduce adverse effects, has been enabled by the magnificent growth in the field of biomedical biotechnology [9, 10]. Fig. (**1**) provides a comprehensive overview of recent research investigating nanotechnology-based approaches for diagnosing and treating NAFLD. A wide range of nanotechnology-based formulations, including liposomes, nanogels, polymeric nanoparticles, niosomes, dendrimers, and nanosuspensions, as well as quantum dots, have been examined to explore their therapeutic role in NAFLD treatment [11, 12]. However, many ongoing clinical trials for NAFLD/NASH are still focused on small drug molecules, lifestyle interventions, or non-nanoparticle-based biologics [13], with only a limited number of clinical trials directly involving nanocarrier-based systems. For instance, a double-blind, randomized, placebo-controlled trial in overweight/obese NAFLD patients showed that nanocurcumin supplementation (40 mg twice daily for 3 months) significantly improved serum lipids, glucose indices, inflammatory markers, liver transaminases, nystatin levels, and the degree of liver steatosis compared to placebo [15]. Similarly, BMS-986263, a lipid nanoparticle formulation encapsulating siRNA targeting HSP47 (a collagen chaperone), has been assessed in a phase 2 clinical trial in patients with advanced hepatic fibrosis due to NAFLD and shows promise for ameliorating fibrosis [16]. Beyond these clinical studies, several preclinical studies employing *ex vivo*, *in vitro,* and *in vivo* disease models have provided invaluable insights into the development of nanocarrier systems for NAFLD treatment, which are discussed below.

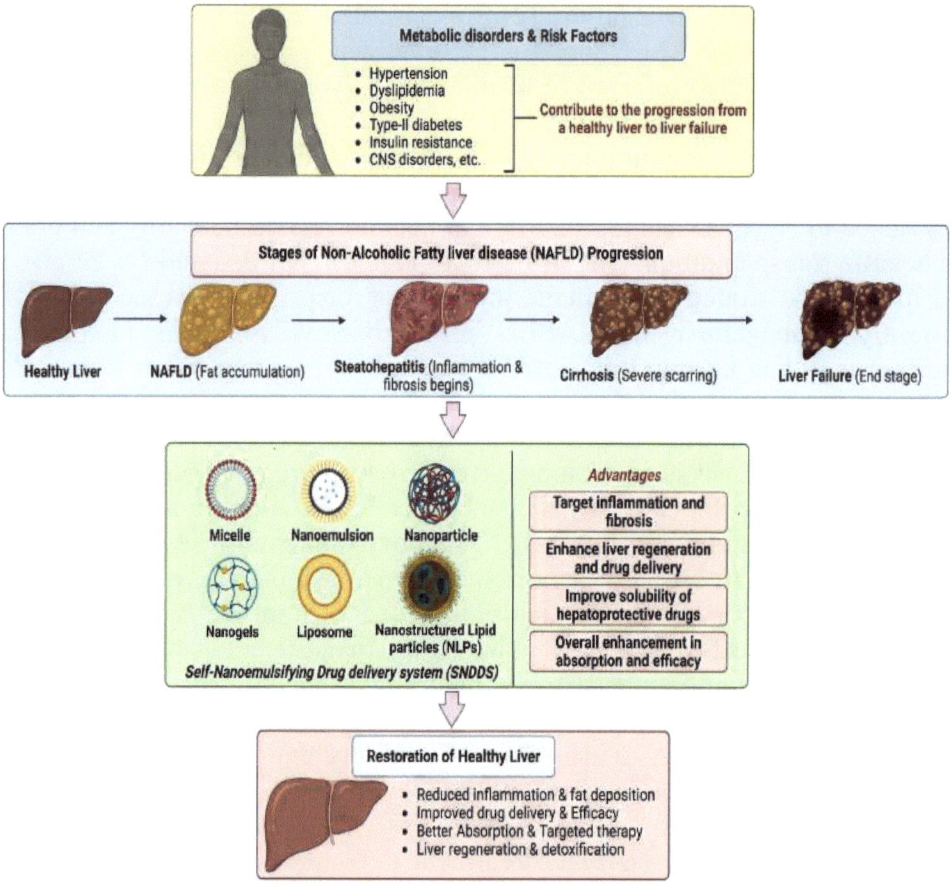

Fig. (1). Summary of various conditions of NAFLD and uses of nanocarriers for NAFLD treatment and diagnosis.

CASE STUDIES ON NANOCARRIER-BASED APPROACHES TO FATTY LIVER DISEASE

The section highlights various case studies on the application of nanocarriers for the management of fatty liver. These studies demonstrate the potential of nanocarrier systems in improving drug delivery, efficacy, and targeting in fatty liver disease.

Case Study 1

One of the chemical constituents of capsicum, capsaicin, helps protect the liver through its anti-swelling properties. This can also protect cells by eliminating harmful elements. However, several factors, such as reduced absorption, high aqueous insolubility, high cellular processing, high rate of metabolism, and restricted absorption in the alimentary tract, can create limitations on the use of capsaicin. There has been significant interest in lignin as a versatile material for pharmaceutical drug delivery devices due to its safety, eco-friendliness, and multifunctionality. As a key regulator of cell defense against harmful stimuli, it has demonstrated significant qualities, including the ability to remove harmful chemicals and regenerate hepatic tissue, which make it a suitable polymer for the development of delivery systems to treat symptoms of NAFLD. A combination of these compounds can effectively enhance the bioavailability and stability of capsaicin and its targeted delivery to hepatic cells. Encapsulation of capsaicin with the combination of lignin has emerged as a smart drug delivery perspective in the treatment of NAFLD. In laboratory research, capsaicin-encapsulated lignin nanoparticles can inhibit lipid formation [13].

Case Study 2

Multiple studies demonstrate that targeted deletion of Rubicon in hepatocytes significantly enhances autophagy, leading to a substantial decrease in liver steatosis and tissue damage. Nonetheless, direct siRNA administration faces hurdles due to its poor absorption, which is attributed to its substantial size and negative charge. A previous study demonstrated that encapsulating siRNA in phospholipid bilayer vesicles is a highly efficient and straightforward method for targeted cellular delivery. Consequently, hepatocyte-targeting RNA interference nanoliposomes demonstrate promise for the safe and effective treatment of NAFLD, as evidenced by autophagy activation, reduced liver fat accumulation, improved insulin sensitivity, and improved histopathological features in mice [14].

Case Study 3

The development of nonalcoholic steatohepatitis (NASH) depends on the inflammatory mediators interleukin-1β (IL-1β) and tumor necrosis factor (TNF), which are primarily secreted by hepatic macrophages. Intravenous exosomes are mostly endocytosed by hepatic macrophages and are mainly found in the liver. Antisense oligodeoxynucleotide for TNF (ASO-TNF) and 2-deoxy-D-glucose (2DG) significantly reduced the amounts of TNF and/or IL1β expression in macrophages. *In vitro* and *in vivo*, exosomes containing ASO-TNF or 2DG significantly suppress macrophage-mediated TNF and/or IL1β production.

Furthermore, treatment with Exo/ASO-TNF or Exo/2DG significantly decreased experimental steatohepatitis in mice fed methionine and choline-deficient (MCD) or choline-deficient amino acid-defined (CDAA) diets. RNA-seq analysis revealed that Exo/ASO-TNF or Exo/2DG therapy significantly downregulated inflammatory signaling processes. Consequently, the administration of drugs that inhibit hepatic swelling represents a promising therapeutic approach for the treatment of NASH [15].

Case Study 4

A hepatic-targeted vesicle system containing fucoxanthin (GA-LpEVs-FX) was successfully developed to target nonalcoholic fatty hepatic disorder. The formulation includes the self-assembly of extracellular vesicles derived from *Lactobacillus paracasei* (LpEVs), modification with glycyrrhetinic acid via an amide reaction to impart liver-targeting capabilities, and the integration of fucoxanthin (FX) via sonication. A laboratory-scale study found that this can help reduce fat deposition in the liver. It also mitigated reactive oxygen species, which are directly linked to lipid deposition ($p<0.05$) [16].

Case Study 5

A nanoscale vesicular system plays a critical role in achieving efficient drug loading and enhances the therapeutic effects of ORI, which is highly effective in NAFLD. Recent studies have shown that it primarily inhibits lipid storage and reduces levels of low- and very-low-density lipoproteins. Notably, ORI/HP---CD/H9-HePC nanoparticles demonstrated targeted hepatic accumulation and improved therapeutic efficacy. This nanodrug delivery system provides a promising strategy for encapsulating ORI to effectively mitigate the progression of NAFLD [17].

Case Study 6

Bile acids and fatty acids can be used to form Lovastatin-loaded nanoemulsions via manual mixing, thereby enhancing the drug's efficacy against NAFLD. In the non-aqueous phase, garlic and ginger oils play a key role in the formulation. Ursodeoxycholic acid and essential fatty acids, such as linoleic acid, act as targeted functional groups. Ex vivo studies of BA/FA-integrated nanoemulsions in isolated rat intestines demonstrated enhanced flux compared to non-integrated formulations. Liver histology, together with in vivo lipid profiles and liver function tests, indicated that these nanoemulsions have therapeutic potential as effective pharmaceutical carriers for NAFLD [18].

Case Study 7

Although graphene oxide can be effectively reduced by the natural and non-toxic molecule naringenin, Nar-RGO is more effective than crude naringenin at reducing the cytotoxicity of HFFD-induced NAFLD. It was employed as a reducing agent in a straightforward experimental setup to create naringenin-reduced graphene oxide nanosheets (Nar-RGO). Electron microscopy (TEM and SEM) and zeta potential analysis were used to verify the incorporation of naringenin into graphene oxide. Compared to pure naringenin, reduced graphene oxide for naringenin encapsulation significantly increased oxidative stress, inflammatory markers, insulin resistance, and hepatic steatosis in HFFD-induced NAFLD. This study demonstrated that Nar-RGO has a significantly higher potency than free naringenin. Consequently, it can potentially be used to treat NAFLD caused by a high-fat, high-fructose diet (HFFD) [19].

Case Study 8

Silibinin (Sil), a naturally derived compound, has demonstrated significant therapeutic potential for NAFLD treatment and is widely used in the clinical management of hepatic disorders. Nevertheless, since Sil exhibits low bioavailability and poor absorption, further investigation is required to determine whether it is appropriate for the treatment of NAFLD. A study aimed to develop a Sil-loaded liposome (Sil-Lip) to address its pharmacokinetic elimination and improve its therapeutic potential on NAFLD. It also investigated the mechanisms underlying Sil-Lip action. It was created using the Bangham method. It was found that Sil-Lip plays a significant role in gastroprotection and enhances permeation and intestinal uptake. Laboratory testing on NAFLD models revealed that Sil-Lip was more effective than Sil alone in reducing lipid metabolic disorders, insulin resistance, and inflammation. Further mechanistic investigations showed that the positive effects of Sil-Lip were influenced by modifications in intrahepatic insulin resistance-related and nuclear factor-kappa B (NF-κB) signaling pathways, as well as alterations in the extrahepatic gut microbiota. Our results showed that Sil-Lip significantly improved the absorption rate of Sil and enhanced its beneficial effects on NAFLD by modulating liver insulin resistance pathways [20].

Case Study 9

Nanocarriers targeting hepatic parenchymal cells and mitochondria were made to deliver astaxanthin (AST) to hepatic tissue, therefore augmenting the efficacy of AST intervention. Hepatic parenchymal cells were targeted by conjugating galactose (Gal) to whey protein isolate (WPI) through the Maillard reaction, thereby selectively recognizing asialoglycoprotein receptors found solely in hepatocytes. The amidation reaction of triphenylphosphonium (TPP) with glycosylated whey protein isolate (WPI) enabled the formation of nanocarriers (AST@TPP-WPI-Gal) with dual targeting capabilities. The AST@TPP-WPI-Gal nanocarriers efficiently targeted mitochondria in steatotic HepG2 cells, demonstrating enhanced antioxidative and anti-adipogenic characteristics. The ability of AST@TPP-WPI-Gal to target hepatic tissue was validated using a NAFLD animal model, revealing that AST@TPP-WPI-Gal can modify dyslipidemia, protect hepatic function, and reduce hepatic lipid accumulation by 40% compared to free AST. AST@TPP-WPI-Gal has the potential to serve as a dual-targeting hepatic agent for nutritional management in NAFLD [21].

Case Study 10

The Lycopene formulation has shown efficacy in preventing insulin resistance and weight gain, two major risk factors associated with NAFLD. A distinct cohort of sixteen non-obese rats received therapy with or without Lip-Lyco, serving as a control group for comparison. The rats were fed a high-calorie diet, which increased the weight-to-height ratio and induced insulin resistance. The study demonstrated that Lip-Lyco has considerable therapeutic potential for mitigating NAFLD-related metabolic disturbances [22].

Case Study 11

Celastrol (CEL), a bioactive phytoconstituent derived from plant sources, has demonstrated significant anti-inflammatory and anti-obesity activity; however, its clinical use has been limited by inadequate oral bioavailability. To address this limitation, biodegradable albumin-based nanoparticles were designed to target hepatic delivery of CEL for treating NAFLD. CEL encapsulated within lactosylated bovine serum albumin (Lac-BSA) was combined with high-pressure homogenization to produce CEL-loaded Lac-BSA nanoparticles (CEL-Lac-BSA). CEL-Lac-BSA exhibited enhanced hepatocyte absorption and hepatic accumulation relative to free CEL, while also effectively reducing lipid accumulation, enhancing liver function, and increasing insulin sensitivity in a murine model of diet-induced NAFLD. Western blot analysis verified that CEL-Lac-BSA effectively increased the activation of AMP-activated kinase (AMPK) in mice suffering from NAFLD. Cumulatively, CEL-Lac-BSA has shown enhanced efficacy in the treatment of diet-induced NAFLD [23].

Case Study 12

A modern perspective on the treatment of swelling complexity is offered by ultrasmall copper-based nanoparticles, which mimic the properties of a bio-catalyst for the elimination of reactive oxygen species. The natural polyphenolic compound resveratrol has attracted significant interest due to its potent antioxidant activity in combating oxidative stress. Thus, the initial goal was set to treat NAFLD by combining these two medications. However, to achieve a synergistic effect, a stable and effective carrier had to be introduced because Res is poorly soluble in aqueous media and is readily metabolized in the gut. An improved method of treating NAFLD may be offered by liver-directed nanocarriers loaded with bioactive substances [24].

Case Study 13

By activating the PPARα receptor, Fenofibrate helps reduce the impact of NAFLD by increasing lipolysis. However, due to its low rate of absorption and less aqueous solubility, its use is limited. A study investigated FNB-loaded nanoparticles designed to release FNB upon exposure to reactive oxygen species, molecules frequently found in conditions such as non-alcoholic fatty liver disease (NAFLD). The release of FNB was significantly accelerated when nanoparticles were placed in a medium containing higher H2O2 concentrations. Additionally, it was discovered that the FNB-NP formulation was extremely steady in the bloodstream and during accumulation [25].

Case Study 14

The amalgamation of berberine (BER) and curcumin (CUR) is inadequate due to the potential toxicity linked to elevated dosages, especially the gastrointestinal tract (GIT) damage induced by BER at doses surpassing fifty mg per kg in rats through enteral administration. The limited oral bioavailability of BER and CUR, attributable to poor absorption, rapid metabolism, and heightened excretion, diminishes their pharmacological efficacy when administered together. Thus, a co-delivery nanoplatform for the simultaneous administration of BER and CUR is crucial for improving therapeutic efficacy in NAFLD by reducing oral dosage, enhancing oral absorption, increasing distribution rate, and ensuring proper activity in the hepatic region. Multilayer nanovesicles show significant potential for protecting and delivering pharmaceutical combinations orally. Since bile salts are encapsulated within liposomes, bilosomes also exhibit improved permeability across the small intestine and a longer GIT residence time. Bilosomes significantly extended the circulation half-life and enhanced the oral absorption of both BER and CUR, as indicated by *in vivo* pharmacokinetic analysis. Coordinated biodistribution of BER and CUR, with the highest levels in the hepatic region, can be demonstrated by DEAE-DEX@LSDBC, resulting in significant therapeutic benefit in NAFLD. It was later confirmed to be primarily driven by antioxidant and anti-inflammatory processes. The DEAE-DEX-coated bilosome demonstrated improved oral absorption, increased transmucosal capacity, prolonged hemodynamic effects, enhanced pharmacokinetic activity, and improved therapeutic efficacy for non-alcoholic fatty liver disease compared to the free mixture of BER and CUR [26].

Case Study 15

A glycogen-based nanoparticle designed for hepatic targeting and redox responsiveness, intended to effectively deliver resveratrol, was developed to improve NAFLD. In a study, glycogen, α-lipoic acid, and lactobionic acid were combined to synthesize a complex polymer through glycogen modification and conjugation with lipoic acid. The resulting polymer was amphoteric in nature. Ex vivo experiments demonstrated that this novel drug delivery system significantly enhanced the cellular absorption of Res and preserved redox-responsive properties, while also maintaining anti-inflammatory activity through modulation of the NF-κB (nuclear factor kappa-light-chain-enhancer of activated B cells) signaling pathway via receptor 4. This innovative approach introduces a potential method for addressing NAFLD [27].

Case Study 16

In Western countries, long-term liver damage is common and currently has no definitive cure. Hydroxytyrosol provides protection against liver damage through its antilipidemic effects, removal of harmful cellular moieties, and inhibition of cellular swelling. A critical factor in its efficacy is efficient delivery to hepatocytes, and the development of smart nanogels represents a promising strategy to enhance intracellular uptake. HT-loaded nanoscale scaffolds significantly reduced intracellular triglyceride levels, improved cell viability, and outperformed non-encapsulated hydroxytyrosol. Additionally, these nanogels are biosafe, as they do not impair cellular oxygen flow. This novel nanogel technology offers a viable approach for treating NAFLD, demonstrating greater effectiveness than conventional drug delivery methods [28].

Case Study 17

Rapamycin-loaded nanoparticles were synthesized using the mPEG-PLGA polymer via an eco-friendly emulsion/solvent evaporation process, yielding a narrow size distribution and superior dispersion stability. The therapeutic effectiveness of the NP-RP was evaluated using in vitro HepG2 cells models of NAFLD treated with oleic acid and *in-vivo* mouse models for treating NAFLD induced by a high-fat diet [29].

Case Study 18

A study demonstrated that ZnO nanoparticles (ZnONPs) downregulate de novo lipogenesis compared to wild-type hepatocytes. The findings indicated that SIRT1 promotes AMPK activation via an LKB1-dependent mechanism, thereby mediating the beneficial effects of ZnONPs on hepatocyte lipid metabolism. Treatment with ZnONPs increased intracellular Zn^{2+} availability, which enhanced SIRT1 binding to Zn^{2+}, stabilizing the protein and activating AMPK through LKB1. The study also revealed that ZnONP administration influences the subcellular localization of SREBP-1c and modulates its transcriptional activity. Ultimately, ZnONP treatment mitigates hepatic steatosis and hepatotoxicity while improving glucose tolerance in diet-induced obese mice. These findings may have direct implications for improving insulin sensitivity, maintaining glucose homeostasis, and alleviating liver steatosis in individuals with T2DM [30].

Case Study 19

Hepatic-targeted oxidized starch-lysozyme nanocarriers have been developed for the targeted delivery of resveratrol (Res) to liver tissue, aiming to enhance its therapeutic efficacy in liver-related disorders. Hepatic targeting was conferred by covalent conjugation to galactose, a ligand specifically recognized by asialoglycoprotein receptors on hepatocytes. In a steatotic HepG2 process, the novel delivery method helps reduce lipid formation and triglyceride accumulation. It also helps maintain insulin responsiveness. Moreover, Gal-OSL/Res demonstrated a potent capacity to ameliorate hepatic steatosis and insulin resistance by modulating the AMPK/SIRT1/FAS/SREBP1c signaling network and decreasing the phosphorylation of insulin receptor substrate at serine 307 in the liver. This process plays a vital role in the treatment of hepatic disease, especially NAFLD [31].

Case Study 20

Cerium oxide nanoparticles have shown hepatoprotective effects in experimental liver injury by acting as multi-enzyme mimetics and scavengers of harmful moieties. An experimental model of NAFLD was used to determine whether CeO2 NPs have therapeutic effects. A methionine and choline-deficient diet (MCDD) was administered to fifteen Wistar rats for a duration of six weeks. CeO2NPs were administered intravenously during the third and fourth weeks of the dietary regimen. Serum biochemistry, hepatic fatty acid composition, inflammation, hepatic steatosis, and the expression of genes associated with lipid metabolism and ROS regulation were assessed. The MCDD regimen induced significant hepatic inflammation, increased the accumulation of both saturated and unsaturated fatty acids, and upregulated genes implicated in NAFLD pathogenesis. CeO2NPs treatment markedly diminished the size and quantity of lipid droplets in hepatocytes, along with decreasing hepatic triglyceride- and cholesterol ester-derived fatty acids levels. Furthermore, CeO2NP administration downregulated the expression of various genes involved in cytokine, adipokine, and chemokine signaling pathways, indicating an anti-inflammatory effect. These findings imply that CeO2NPs have the potential to be used as therapeutic agents for the treatment of NAFLD [32].

CONCLUSION

Given the rising incidence and severity of this disease, the pursuit of innovative treatment methods has become increasingly urgent. An explicit understanding of nanotechnology, an emerging frontier in medicine, is essential, as it offers new optimism for addressing this formidable challenge. It helps with precise medication and reduces any toxic effects. Various nanoformulations have demonstrated encouraging results when applied to humans for the treatment of NAFLD. The distinctive feature of this method enables its interaction at a very small level and facilitates substantial progress in the diagnosis and treatment of NAFLD. However, in conjunction with these promising prospects, it is crucial not to overlook the obstacles confronting nanotechnology. Challenges include technical difficulties, potential toxicity, issues with targeted medication delivery, lack of standardized protocols, and ethical considerations that must be addressed before the complete potential of nanotechnology in the management of NAFLD can be achieved. The elevated expense of treatments may impede their wider adoption, particularly in resource-limited environments. Consequently, researchers, doctors, ethicists, and politicians must collaborate as we advance on this path. In summary, although conventional management options for NAFLD, such as lifestyle changes and current pharmacological treatments, remain crucial, the direction of treatment in the near future will be more advanced and more accurate with the development of novel drug delivery systems. The journey is not yet complete, but progress in nanotechnology offers a promising prospect in our battle against this concern. This chapter explores advanced nanocarrier-based delivery systems currently under investigation for NAFLD treatment, highlighting their potential for treating hepatic diseases. Nanotechnology may significantly improve the bioavailability of therapeutic agents, offering promising outcomes. Recent breakthroughs in laboratory research will enhance the application of nanocarrier-based delivery methods in the treatment of hepatic diseases. Nevertheless, the large-scale production of nanoparticles remains a significant challenge. Therefore, progress in large-scale manufacturing will progressively facilitate the therapeutic application of nanoparticle delivery systems.

LIST OF ABBREVIATIONS

NAFLD	Non-alcoholic fatty liver disease
NPs	Nanoparticles
MAFLD	Metabolic Associated Fatty Liver Disease
NASH	Nonalcoholic Steatohepatitis
ASO	Antisense Oligonucleotide
2DG	2-Deoxy-D-glucose
MCD	Methionine and Choline-Deficient
FX	Fucoxanthin
ORI	Oridonin
TNF	Tumor Necrosis Factor
BA/FA	Biliary Acid/Fatty Acid
NES	Nano Emulsions
Nar-RGO	Naringenin-reduced graphene oxide nanosheets
TEM	Transmission electron microscopy
SEM	Scanning electron microscopy
HFFD	High-Fructose Fatty Diet
AST	Astaxanthin
WPI	Whey Protein Isolate
CEL	Celastrol
AMPK	AMP-activated kinase
PPAR	Peroxisome Proliferator-Activated Receptor
FNB-NP	Fenofibrate-loaded Nanoparticles
BER	Berberine
CUR	Curcumin
GIT	Gastrointestinal Tract
DEAE-DEX	Diethyl amino ethyl Dextran
T2DM	Type-2 Diabetes Mellitus
SIRT	Sirtuin
Res	Resveratrol
ROS	Reactive Oxygen Species

REFERENCES

[1] Thapa K, Grewal AS, Kanojia N, Rani L, Sharma N, Singh S. Alcoholic and non-alcoholic liver diseases: promising molecular drug targets and their clinical development. Curr Drug Discov Technol 2021; 18(3): 333-53.
[http://dx.doi.org/10.2174/1570163817666200121143959] [PMID: 31965945]

[2] Han SK, Baik SK, Kim MY. Non-alcoholic fatty liver disease: Definition and subtypes. Clin Mol Hepatol 2023; 29 (Suppl.): S5-S16.
[http://dx.doi.org/10.3350/cmh.2022.0424] [PMID: 36577427]

[3] Younossi ZM, Golabi P, Paik JM, Henry A, Van Dongen C, Henry L. The global epidemiology of nonalcoholic fatty liver disease (NAFLD) and nonalcoholic steatohepatitis (NASH): a systematic review. Hepatology 2023; 77(4): 1335-47.
[http://dx.doi.org/10.1097/HEP.0000000000000004] [PMID: 36626630]

[4] Gupta M, Kaur A, Singh TG, Arora S, Bedi O. Investigational study on awareness of non-alcoholic fatty liver disease (NAFLD) among people of Zirakpur (Punjab) region. Plant Arch 2019; 19(2): 1378-84.

[5] Godoy-Matos AF, Silva Júnior WS, Valerio CM. NAFLD as a continuum: from obesity to metabolic syndrome and diabetes. Diabetol Metab Syndr 2020; 12(1): 60.
[http://dx.doi.org/10.1186/s13098-020-00570-y] [PMID: 32684985]

[6] Byrne CD, Armandi A, Pellegrinelli V, Vidal-Puig A, Bugianesi E. Metabolic dysfunction-associated steatotic liver disease: a condition of heterogeneous metabolic risk factors, mechanisms and comorbidities requiring holistic treatment. Nat Rev Gastroenterol Hepatol 2025; 22(5): 314-28.
[http://dx.doi.org/10.1038/s41575-025-01045-z]

[7] Eslam M, Newsome PN, Sarin SK, *et al.* A new definition for metabolic dysfunction-associated fatty liver disease: An international expert consensus statement. J Hepatol 2020; 73(1): 202-9.
[http://dx.doi.org/10.1016/j.jhep.2020.03.039] [PMID: 32278004]

[8] Ben MD, Polimeni L, Baratta F, Pastori D, Loffredo L, Angelico F. Modern approach to the clinical management of non-alcoholic fatty liver disease. World J Gastroenterol 2014; 20(26): 8341-50.
[http://dx.doi.org/10.3748/wjg.v20.i26.8341] [PMID: 25024593]

[9] Li F, Yuan R, Zhang J, Su B, Qi X. Advances in nanotechnology for the diagnosis and management of metabolic dysfunction-associated steatotic liver disease. Asian Journal of Pharmaceutical Sciences 2025; 20(2): 101025.
[http://dx.doi.org/10.1016/j.ajps.2025.101025] [PMID: 40182137]

[10] Abou Assi R, Abdulbaqi IM, Siok Yee C. The evaluation of drug delivery nanocarrier development and pharmacological briefing for metabolic-associated fatty liver disease (MAFLD): an update. Pharmaceuticals (Basel) 2021; 14(3): 215.
[http://dx.doi.org/10.3390/ph14030215] [PMID: 33806527]

[11] Liang C, Liu X, Sun Z, *et al.* Lipid nanosystems for fatty liver therapy and targeted medication delivery: a comprehensive review. Int J Pharm 2025; 669: 125048.
[http://dx.doi.org/10.1016/j.ijpharm.2024.125048] [PMID: 39653287]

[12] Böttger R, Pauli G, Chao PH, AL Fayez N, Hohenwarter L, Li SD. Lipid-based nanoparticle technologies for liver targeting. Adv Drug Deliv Rev 2020; 154-155: 79-101.
[http://dx.doi.org/10.1016/j.addr.2020.06.017] [PMID: 32574575]

[13] Mehta J, Kumar P, Pawar SV. Exploration of capsaicin-encapsulated lignin nanoparticles for alleviating non-alcoholic fatty liver disease: In-vitro study. Int J Biol Macromol 2025; 303: 140616.
[http://dx.doi.org/10.1016/j.ijbiomac.2025.140616] [PMID: 39909244]

[14] Zhang Y, Wang H, Xu C, *et al.* Rubicon siRNA-encapsulated liver-targeting nanoliposome is a promising therapeutic for non-alcoholic fatty liver disease. Int J Pharm 2025; 672: 125291.
[http://dx.doi.org/10.1016/j.ijpharm.2025.125291] [PMID: 39880145]

[15] He F, Du W, Liu Y, *et al.* Exosome-equipped TNF antisense oligodeoxynucleotide or 2-deoxy-D-glucose ameliorated nonalcoholic steatohepatitis by modulating superoxide dismutase 1 in mice. Redox Biol 2025; 80: 103488.
[http://dx.doi.org/10.1016/j.redox.2025.103488] [PMID: 39778469]

[16] Wu C, Xiang S, Wang H, *et al.* Orally deliverable sequence-targeted fucoxanthin-loaded biomimetic

extracellular vesicles for alleviation of nonalcoholic fatty liver disease. ACS Appl Mater Interfaces 2024; 16(8): 9854-67.
[http://dx.doi.org/10.1021/acsami.3c18029] [PMID: 38375789]

[17] Zhang L, Yu Y, Wang Q, Huang X, Feng Z, Li Z. Oridonin loaded peptide nanovesicles alleviate nonalcoholic fatty liver disease in mice. Pharm Dev Technol 2024; 29(2): 123-30.
[http://dx.doi.org/10.1080/10837450.2024.2315460] [PMID: 38327230]

[18] Faran SA, Hussain T, Khalid SH, *et al.* Bile acid/fatty acid integrated nanoemulsomes for nonalcoholic fatty liver targeted lovastatin delivery: stability, *in-vitro, ex-vivo*, and *in-vivo* analyses. Expert Opin Drug Deliv 2024; 21(5): 779-96. Epub ahead of print
[http://dx.doi.org/10.1080/17425247.2024.2361117] [PMID: 38795359]

[19] Abdelmoneim D, Eldomany EB, El-Adl M, Farghali A, El-Sayed G, El-Sherbini ES. Possible protective effect of natural flavanone naringenin-reduced graphene oxide nanosheets on nonalcoholic fatty liver disease. Naunyn Schmiedebergs Arch Pharmacol 2024; 397: 1-16.
[PMID: 39414698]

[20] Yan B, Zheng X, Wang Y, *et al.* Liposome-based silibinin for mitigating nonalcoholic fatty liver disease: dual effects via parenteral and intestinal routes. ACS Pharmacol Transl Sci 2023; 6(12): 1909-23.
[http://dx.doi.org/10.1021/acsptsci.3c00210] [PMID: 38093834]

[21] Che T, Song Y, Su W, Xing S, Wang H, Tan M. Hepatic parenchymal cell and mitochondrial-targeted astaxanthin nanocarriers for relief of high fat diet-induced nonalcoholic fatty liver disease. Food Funct 2023; 14(6): 2908-20.
[http://dx.doi.org/10.1039/D2FO04036K] [PMID: 36883333]

[22] Salem GA, Mohamed AAR, Khater SI, *et al.* Enhancement of biochemical and genomic pathways through lycopene-loaded nano-liposomes: Alleviating insulin resistance, hepatic steatosis, and autophagy in obese rats with non-alcoholic fatty liver disease: Involvement of SMO, GLI-1, and PTCH-1 genes. Gene 2023; 883: 147670.
[http://dx.doi.org/10.1016/j.gene.2023.147670] [PMID: 37516284]

[23] Fan N, Zhao J, Zhao W, *et al.* Celastrol-loaded lactosylated albumin nanoparticles attenuate hepatic steatosis in non-alcoholic fatty liver disease. J Control Release 2022; 347: 44-54.
[http://dx.doi.org/10.1016/j.jconrel.2022.04.034] [PMID: 35483638]

[24] Guo X, Huang Z, Chen J, *et al.* Synergistic delivery of resveratrol and ultrasmall copper-based nanoparticles by aptamer-functionalized ultrasound nanobubbles for the treatment of nonalcoholic fatty liver disease. Front Physiol 2022; 13: 950141.
[http://dx.doi.org/10.3389/fphys.2022.950141] [PMID: 36160874]

[25] Du K, Huang X, Peng A, *et al.* Engineered fenofibrate as oxidation-sensitive nanoparticles with ROS scavenging and PPARα-activating bioactivity to ameliorate nonalcoholic fatty liver disease. Mol Pharm 2023; 20(1): 159-71.
[http://dx.doi.org/10.1021/acs.molpharmaceut.2c00549] [PMID: 36342356]

[26] Chen Y, Jiang Z, Xu J, *et al.* Improving the ameliorative effects of berberine and curcumin combination via dextran-coated bilosomes on non-alcohol fatty liver disease in mice. J Nanobiotechnology 2021; 19(1): 230.
[http://dx.doi.org/10.1186/s12951-021-00979-1] [PMID: 34348707]

[27] Li X, Chen XX, Xu Y, *et al.* Construction of glycogen-based nanoparticles loaded with resveratrol for the alleviation of high-fat diet-induced nonalcoholic fatty liver disease. Biomacromolecules 2022; 23(1): 409-23.
[http://dx.doi.org/10.1021/acs.biomac.1c01360] [PMID: 34964604]

[28] Mauri E, Gori M, Giannitelli SM, *et al.* Nano-encapsulation of hydroxytyrosol into formulated nanogels improves therapeutic effects against hepatic steatosis: An in vitro study. Mater Sci Eng C 2021; 124: 112080.

[http://dx.doi.org/10.1016/j.msec.2021.112080] [PMID: 33947572]

[29] Zhao R, Zhu M, Zhou S, Feng W, Chen H. Rapamycin-loaded mPEG-PLGA nanoparticles ameliorate hepatic steatosis and liver injury in non-alcoholic fatty liver disease. Front Chem 2020; 8: 407. [http://dx.doi.org/10.3389/fchem.2020.00407] [PMID: 32548088]

[30] Dogra S, Kar AK, Girdhar K, *et al.* Zinc oxide nanoparticles attenuate hepatic steatosis development in high-fat-diet fed mice through activated AMPK signaling axis. Nanomedicine 2019; 17: 210-22. [http://dx.doi.org/10.1016/j.nano.2019.01.013] [PMID: 30708053]

[31] Teng W, Zhao L, Yang S, *et al.* The hepatic-targeted, resveratrol loaded nanoparticles for relief of high fat diet-induced nonalcoholic fatty liver disease. J Control Release 2019; 307: 139-49. [http://dx.doi.org/10.1016/j.jconrel.2019.06.023] [PMID: 31233775]

[32] Carvajal S, Perramón M, Oró D, *et al.* Cerium oxide nanoparticles display antilipogenic effect in rats with non-alcoholic fatty liver disease. Sci Rep 2019; 9(1): 12848. [http://dx.doi.org/10.1038/s41598-019-49262-2] [PMID: 31492960]

CHAPTER 14

Challenges and Opportunities in Nanocarrier-based Drug Delivery for Fatty Liver Disease

Saksham Sharma[1], **Shushank Mahajan**[1], **Sanchit Dhankhar**[1,*], **Sabina Yasmin**[2], **Monika Saini**[3] and **Samrat Chauhan**[1]

[1] *Chitkara College of Pharmacy, Chitkara University, Rajpura, Punjab, India*

[2] *Department of Pharmaceutical Chemistry, College of Pharmacy, King Khalid University, Abha, Saudi Arabia*

[3] *MM College of Pharmacy, Maharishi Markandeshwar (Deemed to be University), Mullana, Haryana, India*

Abstract: Fatty liver disease (FLD), ranging from benign hepatic steatosis to non-alcoholic steatohepatitis (NASH), is becoming the most common chronic liver disease globally, largely propelled by the global epidemic of obesity, type 2 diabetes, and metabolic syndrome. Although it has a growing burden and potential for progression to cirrhosis and hepatocellular carcinoma, no pharmacotherapy is universally agreed upon, and lifestyle changes alone are frequently insufficient to prevent further disease progression. Successful treatment is hindered by the multifactorial etiology of FLD and by the limitations of systemic drug administration, such as low solubility, fast degradation, and off-target toxicity. Targeted drug delivery systems, especially nanocarrier-based platforms, have emerged as a promising solution to overcome these limitations. Nanocarriers enhance drug stability and solubility, and facilitate liver-specific uptake via passive and active targeting mechanisms. In addition, they facilitate the controlled release of drugs, the simultaneous co-delivery of dual therapeutic agents, and the minimization of systemic side effects, all of which are vital for the treatment of chronic liver diseases. In this chapter, the therapeutic application, existing limitations, and novel approaches of nanocarrier-mediated drug delivery in FLD are discussed with emphasis on its revolutionary role in the formulation of more efficient and safer long-term treatment protocols.

Keywords: Controlled release, Fatty liver disease, Liver fibrosis, Metabolic syndrome, Non-alcoholic steatohepatitis, Nanocarriers.

* **Corresponding author Sanchit Dhankhar:** Chitkara College of Pharmacy, Chitkara University, Rajpura, Punjab, India; E-mail: sanchitdhankar@gmail.com

INTRODUCTION

Fatty liver disease (FLD) is arguably the most common chronic liver condition globally, fueled by the rising incidence of obesity, type 2 diabetes mellitus, and metabolic syndrome. FLD represents a heterogeneous group of liver disorders, ranging from simple hepatic steatosis (fatty infiltration of hepatocytes) to non-alcoholic steatohepatitis (NASH), which is characterized by inflammation, hepatocellular injury, and varying degrees of fibrosis. Untreated NASH will progress to cirrhosis, liver failure, and finally hepatocellular carcinoma [1, 2]. Unlike alcohol-induced liver disease, FLD occurs in patients regardless of alcohol consumption, and its occult, insidious progression often results in delayed presentation at an advanced stage. Despite increasing FLD global load, no universally accepted pharmacotherapy exists for this entity; the cornerstone of management remains lifestyle modifications. However, lifestyle modification is itself typically not sufficient to stop disease progression in patients with NASH and fibrosis. This underscores the need for practical therapeutic measures that can influence the multifactorial pathological processes underlying FLD, such as hepatic steatosis, insulin resistance, inflammation, and fibrogenesis [1]. Drug delivery to the liver, specifically to cell types, such as hepatocytes, hepatic stellate cells, or Kupffer cells, without inducing side effects in other organs, remains one of the greatest challenges in developing effective treatments for FLD. Most candidate therapeutic compounds, including antioxidants, anti-inflammatory drugs, and anti-fibrotic agents, are plagued by low water solubility, rapid degradation, short circulation half-lives, and off-target toxicity following systemic administration. In addition, the complex architecture of the liver and the altered microenvironment in FLD, *i.e.*, steatosis and fibrosis, may interfere with drug penetration and action. These constraints emphasize the value of targeted drug-delivery systems that can improve the bioavailability of the therapeutic agent, selectively target diseased liver tissues, and reduce systemic side effects [2]. Targeted delivery systems would not only improve the therapeutic index of drugs but also enable low-dose therapy and less treatment-related toxicity, an important factor in chronic diseases like FLD that need to be treated for many years. Nanocarrier-based drug delivery systems present a promising solution to these problems. Taking advantage of the desirable properties of nanoscale materials, *i.e.*, their size-controllable dimensions, surface properties, and drug-loading ability, nanocarriers are able to deliver drugs in a stabilized state, increase their solubility and stability, and allow them to accumulate in the liver through passive or active targeting mechanisms [3]. Passive targeting leverages the liver's natural filtering capacity and fenestrated vasculature to increase nanoparticle uptake, whereas active targeting entails surface modification of the nanocarrier with ligands that bind receptors overexpressed on liver cells, *i.e.*, the glycoprotein receptor of hepatocytes or the mannose receptor of Kupffer cells [4]. In addition, nanocarriers can be designed to release drugs in a sustained, controlled manner, prolonging therapeutic action with fewer doses. Nanocarrier systems are also highly versatile for the co-delivery of two or more drugs, which can treat the multifactorial pathogenesis of FLD more effectively. With future advancements in materials science and nanotechnology, nanocarrier-based therapy is poised to revolutionize the therapeutic paradigm for FLD, offering new hope of halting or even reversing the disease process [5]. This chapter presents the potential, challenges, and novel applications of nanocarrier-based drug delivery methods for the treatment of fatty liver disease.

PATHOPHYSIOLOGY OF FATTY LIVER DISEASE

Fatty liver disease (FLD) is generally classified into two categories based on its etiology: alcoholic fatty liver disease (AFLD) and non-alcoholic fatty liver disease (NAFLD). Even though they share histological features, such as hepatic steatosis, inflammation, and fibrosis, their etiologies are quite distinct [6]. AFLD is a consequence of long-standing and excessive alcohol use, and the subsequent hepatic accumulation of fat is a result of dysfunctional oxidation of fatty acids, augmented lipogenesis, and oxidative damage induced by ethanol. NAFLD, by contrast, affects patients with little or no alcohol use and is very much related to metabolic risk factors, including obesity, type 2 diabetes, dyslipidemia, and insulin resistance. NAFLD has emerged as the world's leading liver disease after the increasing epidemic of metabolic syndrome. Both types of FLD tend to progress through similar pathological phases: simple steatosis (steatosis and inflammatory liver) to steatohepatitis (hepatocytic injury and inflammation), followed by fibrosis, cirrhosis, and, finally, hepatocellular carcinoma [7]. The non-alcoholic form, however, is more insidious in its course and would remain undetected until late because it is usually asymptomatic. At the molecular level, the pathogenesis of FLD is multifactorial and further exacerbated by a cascade of fibrotic remodeling, inflammatory reactions, and metabolic derangements. In NAFLD, insulin resistance is the primary driver of excess lipid deposition in the liver by enhancing rapid free fatty acid flux from adipose tissue, promoting de novo lipogenesis, and inhibiting fatty acid oxidation [8]. This excess lipid triggers lipotoxicity and hepatocyte injury and activates stress signaling pathways, including oxidative stress, ER stress, and mitochondrial dysfunction. Cellular stresses induce the release of pro-inflammatory cytokines (*e.g.*, TNF-α, IL-6) and chemokines, leading to recruitment of immune cells and sustenance of hepatic inflammation. In addition, the gut-liver axis plays a role; dysbiosis and elevated gut permeability facilitate endotoxin (*e.g.*, lipopolysaccharide) translocation to the liver and contribute to enhanced inflammation [9]. In AFLD and in NAFLD, ongoing hepatocellular tissue damage induces hepatic stellate cells to undergo transdifferentiation into activated myofibroblasts that secrete more extracellular matrix components to accumulate and induce fibrosis in the liver. Progressive fibrosis induces loss of the liver architecture and function, leading to cirrhosis and hepatocellular carcinoma risk. Aside from that, genetic predispositions (*e.g.*, PNPLA3 and TM6SF2 polymorphisms) also play a role in disease progression susceptibility [10].

As knowledge of the molecular mechanisms of FLD increases, current therapeutic approaches remain infrequent and, in most cases, insufficient. For NAFLD and NASH, there are no drugs that have been approved for their specific use. Treatment is largely limited to lifestyle changes, including weight reduction, diet, and physical exercise, which have been partially effective in improving liver histology [11]. Pharmacological treatments, such as insulin sensitizers (*e.g.*, pioglitazone), antioxidants (*e.g.*, vitamin E), and lipid-lowering drugs (*e.g.*, statins), have yielded conflicting results and are not consistent across all studies, and they carry the potential for adverse effects. Avoidance of alcohol is still the mainstay of AFLD treatment, but it is difficult to practice in the long term and results in substantial liver injury following alcohol withdrawal. The multifactorial etiology of FLD, which includes metabolic, inflammatory, and fibrotic processes, impedes the development of pharmacotherapy targeting a single factor [12]. Furthermore, reduced drug bioavailability, off-target toxicities, and reduced efficacy in cirrhosis or advanced fibrosis further restrict treatment. Such types of therapeutic challenges underscore the need for new approaches, including targeted drug delivery systems, with the ability to effectively modulate multiple pathological pathways in the liver without causing systemic toxicity (Fig. **1**) [13].

NANOCARRIERS IN DRUG DELIVERY

Nanocarriers represent a technological innovation in drug delivery, offering novel solutions to age-old challenges in traditional pharmaceutical formulations. Nanocarriers are typically nanoscale carriers, usually 1-1000 nanometers in diameter, designed to carry, protect, and deliver therapeutic agents to specific sites within the body [14]. These carriers can entrap a variety of payloads, ranging from small-molecule therapeutics to proteins, nucleic acids, and imaging agents, and are designed to enhance pharmacokinetics, bioavailability, and therapeutic benefit. Depending on their structure, architecture, and biological properties, nanocarriers can be classified into various categories, such as lipid-based carriers (liposomes, solid lipid nanoparticles, nanostructured lipid carriers), polymer-based carriers (polymeric nanoparticles, dendrimers, micelles), inorganic nanoparticles (gold nanoparticles, silica nanoparticles), and biologically derived

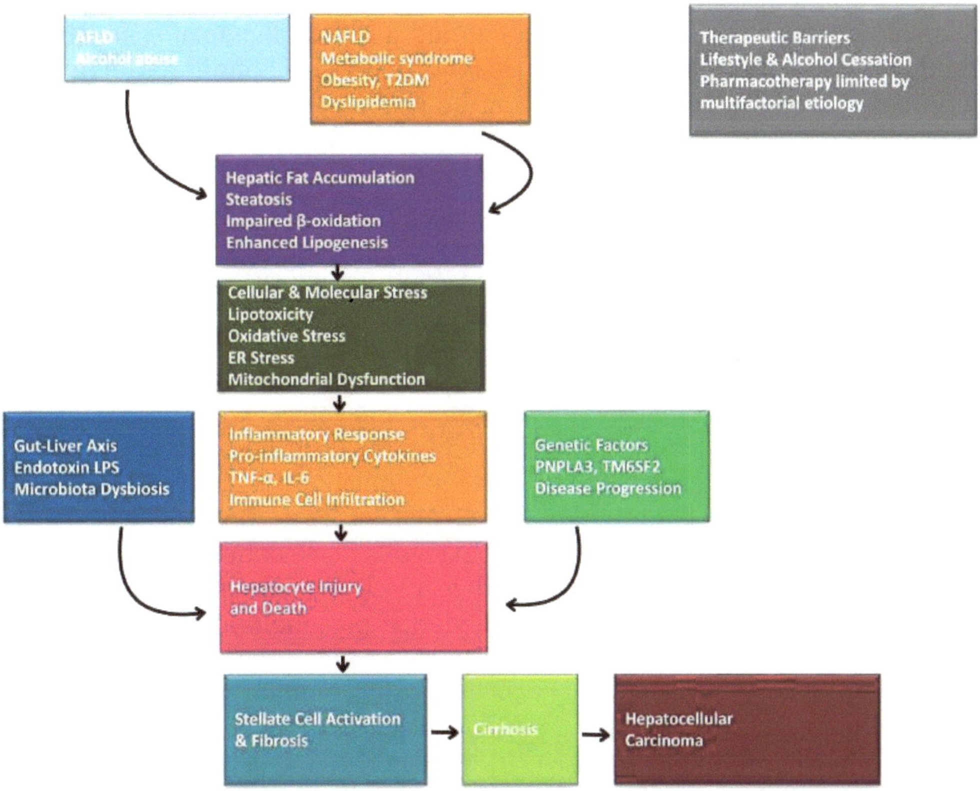

Fig. (1). Pathophysiology of fatty liver disease.

vesicles (exosomes) [15]. In contrast to traditional drug delivery systems, such as oral tablets, capsules, and plain IV infusions, nanocarrier-based systems offer distinct advantages that make them highly preferable for the treatment of complex and chronic diseases like fatty liver disease. Firstly, nanocarriers can improve the solubility and stability of poorly water-soluble or unstable drugs. Most therapeutic agents with good *in vitro* activity have also clinically failed because they are compromised by low solubility, drug degradation, or poor pharmacokinetics. Nanocarriers can shield drugs from enzymatic degradation and chemical breakdown, extend their half-life in the circulation, and enhance bioavailability [16]. Second, nanocarriers enable targeted delivery. They can be designed to selectively accumulate in particular tissues or cells, either passively by exploiting phenomena such as increased permeability and retention (EPR) in tumors or in the fenestrated liver vasculature, or actively by ligand-dependent delivery to overexpressed receptors. Targeting prevents off-target drug release and systemic toxicity, which are important in diseases such as fatty liver disease, where prolonged drug release is needed [17]. Third, nanocarriers can deliver drugs in a sustained and controlled manner, maintaining a steady therapeutic level for an extended period, thereby reducing dosing intervals. Fourth, co-delivery of multiple drugs or therapeutic agents can be achieved using nanocarriers. Since two or more drugs are loaded into a single carrier, there is space for synergism, which can be invaluable for multifactorial disease conditions when more than a single pathological pathway needs to be addressed simultaneously [18]. Nanocarriers can be further functionalized with imaging agents to create theranostic effects, co-packaging therapy and diagnosis so that, in theory, clinicians can monitor treatment response in real time.

Several nanocarrier platforms have been widely investigated and applied in drug delivery research and clinical applications. Liposomes, which are spherical-shaped vesicles composed of one or more phospholipid bilayers, are one of the most investigated nanocarriers due to their biocompatibility, ability to encapsulate both hydrophobic and hydrophilic drugs, and ease of functionalization with targeting groups or PEGylation for extended circulation half-lives [19]. Liposomes have been successfully used in clinical settings, including cancer treatment and infectious disease therapy, and their potential for liver-targeted drug delivery has been widely documented. Polymeric nanoparticles, by definition, are composed of biodegradable polymers such as polylactic-co-glycolic acid (PLGA) or polyethylene glycol (PEG)-based systems, which offer high flexibility for drug encapsulation and prolonged release [20]. Polymeric nanoparticles are engineered with surface modulation to function as liver targeting and cellular uptake. Solid lipid nanoparticles (SLNs) and nanostructured lipid carriers (NLCs) are lipid-based delivery systems that share the benefits of polymeric nanoparticles and liposomes, with good biocompatibility, high loading capacity, and physical stability. They are especially valuable for encapsulation of low-solubility lipophilic drugs. Dendrimers are densely branched, treelike polymeric architectures with high surface functionality and interior volume to accommodate high drug loading and proper size and shape control [21]. Their multivalency provides simultaneous drug loading and attachment of targeting ligands or imaging moieties. Although they require complex preparation and are toxic, dendrimers remain an intriguing family of nanocarriers. Inorganic nanoparticles, *e.g.*, gold nanoparticles and mesoporous silica nanoparticles, possess specific optical, magnetic, and structural properties that can be leveraged for drug delivery and imaging, although long-term biocompatibility remains under investigation. Natural extracellular vesicles secreted by cells, including exosomes, have become preferred owing to their biocompatibility, cell-targeting ability, and ability to deliver nucleic acids and proteins [22]. Their endogenous origin reduces immunogenicity, making them ideal for liver-targeted use.

APPLICATION OF NANOCARRIERS IN FLD MANAGEMENT

Nanocarrier-mediated drug delivery systems have been utilized in the treatment of fatty liver disease (FLD) and have been shown to provide a novel method of treating the multi-component pathophysiology of the syndrome, *e.g.*, hepatic steatosis, inflammation, and fibrosis [23]. A major advantage of nanocarriers for the treatment of FLD is that they can deliver drugs to hepatocytes in a target-directed manner, the key cell population involved in alcoholic and non-alcoholic fatty liver disease [24]. The liver, as a result of its anatomical and physiological peculiarities, is also a readily accessible target organ for nanoparticles. It is extremely rich in blood and has a fenestrated, sinusoidal endothelial lining, so nanoparticles of any dimension, up to a point, can move through and come into contact with liver cells [25]. Target delivery is further improved through active delivery mechanisms, in which nanocarriers are conjugated to ligands that bind preferentially to receptors highly expressed in hepatocytes. Among the most significant targets is the Asialoglycoprotein receptor (ASGPR), which is highly expressed on the surface of hepatocytes and binds to galactose or N-acetylgalactosamine moieties. Conjugation of these ligands to nanocarriers has enabled researchers to trigger receptor-mediated endocytosis, thereby delivering therapeutic payloads to hepatocytes while sparing non-hepatic tissues. Similarly, mannose-targeted nanoparticles may target Kupffer cells (liver macrophages), which are responsible for hepatic inflammation. Such targeting mechanisms not only enhance therapeutic efficacy but also reduce systemic toxicity, a significant concern with prolonged FLD treatment [26].

Apart from enhancing drug delivery to hepatocytes, nanocarrier systems are also critical in minimizing hepatic inflammation, fibrosis, and steatosis, the core pathological processes that dictate disease establishment [27]. Nanocarriers can encapsulate and deliver anti-inflammatory drugs, antioxidants, and anti-fibrotic agents directly to the liver, thereby resulting in elevated local concentrations and long-term therapeutic effects. For example, oxidative stress is a primary cause of hepatocellular damage and inflammation in FLD. Antioxidant encapsulation, such as curcumin, resveratrol, or silymarin, in lipid nanoparticles or polymer carriers improves solubility, prevents degradation, and facilitates hepatic uptake [28]. Research has found that solid lipid nanoparticles loaded with curcumin improve curcumin bioavailability and reduce hepatic lipid accumulation, oxidative stress markers, and inflammatory cytokines by substantial amounts in animal models of NASH [29]. Additionally, nanocarriers can deliver anti-fibrotic drugs, such as siRNA or small-molecule inhibitors, directly to hepatic stellate cells (HSCs), the major effector cells of liver fibrosis. Nanoparticle-mediated delivery of TGF-β- or CTGF-specific siRNA has been shown to inhibit fibrogenic gene expression, decrease collagen deposition, and regulate fibrosis in preclinical models [5]. Moreover, co-delivery approaches that simultaneously deliver anti-inflammatory and anti-fibrotic drugs within a single nanocarrier can synergistically regulate multiple disease mechanisms and exert broad therapeutic effects in FLD [30].

Some nanocarrier-formulated therapeutic drugs are in use for their potential application in the management of FLD, which have provided promising preclinical results. Galactosylated liposomes containing silymarin, a strong antioxidant and hepatoprotective drug isolated from milk thistle, were shown to accumulate to a larger extent in hepatocytes, leading to increased liver function and decreased oxidative injury in animal models of NAFLD [31]. No less impressive is the formulation of mannose-conjugated chitosan nanoparticles that target siRNA against tumor necrosis factor-alpha (TNF-α) to specifically modulate Kupffer cell activity and thereby suppress liver inflammation. Another good example is curcumin delivery using nanostructured lipid carriers (NLCs) [32]. The NLCs have been shown to possess enhanced loading capacity, stability, and prolonged release compared with traditional vehicles, resulting in significant improvements in liver histology and metabolic parameters in rodent models of NASH. Polymeric nanoparticles, such as PLGA nanoparticles, have also been used to deliver pioglitazone, a PPARγ agonist with insulin-sensitizing and anti-inflammatory activity [33]. Pioglitazone encapsulated in PLGA nanoparticles has been shown to improve its hepatic bioavailability and therapeutic action, significantly lowering steatosis, inflammation, and fibrosis compared with free drug delivery. Exosome delivery systems have also emerged as a new modality in the management of FLD. Exosomes derived from MSCs, for instance, have intrinsic anti-inflammatory and regenerative properties. Naturally secreted exosomes can deliver bioactive molecules, such as microRNAs (*e.g.*, miR-122) and proteins, to hepatocytes and other liver cells to influence lipid metabolism and inflammatory signaling [34]. Preclinical research indicates that exosome therapies can decrease hepatic lipid deposition, inhibit pro-inflammatory cytokine expression, and enhance tissue repair in FLD models.

CHALLENGES IN NANOCARRIER-BASED FLD THERAPY

Biological Barriers in Liver Targeting

Despite the broad therapeutic potential of nanocarrier-based drug delivery systems for treating fatty liver disease (FLD), several important challenges hinder their seamless translation from bench to bedside. Some of these include biological obstacles and restrictions on targeting specificity, nanocarrier stability problems, toxicity, biocompatibility, manufacturing scale-up, and regulatory approval. One of the most challenging tasks is overcoming biological barriers and achieving precise targeting specificity within the liver's complex microenvironment. Even though the fenestrated liver vasculature allows for nanoparticle uptake, efficiently targeting nanocarriers to specific cell types, *e.g.*, hepatocytes, hepatic stellate cells, or Kupffer cells, is difficult. After systemic administration, nanocarriers are immediately engaged with plasma proteins (opsonization), resulting in rapid clearance by the reticuloendothelial system (RES), mainly via Kupffer cells in the liver and splenic macrophages [35, 36].

Impact of Disease-related Liver Architecture

Although this native hepatic uptake is useful for targeting the liver as a whole, it compromises the potential to target therapies to specific cell populations, *e.g.*, hepatic stellate cells involved in fibrosis or hepatocytes involved in lipid metabolism. Additionally, disrupted liver architecture in advanced FL steatosis and fibrosis can impede nanoparticle delivery and penetration, blemishing the effectiveness of therapy [37]. Despite surface functionalization *via* ligand-targeting (*e.g.*, mannose for Kupffer cells or galactose for hepatocytes), receptor-mediated uptake is increased, but achieving ligand specificity, optimal ligand loading, and avoiding off-target binding remains technologically demanding [38]. Furthermore, patient-to-patient or stage-to-stage variability in receptor expression levels also affects targeting, reducing consistency and reliability in clinical practice.

Stability and Toxicity Concerns

The second most dominant challenge in nanocarrier therapy is biocompatibility, especially stability and toxicity. The physicochemical stability of nanocarriers during storage and throughout their shelf life after administration is critical to ensure sustained drug activity [39]. Nanoparticles are susceptible to agglomeration, drug loss from them, and physical degradation in the body, which can destabilize prolonged release and targeted drug activity. In addition, nanocarrier-forming materials, whether lipids, polymers, metals, or surfactants, should be biocompatible and non-immunogenic. Some nanocarriers, particularly inorganic nanoparticles, such as gold or silica, tend to accumulate in tissues and cause chronic toxicity or inflammation due to slow degradation or clearance [40]. Even biocompatible carriers, such as liposomes and polymeric nanoparticles, can trigger undesirable immune responses or complement activation-related pseudoallergy (CARPA) reactions. Furthermore, breakdown products of some polymers or surfactants can be cytotoxic or can affect cellular function [41]. Dose-related toxicity, particularly when extended administration is needed for chronic illnesses, such as FLD, also poses additional safety concerns. Characterization of the pharmacokinetics, biodistribution, metabolism, and excretion (ADME) of nanocarriers is therefore crucial to prevent these hazards. Notably, size, shape, surface charge, and heterogeneity in functionalization of nanoparticles can give rise to unpredictable biological interactions, making it difficult to predict *in vivo* behavior and therapeutic effects.

Manufacturing Scalability Challenges

In addition to safety and biological issues, manufacturing scalability and regulatory barriers are significant barriers to clinical translation of nanocarrier-based therapy. Manufacturing scalable, consistent, and reproducible nanocarriers is challenging [42]. A slight change in synthesis conditions leads to batch-to-batch variability in particle size, drug loading, surface modification, and release profiles. Scale-up manufacturing with rigorous control over these parameters is needed to meet Good Manufacturing Practice (GMP) standards required for clinical applications. Also, the complexity of nanocarrier formulations often entails multi-step syntheses, purification, and characterization, thereby increasing production costs and reducing commercial attractiveness [43]. Regarding regulatory issues, approval of nanomedicines is particularly problematic. Existing regulatory guidelines, such as those from the U.S. Food and Drug Administration (FDA) and the European Medicines Agency (EMA), were originally formulated for traditional drugs and may not be entirely suitable for the complexity of nanocarriers [44]. Regulatory authorities need detailed characterization of nanocarrier physicochemical properties, toxicology, pharmacokinetics, and long-term safety data. Guidelines and standardized protocols for assessing these parameters in nanomedicines continue to evolve [45]. In addition, proving clear-cut clinical advantages over available treatments, especially where no licensed medicines for FLD exist, introduces further regulatory complexity.

STRATEGIES TO OVERCOME CHALLENGES

To achieve the maximum therapeutic effectiveness of nanocarrier-based drug delivery systems for treating fatty liver disease (FLD) and to address relevant issues, several advanced strategies have been developed [46]. They are intended to improve targeting specificity, optimize biological stability, reduce toxicity, and facilitate clinical translation. Some of the most promising approaches include surface modification and ligand conjugation, stimulus-responsive and intelligent nanocarrier development, and hybrid and multi-functional delivery system design [47]. Surface modification and ligand conjugation are among the most widely used strategies to enhance targeting specificity and prevent premature clearance of nanocarriers [48]. By surface-coating nanoparticles with hydrophilic polymers, such as polyethylene glycol (PEG), a process known as PEGylation, the nanocarrier can avoid opsonization by serum proteins and subsequent phagocytosis by macrophages of the reticuloendothelial system (RES) [49]. Circulation time is increased, bioavailability is improved, and there is a greater likelihood that nanocarriers will reach target cells in the liver. In addition to PEGylation, active targeting can be achieved by conjugating ligands to nanocarriers that specifically bind overexpressed receptors on targeted liver cell types. Galactose and N-acetylgalactosamine (GalNAc) ligands, for instance, target asialoglycoprotein receptor (ASGPR) on hepatocytes, whereas mannose ligands target mannose receptors on Kupffer cells [50]. Additional ligands, including peptides, aptamers, or antibodies, can be designed to target activated hepatic stellate cells involved in fibrosis. Carefully tuning ligand density, spatial distribution, and binding affinity can optimize receptor-mediated uptake and avoid off-target effects. Zwitterionic or polysaccharide coatings, such as chitosan or hyaluronic acid, also provide biocompatible alternatives to PEG to improve nanoparticle stability and reduce immunogenicity [51].

Another emerging method is the formulation of stimuli-responsive and intelligent nanocarriers that release the drug payload in response to specific environmental triggers present in affected liver tissue. The stimuli are either internal, such as pH, redox potential, or enzymatic activity, or external, such as temperature, light, or magnetism [52]. For example, the microenvironment of fibrotic or inflammatory liver tissue has a lower pH than that of normal tissue. pH-sensitive nanocarriers can be formulated to be circulation-stable while undergoing structural alteration or degradation in acidic microenvironments, leading to preferential drug release at the disease site [53]. Redox-sensitive nanoparticles have been prepared using disulfide linkages that are reducible under high intracellular glutathione conditions, thereby inducing controlled drug release within target cells. Enzyme-activated nanocarriers can utilize overexpressed enzymes, such as matrix metalloproteinases (MMPs), in fibrotic tissues to aid site-specific drug release [54]. Therapeutic responsiveness is improved by sequestering the drug to be released almost fully at the delivery site, curbing systemic toxicity. Additionally, external activation via near-infrared (NIR) irradiation or magnetic fields enables on-demand release, further enhancing treatment precision. Hybrid and multifunctional delivery systems integrate multiple functions and materials into a single nanocarrier to resolve multiple issues at once [55]. Hybrid nanoparticles, made up of both organic and inorganic matter, can capitalize on the best features of both types of material. For instance, lipid-polymer hybrid nanoparticles integrate the drug-loading capability and biocompatibility of liposomes with the structural strength and programmed release of polymeric nanoparticles [56]. In a similar vein, polymer- or lipid-coated gold nanoparticles can be employed for the delivery of drugs and imaging agents for theranostic use, integrating therapy and diagnostics. Multifunctional nanocarriers can be designed to co-deliver drugs in combination, *i.e.*, an anti-inflammatory drug and an anti-fibrotic siRNA, to target multiple disease pathways in FLD [57]. Surface modification is also used to accommodate both stealth coatings (*e.g.*, PEG) and targeting ligands, thereby providing a cocktail of drugs for synergy. The hybrid and multifunctional systems are modular in design, making them highly flexible and adaptable to the phase of the disease or patient profiles, opening the way to personalized approaches to medicine [58].

RECENT ADVANCES IN NANOCARRIER-BASED DRUG DELIVERY FOR FATTY LIVER DISEASE

Recent advances in nanocarrier-based drug delivery systems for fatty liver disease (FLD) have significantly expanded the treatment landscape, with numerous preclinical and ongoing clinical trials highlighting their potential to modulate key pathogenic processes, including steatosis, inflammation, and fibrosis. Building on the advantages of sophisticated nanoparticle engineering and innovative targeting mechanisms, some case studies and model systems have made tremendous strides in treating the multifaceted pathophysiology of FLD, opening the way for final clinical translation [59]. One of the most potent preclinical accounts is the use of curcumin-loaded nanostructured lipid carriers (NLCs) in rodent models of non-alcoholic steatohepatitis (NASH). Curcumin, a phytochemical polyphenol with strong anti-inflammatory and antioxidant properties, is hampered by low bioavailability and increased metabolism following oral administration [60]. Encapsulating curcumin in lipid nanoparticles enhanced its solubility, prolonged its circulation time, and increased liver accumulation [61]. Model studies of high-fat diet-induced NASH confirmed that curcumin-loaded NLCs significantly decreased hepatic lipid content, inhibited pro-inflammatory cytokines TNF-α and IL-6, lowered markers of oxidative stress, and promoted liver histological recovery. Likewise, silymarin nanoparticles, employing liposomes and polymeric carriers, have been reported to exhibit hepatoprotective activity by enhancing markers of liver function and inhibiting lipid accumulation in animal models of NAFLD [62]. Silymarin, which is of milk thistle origin, possesses antioxidant and anti-fibrotic action but suffers from the same limitation of bioavailability as curcumin, against which nanocarrier systems are amply capable.

A great example is also that of fibrogenic-targeting siRNA-nanoparticle complexes. In research, siRNA directed against TNF-α was transfected into Kupffer cells in fibrotic livers using mannose-modified chitosan nanoparticles [63]. This procedure significantly reduced liver inflammation, collagen accumulation, and fibrotic biomarkers in carbon tetrachloride (CCl_4)-induced models of liver fibrosis. In parallel, delivery of siRNA *via* polymeric nanoparticles against anti-transforming growth factor-beta (TGF-β), a master activator of hepatic stellate cells, also inhibited profibrotic gene expression and reduced fibrosis in animal models. These findings emphasize the potential of gene-silencing nanotherapies for the treatment of FLD by targeting primary pathogenic mechanisms [64]. Emerging evidence with exosome-based treatments is also of significant translational significance. MSC-derived exosomes have also been studied for their inherent anti-inflammatory, regenerative, and anti-fibrotic activities. In murine models of NASH, MSC-derived exosome treatment was correlated with decreased hepatic lipid deposition, decreased inflammatory infiltration, and enhanced insulin sensitivity [65]. These inherent nanovesicles are extremely biocompatible, low in immunogenicity, and have inherent targeting abilities, making them an exciting future FLD therapy candidate. Besides these model systems, the translational value and current clinical trials of nanocarrier-based therapies for FLD are slowly gaining momentum [66]. While the majority of uses of nanocarriers in FLD are still at preclinical levels, efficacy in other FLD-associated liver diseases like hepatitis, liver cancer, and fibrosis provides a strong basis for clinical progress. As an illustration, GalNAc-conjugated siRNA drugs, taken up by hepatocytes *via* ASGPR-mediated endocytosis, have already demonstrated clinical value in the treatment of hereditary transthyretin-mediated amyloidosis and hypercholesterolemia [67]. Clinical clearance of patisiran and givosiran, GalNAc-siRNA conjugates, confirms the feasibility and therapeutic potential of ligand-modified nanocarriers for liver targeting. Such observations indicate that the same method could be modified to silence genes involved in the progression of FLD, including those involved in lipid metabolism, inflammation, or fibrosis [68].

Although there are few direct clinical trials of FLD with nanocarrier-based therapies, many nanomedicines for liver disorders in general are in clinical trials and can provide insight into future FLD interventions. Lipid nanoparticle (LNP)-based therapies, such as those used in mRNA vaccines and RNA therapeutics, have demonstrated scalable manufacturing and clinical feasibility, establishing precedence for analogous delivery platforms in liver-targeted therapies [69]. Furthermore, GalNAc–siRNA conjugates, which are already in advanced clinical trials for the treatment of liver fibrosis and metabolic liver diseases, are of particular interest for FLD, as these conditions share overlapping pathological mechanisms. Translational research is further supported by advancements in *in vivo* and *in vitro* experimental models that more accurately recapitulate human FLD. Three-dimensional liver organoids, humanized mouse models, and diet-induced NASH models exhibit human-relevant metabolic comorbidities (*e.g.*, insulin resistance and obesity) and are increasingly used to assess nanocarrier activity, biodistribution, and toxicity [70]. Such advanced models bridge the gap between preclinical results and human disease, improving the translatability of preclinical data and the design of clinical trials.

Nevertheless, there are some obstacles ahead of nanocarrier-based treatments for FLD before they reach common clinical practice. Reliable and reproducible manufacturing processes, long-term safety information, and proof of unequivocal clinical advantages over existing lifestyle or pharmacologic regimens are necessary [71]. In addition, FLD is a polygenic disease with a wide range from mild steatosis to NASH and cirrhosis, requiring individualized treatment that nanocarriers are uniquely capable of delivering. The ability to customize drug combinations, release rates, and targeting approaches renders nanocarrier systems highly versatile to the heterogeneous clinical manifestations of FLD [72]. Advances in nanocarrier-based drug delivery over the past few years have provided a solid foundation for the establishment of effective, targeted therapies for fatty liver disease. Preclinical studies in animal models have shown unprecedented efficacy in reducing steatosis, inflammation, and fibrosis, whereas early clinical efficacy in corresponding liver disease provides a template for translation [73]. Interdisciplinary research, the inclusion of sophisticated disease models, and well-designed clinical trials will be crucial to fulfilling the promise of nanocarrier-based therapies for the treatment of FLD. As the science continues to evolve, such new strategies could revolutionize treatment paradigms for FLD, offering a glimmer of hope to millions of individuals who suffer from this rapidly growing worldwide health burden [74].

Nanocarrier-based drug delivery systems have become a promising way to treat fatty liver diseases like NAFLD and MAFLD by making drugs more stable, available, and targeted. These systems work by targeting the liver specifically, controlling and responding to stimuli that trigger drug release, and increasing drug accumulation at disease sites, thereby reducing systemic side effects [75]. Recent developments include lipid-based nanocarriers, hybrid polymer-lipid systems, and gene therapy techniques, such as siRNA delivery to control fibrosis and inflammation. There are still issues with scaling them, getting them approved by regulators, and ensuring they are safe in the long run, even though they have a lot of potential. Ongoing clinical trials, including those evaluating BMS-986263, highlight the translational potential of these nanocarriers, offering prospects for personalized therapies and combination treatments to more effectively tackle fatty liver disease [76].

REGULATORY AND COMMERCIALIZATION ASPECTS

As nanocarrier drug delivery systems move towards clinical translation in fatty liver disease (FLD), commercialization and regulatory affairs are now the frontiers of their successful translation. Although the therapeutic promise of nanomedicines cannot be overlooked, the journey through the mature ecosystem of set guidelines, approval pathways, and challenges to clinical translation and market access is challenging. These commercial and regulatory issues must be addressed for effective, safe, and scalable nanocarrier-based therapeutics to ultimately reach patients. Worldwide, regulatory agencies, such as the United States' Food and Drug Administration (FDA), the European Medicines Agency (EMA), and country-specific agencies, are responsible for regulating the assessment, approval, and oversight of nanomedicines [77]. While no nanocarrier-based therapy is currently approved to treat FLD, regulatory guidelines for other nanomedicines, such as liposomal formulations, polymeric nanoparticles, and lipid-based RNA therapeutics, provide a general framework. The FDA does not consider "nanotechnology" or "nanomedicine" as a distinct regulatory category; nanocarrier-based pharmaceuticals are reviewed under the same processes as conventional drugs or biologics, with additional scrutiny for nanoscale features. The FDA Nanotechnology Task Force and companion guide documents highlight detailed characterization of the nanocarrier's physicochemical properties, including size distribution, surface charge, morphology, drug-loading efficacy, release profiles, and stability [78]. Furthermore, *in vitro* and *in vivo* pharmacokinetic, biodistribution, immunogenicity, and toxicity studies must be performed to determine how biological behavior is regulated by nanoscale properties.

Consequently, the EMA, in its Reflection Paper on Nanotechnology-based Medicinal Products, promotes pre-notification to regulatory authorities in light of product-specific issues. Many organizations believe in applying Quality by Design (QbD) principles to design robust, reproducible manufacturing processes. From the regulatory pathways' perspective, drug delivery systems mediated by nanocarrier-delivery would be new molecular entities (NMEs), generic nanomedicines (nanosimilars), or combination products, each with different regulatory requirements. For example, the 505(b)(2) pathway under US conditions provides a quick track for nanocarrier-based formulations of already approved drugs, and this could be beneficial for reformulation of established FLD treatments, such as pioglitazone or vitamin E as nanoparticle-mediated systems [79]. Nevertheless, several issues render clinical translation and market entry for FLD nanocarrier-based treatments problematic. Firstly, the inherent formulation complexity of nanocarriers impedes standardization, quality control, and scalability. Unlike small-molecule pharmaceuticals with clearly defined chemical structures, nanocarriers tend to be heterogeneous batches of particles, with size, shape, and surface chemistry liable to vary with slight modifications in the conditions used for production [80]. Batch-to-batch consistency is especially challenging but essential to regulatory compliance and patient safety. Scaling from laboratory to industrial scales while tightly controlling these parameters is technologically and resource-intensive.

Second, the long-term safety of nanoparticles is a regulatory issue. Chronic long-term diseases, such as FLD, might involve prolonged or repeated dosing, raising concerns of nanoparticle accumulation, biodegradation, and long-term potential toxicity. Regulatory agencies demand extensive long-term animal studies and finally human data to establish safety, leading to slow development and higher costs [81]. Furthermore, there is regulatory ambiguity regarding the classification of multifunctional or hybrid nanocarriers that combine therapeutic, diagnostic, or imaging functionalities (theranostics). These combination products can be regulated under several paradigms simultaneously, thereby posing a challenge to approval. From a commercialization perspective, manufacturing is costly, specialized equipment is required, and rigorous quality control renders nanomedicines more costly to produce than traditional drug products. Intellectual property (IP) is also multifaceted, as nanocarriers often involve more than one patented element, materials, targeting ligands, and encapsulating drugs, potentially involving companies in licensing issues or creating entry barriers. Additionally, clinician uptake and market acceptance depend on the provision of transparent clinical advantages, such as enhanced efficacy, improved safety profiles, or increased patient compliance compared to current therapies [82]. Since lifestyle interventions and low-cost oral therapies are now leading the treatment of FLD, payers and healthcare organizations will only be persuaded to pay more for more costly nanocarrier-based therapies by strong health-economic evidence.

MECHANISTIC CHALLENGES AND TRANSLATIONAL OPPORTUNITIES IN NANOCARRIER-BASED THERAPY FOR FATTY LIVER DISEASE

Fatty liver disease presents unique challenges for nanocarrier-based treatment because lipotoxicity, a pro-inflammatory environment, and growing fibrosis obstruct targeted delivery and therapeutic efficacy. Mechanistic developments targeting these specific pathophysiological features could significantly improve *in vivo* stability, site-specific drug release, and clinical translation.

Lipotoxicity

Excessive lipid accumulation in hepatocytes is a hallmark of fatty liver disease, triggering cellular stress pathways, mitochondrial dysfunction, and cell death, all of which significantly affect liver function. This pathological state may interfere with intracellular trafficking, controlled drug release, and nanocarrier uptake. Using nanocarriers with lipid-responsive release mechanisms, antioxidant co-therapies, or hepatocyte-targeting ligands, therapeutic medicines that reduce lipotoxic stress while preserving healthy liver cells can be selectively delivered to overcome these challenges.

Inflammatory Microenvironment

Chronic low-grade inflammation in FLD is characterized by immune cell recruitment, Kupffer cell activation, and elevated pro-inflammatory cytokines, creating a milieu that is not conducive to conventional medication delivery. Nanocarriers can deliver medications to specific sites, modulate immune responses, and reduce systemic side effects by responding to inflammatory cues, such as pH, reactive oxygen species, and cytokine gradients. Additionally, inflammatory-responsive or immune-cell-targeted nanocarriers enhance retention in disease sites, increasing therapy efficacy.

Fibrotic Progression

Physical and metabolic hurdles that prevent nanocarrier penetration and uniform drug distribution are driven by excessive extracellular matrix deposition and architectural distortion associated with increasing liver fibrosis. Mechanistic strategies, such as conjugation with fibrosis-targeting ligands, matrix metalloproteinase-responsive carriers, or nanocarriers that can remodel fibrotic tissue, can ultimately slow the disease's progression by increasing the bioavailability of therapeutic agents and enabling deeper tissue penetration.

Clinical Translation Opportunities

By designing nanocarriers with disease-specific pathophysiological cues, such as fibrosis, inflammation, and lipotoxicity, these technologies can deliver improved pharmacokinetics, controlled release, and greater specificity. In fatty liver disease, such rationally engineered carriers could enable precision therapeutics by reducing off-target toxicity, addressing *in vivo* stability issues, and bridging the gap between preclinical success and clinical use.

FUTURE PERSPECTIVES AND OPPORTUNITIES

The future of nanocarrier-mediated drug delivery for fatty liver disease (FLD) will be defined by pioneering innovations that can potentially enhance precision, efficacy, and personalization in treatment protocols. As heterogeneity in FLD becomes better appreciated, personalized nanomedicine offers a compelling prospect to optimize therapeutic interventions based on patients' individual profiles. Since FLD is etiologically multifactorial, from simple steatosis to non-alcoholic steatohepatitis (NASH), fibrosis, and cirrhosis, the patients can present with heterogeneous metabolic, genetic, and inflammatory contexts [83]. Nanocarriers enable the loading of multiple drugs, siRNAs, or therapeutic molecules into a single delivery system that can be tailored to the molecular and pathological characteristics of an individual patient. Advances in omics technologies (genomics, proteomics, and metabolomics) and in biomarkers associated with FLD development can guide the rational design of nanocarrier-based drug delivery systems, enabling the targeted delivery of therapeutics that address the specific pathological mechanisms involved in a given patient, such as lipid dysregulation, inflammation, or fibrosis. This approach maximizes therapeutic efficacy while minimizing off-target toxicity and redundant drug exposure, in accordance with the principles of precision medicine [84].

One promising field is combining diagnostics with nanotechnology to create theranostic systems that combine therapeutic and diagnostic capabilities within a single nanocarrier. Theranostic nanoparticles can deliver therapeutic agents while simultaneously enabling imaging or biomarker detection, thereby allowing real-time monitoring of disease progression, drug delivery, and treatment response. In FLD, this is possible using nanoparticles that can deliver anti-fibrotic drugs and visualize fibrotic tissue via magnetic resonance imaging (MRI) or fluorescent imaging [85]. Some of these include gold and iron oxide nanoparticles, which have imaging properties and can be functionalized for targeting specific liver cell populations and delivering therapeutic cargos. This dual role enables clinicians to make evidence-based decisions, *e.g.*, dose adjustments or between-therapy changes, based on dynamic feedback, thereby improving patient outcomes and minimizing trial-and-error in treatment regimens. Theranostic nanomedicine can be especially valuable for monitoring subtle progression from NAFLD to NASH, or for assessing fibrosis reversal during treatment [60]. Future-oriented, some upcoming trends have the potential to further propel nanocarrier-based therapeutics in FLD. The integration of machine learning and artificial intelligence can expedite the optimization, design, and forecasting of nanocarrier behavior. AI models can simulate intricate data to predict favorable nanoparticle composition, release profiles, and surface functionality, advancing towards improved, safer formulations with greater efficiency. Concurrently, nanobiointerfaces, the field of study that examines interfaces between nanomaterials and living systems, will provide further insights into nanoparticle-cell interactions, immune responses, and biodistribution patterns, enabling the rational design of highly targeted and biocompatible nanocarriers [86]. Emerging materials, such as stimuli-responsive polymers, biodegradable nanocomposites, and engineered exosomes, pave the way for more effective and adaptive delivery systems. Furthermore, the coupling between nanotechnology and 3D bioprinting is expected to enable the printing of personalized liver tissue models for patients, which may serve as sophisticated platforms for assessing nanocarrier performance and toxicity ex vivo. The integration of nanotechnology with personalized medicine, diagnostics, and emerging technologies promises significant advances for the future of FLD management. With more intradisciplinary studies on the horizon, nanocarrier-based systems are poised to provide not only more efficient treatments but also devices for accurate monitoring and tailored care, revolutionizing the treatment of liver disease at its very foundation [87].

DISCUSSION

Nanocarrier-based drug delivery systems are designed to address the complex pathophysiology of fatty liver disease (FLD), which poses distinct challenges not encountered in standard liver or tumor settings. FLD is characterized by hepatocellular lipotoxicity resulting from excessive lipid accumulation, which induces oxidative and endoplasmic reticulum stress. Nanocarriers can mitigate these effects by delivering antioxidants and metabolic modulators directly to hepatocytes [88]. The chronic inflammatory environment is mitigated by engineering nanocarriers that specifically transport anti-inflammatory agents to Kupffer cells and hepatocytes via receptor-mediated targeting, thereby reducing systemic toxicity. To fight progressive fibrosis, nanocarriers are modified to deliver antifibrotic agents, such as siRNA, to hepatic stellate cells, thereby directly targeting pathways that drive matrix deposition. Advanced nanocarriers also exhibit microenvironment-responsive release triggered by pH, redox states, or enzyme activity, which is typical of diseased liver tissue. This makes precision therapy possible. Combining genetic information about specific diseases enables the design of personalized nanocarriers that work better for treatment. This customized approach guarantees that nanocarriers enhance drug stability and bioavailability while precisely regulating the unique metabolic, inflammatory, and fibrotic processes in FLD, thereby optimizing therapeutic outcomes and minimizing off-target effects [89].

Nanocarrier-based drug delivery systems are specifically engineered to target the distinctive, multifactorial pathophysiology of fatty liver disease (FLD), characterized by hepatocellular lipotoxicity, a pro-inflammatory microenvironment, and advancing fibrosis. FLD nanocarriers differ from generic liver or tumor contexts because they use antioxidant-loaded carriers to reduce oxidative and ER stress in hepatocytes with excessive fat. They are designed to deliver anti-inflammatory drugs to Kupffer cells and hepatocytes via receptor-mediated targeting, thereby reducing systemic toxicity. Nanocarriers are also designed to target hepatic stellate cells to halt the progression of fibrosis using siRNA or antifibrotic drugs. Advanced nanocarriers can also respond to microenvironmental changes specific to FLD, such as pH or redox conditions. This makes it possible for drugs to be released at specific sites. Adding genetic predispositions (such as PNPLA3 and TM6SF2) to therapy makes it even more personalized, increasing its effectiveness while reducing side effects. This targeted design addresses the metabolic, inflammatory, and fibrotic characteristics of FLD, improving therapeutic results beyond broad liver-targeted strategies [90].

CONCLUSION

Nanocarrier-mediated drug delivery systems represent a novel area in the management of fatty liver disease (FLD), and with the assistance of nanoscale engineering, such sophisticated delivery systems have been shown to improve the bioavailability, targeted delivery, and sustained release of drugs and thus rectify the multifactorial pathophysiologic processes of alcoholic as well as non-alcoholic FLD. Preclinical research involving various nanocarriers, from liposomes and polymeric nanoparticles to dendrimers and exosomes, has provided strong evidence for their potential to alleviate hepatic steatosis, inflammation, and fibrosis via targeted hepatocyte delivery, as well as to influence critical molecular processes. Encouraging results from model systems and translational action of nanomedicines in other liver disorders highlight the therapeutic utility of nanocarriers in transforming the treatment paradigm in FLD. Despite such developments, there are real issues of clinical translation. Target specificity, biological barriers, long-term safety, scalability in production, and regulatory hurdles still hold back the clinical translation of FLD therapies based on nanocarriers. However, innovative strategies, including stimulus-responsive systems, surface modification, ligand conjugation, and multifunctional nanocarriers, are progressively overcoming these roadblocks, and safer, more efficient, and clinically translatable formulations are emerging. The evolving regulatory policies of agencies, such as the FDA and EMA, coupled with increasing industry experience in the manufacture of nanomedicines, herald a continued, yet gradual, advance towards commercialization. However, strong evidence of clinical efficacy, safety, and cost-effectiveness remains crucial to securing full-scale market uptake and clinician acceptance. Looking ahead, the fusion of nanotechnology with personal medicine and diagnostic platforms holds unprecedented potential to transform FLD treatment. Personalized nanomedicine, founded on patient-specific biomarkers and omics data, has the potential to deliver individualized regimens optimized for maximal efficacy and minimized side effects. Theranostic nanocarriers that deliver concomitant therapy and enable real-time disease monitoring hold promise for maximizing the specificity and responsiveness of treatment. Rising trends, such as artificial intelligence-based nanocarrier design, sophisticated nanobiointerface studies, and the development of smart, biodegradable, and hybrid delivery systems, will further enhance and extend the functions of nanomedicine. As interdisciplinary collaboration intensifies among scientists, doctors, industry, and regulators, nanocarrier-based therapeutics have the potential to deliver seamless, patient-focused solutions that could revolutionize the prevention, diagnosis, and treatment of fatty liver disease and, in turn, drive better outcomes for patients worldwide.

LIST OF ABBREVIATIONS

FLD	Fatty Liver Disease
NASH	Non-Alcoholic Steatohepatitis
AFLD	Alcoholic Fatty Liver Disease
NAFLD	Non-Alcoholic Fatty Liver Disease
ER	Endoplasmic Reticulum
TNF-α	Tumor Necrosis Factor-Alpha
IL-6	Interleukin-6
PNPLA3	Patatin-like Phospholipase Domain-Containing Protein 3
TM6SF2	Transmembrane 6 Superfamily Member 2
ASGPR	Asialoglycoprotein Receptor
siRNA	Small Interfering RNA
HSCs	Hepatic Stellate Cells
CTGF	Connective Tissue Growth Factor
PPARγ	Peroxisome Proliferator-Activated Receptor Gamma
MSCs	Mesenchymal Stem Cells
CCl_4	Carbon Tetrachloride
RES	Reticuloendothelial System
CARPA	Complement Activation-Related Pseudoallergy
ADME	Absorption, Distribution, Metabolism, Excretion
GMP	Good Manufacturing Practice
FDA	Food and Drug Administration
EMA	European Medicines Agency

QbD	Quality by Design
NME	New Molecular Entity
PEG	Polyethylene Glycol
PEGylation	Modification with Polyethylene Glycol
GalNAc	N-Acetylgalactosamine
MMPs	Matrix Metalloproteinases
NIR	Near-Infrared
MRI	Magnetic Resonance Imaging
AI	Artificial Intelligence
mRNA	Messenger RNA
RNAi	RNA Interference
MAFLD	Metabolic Associated Fatty Liver Disease
LNP	Lipid Nanoparticle
IP	Intellectual Property

REFERENCES

[1] Carrieri P, Mourad A, Marcellin F, *et al.* Knowledge of liver fibrosis stage among adults with NAFLD / NASH improves adherence to lifestyle changes. Liver Int 2022; 42(5): 984-94. [http://dx.doi.org/10.1111/liv.15209] [PMID: 35220673]

[2] Gao J, Karp JM, Langer R, Joshi N. The future of drug delivery. Chem Mater. 2023; 35(2): 359□363 [http://dx.doi.org/10.1021/acs.chemmater.2c03003] [PMID: 37799624]

[3] De R, Mahata MK, Kim KT. Structure□based varieties of polymeric nanocarriers and influences of their physicochemical properties on drug delivery profiles. Adv Sci (Weinh) 2022; 9(10): 2105373. [http://dx.doi.org/10.1002/advs.202105373] [PMID: 35112798]

[4] Meng X, Zhu G, Yang YG, Sun T. Targeted delivery strategies: The interactions and applications of nanoparticles in liver diseases. Biomed Pharmacother 2024; 175: 116702. [http://dx.doi.org/10.1016/j.biopha.2024.116702] [PMID: 38729052]

[5] Zhou L, Li Y, Liang Q, Liu J, Liu Y. Combination therapy based on targeted nano drug co-delivery systems for liver fibrosis treatment: a review. J Drug Target 2022; 30(6): 577-88. [http://dx.doi.org/10.1080/1061186X.2022.2044485] [PMID: 35179094]

[6] Han AL. Association of cardiovascular risk factors and metabolic syndrome with non-alcoholic and alcoholic fatty liver disease: a retrospective analysis. BMC Endocr Disord 2021; 21: 91. [http://dx.doi.org/10.1186/s12902-021-00758-x] [PMID: 33933056]

[7] Lee KC, Wu PS, Lin HC. Pathogenesis and treatment of non-alcoholic steatohepatitis and its fibrosis. Clin Mol Hepatol 2023; 29(1): 77-98. [http://dx.doi.org/10.3350/cmh.2022.0237] [PMID: 36226471]

[8] Palma R, Pronio A, Romeo M, *et al.* The role of insulin resistance in fueling NAFLD pathogenesis: from molecular mechanisms to clinical implications. J Clin Med 2022; 11(13): 3649. [http://dx.doi.org/10.3390/jcm11133649] [PMID: 35806934]

[9] Guan H, Zhang X, Kuang M, Yu J. The gut–liver axis in immune remodeling of hepatic cirrhosis. Front Immunol 2022; 13: 946628. [http://dx.doi.org/10.3389/fimmu.2022.946628] [PMID: 37408838]

[10] Kisseleva T, Brenner D. Molecular and cellular mechanisms of liver fibrosis and its regression. Nat Rev Gastroenterol Hepatol 2021; 18(3): 151-66.
[http://dx.doi.org/10.1038/s41575-020-00372-7] [PMID: 33128017]

[11] Zhang C, Yang M. Current options and future directions for NAFLD and NASH treatment. Int J Mol Sci 2021; 22(14): 7571.
[http://dx.doi.org/10.3390/ijms22147571] [PMID: 34299189]

[12] Qu W, Ma T, Cai J, *et al.* Liver fibrosis and MAFLD: from molecular aspects to novel pharmacological strategies. Front Med (Lausanne) 2021; 8: 761538.
[http://dx.doi.org/10.3389/fmed.2021.761538] [PMID: 34746195]

[13] Wang Q, Jia S, Wang Z, *et al.* Nanogene editing drug delivery systems in the treatment of liver fibrosis. Front Med (Lausanne) 2024; 11: 1418786.
[http://dx.doi.org/10.3389/fmed.2024.1418786] [PMID: 39386741]

[14] Park H, Otte A, Park K. Evolution of drug delivery systems: From 1950 to 2020 and beyond. J Control Release 2022; 342: 53-65.
[http://dx.doi.org/10.1016/j.jconrel.2021.12.030] [PMID: 34971694]

[15] Waheed I, Ali A, Tabassum H, Khatoon N, Lai WF, Zhou X. Lipid-based nanoparticles as drug delivery carriers for cancer therapy. Front Oncol 2024; 14: 1296091.
[http://dx.doi.org/10.3389/fonc.2024.1296091] [PMID: 38660132]

[16] Kumari L, Choudhari Y, Patel P, *et al.* Advancement in solubilization approaches: A step towards bioavailability enhancement of poorly soluble drugs. Life (Basel) 2023; 13(5): 1099.
[http://dx.doi.org/10.3390/life13051099] [PMID: 37240744]

[17] Athanasopoulou F, Manolakakis M, Vernia S, Kamaly N. Nanodrug delivery systems for metabolic chronic liver diseases: advances and perspectives. Nanomedicine (Lond) 2023; 18(1): 67-84.
[http://dx.doi.org/10.2217/nnm-2022-0261] [PMID: 36896958]

[18] Al Bostami RD, Abuwatfa WH, Husseini GA. Recent advances in nanoparticle-based co-delivery systems for cancer therapy. Nanomaterials (Basel) 2022; 12(15): 2672.
[http://dx.doi.org/10.3390/nano12152672] [PMID: 35957103]

[19] Thirumal V, Aravindhan V, Niranjanasree AC. Liposomal carriers: development, evaluation, applications with its regulatory aspects. World J Adv Res Rev 2023; 20(3): 324-44.
[http://dx.doi.org/10.30574/wjarr.2023.20.3.2461]

[20] Matalqah S, Lafi Z, Al-Kabariti AY. A recent review of PLGA-PEG hybrid nanoparticles for anticancer and anti-inflammatory applications. Jordan J Pharm Sci 2025; 18(1): 180-95.
[http://dx.doi.org/10.35516/jjps.v18i1.2737]

[21] Viegas C, Patrício AB, Prata JM, Nadhman A, Chintamaneni PK, Fonte P. Solid lipid nanoparticles *vs.* nanostructured lipid carriers: a comparative review. Pharmaceutics 2023; 15(6): 1593.
[http://dx.doi.org/10.3390/pharmaceutics15061593] [PMID: 37376042]

[22] Al-Thani AN, Jan AG, Abbas M, Geetha M, Sadasivuni KK. Nanoparticles in cancer theragnostic and drug delivery: A comprehensive review. Life Sci 2024; 352: 122899.
[http://dx.doi.org/10.1016/j.lfs.2024.122899] [PMID: 38992574]

[23] Kozlov D, Rodimova S, Kuznetsova D. The role of MicroRNAs in liver functioning: from biogenesis to therapeutic approaches 2023.
[http://dx.doi.org/10.17691/stm2023.15.5.06]

[24] Li J, Chen C, Xia T. Understanding nanomaterial–liver interactions to facilitate the development of safer nanoapplications. Adv Mater 2022; 34(11): 2106456.
[http://dx.doi.org/10.1002/adma.202106456] [PMID: 35029313]

[25] Nie H, Qiu B, Yang QX, *et al.* Effect of gal/GalNAc regioisomerism in galactosylated liposomes on asialoglycoprotein receptor-mediated hepatocyte-selective targeting *in vivo*. J Liposome Res 2021;

31(1): 79-89.
[http://dx.doi.org/10.1080/08982104.2019.1682606] [PMID: 31691619]

[26] Jiang Y, Li Y, Fu X, *et al.* Interplay between G protein-coupled receptors and nanotechnology. Acta Biomater 2023; 169: 1-18.
[http://dx.doi.org/10.1016/j.actbio.2023.07.049] [PMID: 37517621]

[27] Liu J, Liu J, Mu W, *et al.* Delivery strategy to enhance the therapeutic efficacy of Liver Fibrosis *via* Nanoparticle Drug Delivery systems. ACS Nano 2024; 18(32): 20861-85.
[http://dx.doi.org/10.1021/acsnano.4c02380] [PMID: 39082637]

[28] Subroto E, Andoyo R, Indiarto R. Solid lipid nanoparticles: Review of the current research on encapsulation and delivery systems for active and antioxidant compounds. Antioxidants 2023; 12(3): 633.
[http://dx.doi.org/10.3390/antiox12030633] [PMID: 36978881]

[29] Hussain S, Ashafaq M, Alshahrani S, *et al.* Hepatoprotective effect of curcumin nano-lipid carrier against cypermethrin toxicity by countering the oxidative, inflammatory, and apoptotic changes in wistar rats. Molecules 2023; 28(2): 881.
[http://dx.doi.org/10.3390/molecules28020881] [PMID: 36677938]

[30] Molinaro G. Polymeric and lipid-based nanoparticles for anti-inflammatory, anti-fibrotic, and regenerative applications in tendon diseases. 2025. Available from: http://hdl.handle.net/10138/590076

[31] Makouie S, Bryś J, Małajowicz J, *et al.* A comprehensive review of silymarin extraction and liposomal encapsulation techniques for potential applications in food. Appl Sci (Basel) 2024; 14(18): 8477.
[http://dx.doi.org/10.3390/app14188477]

[32] Alanazi A, Nagi MN, Alhareth DY, *et al.* Crosstalk of TNF-α, IFN-γ, NF-kB, STAT1 and redox signaling in lipopolysaccharide/d-galactosamine/dimethylsulfoxide-induced fulminant hepatic failure in mice. Saudi Pharm J 2023; 31(3): 370-81.
[http://dx.doi.org/10.1016/j.jsps.2023.01.005] [PMID: 37026046]

[33] Mariadoss AVA, Sivakumar AS, Lee CH, Kim SJ. Diabetes mellitus and diabetic foot ulcer: Etiology, biochemical and molecular based treatment strategies via gene and nanotherapy. Biomed Pharmacother 2022; 151: 113134.
[http://dx.doi.org/10.1016/j.biopha.2022.113134] [PMID: 35617802]

[34] Lu X, Guo H, Wei X, *et al.* Current status and prospect of delivery vehicle based on mesenchymal stem cell-derived exosomes in liver diseases. Int J Nanomedicine 2023; 18: 2873-90.
[http://dx.doi.org/10.2147/IJN.S404925] [PMID: 37283714]

[35] Shi J, Zhu X, Yang JB. Advances and challenges in molecular understanding, early detection, and targeted treatment of liver cancer. World J Hepatol 2025; 17(1): 102273.
[http://dx.doi.org/10.4254/wjh.v17.i1.102273] [PMID: 39871899]

[36] Ezhilarasan D, Shree Harini K. Nanodrug delivery: Strategies to circumvent nanoparticle trafficking by Kupffer cells in the liver. J Drug Deliv Sci Technol 2023; 86: 104731.
[http://dx.doi.org/10.1016/j.jddst.2023.104731]

[37] Sahoo PK, Mishra AK, Pandey M, Dewangan HK, Sl N. A comprehensive review on liver targeting: Emphasis on nanotechnology-based molecular targets and receptors mediated approaches. Curr Drug Targets 2022; 23(15): 1381-405.
[http://dx.doi.org/10.2174/1389450123666220906091432] [PMID: 36065923]

[38] Tafech B, Mohabatpour F, Hedtrich S. Surface modification of lipid nanoparticles for gene therapy. J Gene Med 2024; 26(1): e3642.
[http://dx.doi.org/10.1002/jgm.3642] [PMID: 38043928]

[39] Oladipo AO, Lebelo SL, Msagati TAM. Nanocarrier design–function relationship: The prodigious role of properties in regulating biocompatibility for drug delivery applications. Chem Biol Interact 2023; 377: 110466.

[http://dx.doi.org/10.1016/j.cbi.2023.110466] [PMID: 37004951]

[40] Pradhan R, Dey A, Taliyan R, Puri A, Kharavtekar S, Dubey SK. Recent advances in targeted nanocarriers for the management of triple negative breast cancer. Pharmaceutics 2023; 15(1): 246. [http://dx.doi.org/10.3390/pharmaceutics15010246] [PMID: 36678877]

[41] Saxena S, Sharma S, Kumar G, Thakur S. Unravelling the complexity of CARPA: a review of emerging advancements in therapeutic strategies. Arch Dermatol Res 2025; 317(1): 439. [http://dx.doi.org/10.1007/s00403-025-03971-z] [PMID: 39971823]

[42] Kardani SL. Nanocarrier-based formulations: Regulatory Challenges, Ethical and Safety Considerations in Pharmaceuticals. Asian J Pharm 2024; 18(2) [http://dx.doi.org/10.22377/ajp.v18i02.5444]

[43] Bilal M, Qamar SA, Ashraf SS, Rodríguez-Couto S, Iqbal HMN. Robust nanocarriers to engineer nanobiocatalysts for bioprocessing applications. Adv Colloid Interface Sci 2021; 293: 102438. [http://dx.doi.org/10.1016/j.cis.2021.102438] [PMID: 34023567]

[44] Çetintaş HC, Tonbul H, Şahin A, Çapan Y. Regulatory guidelines of the US Food and Drug Administration and the European Medicines Agency for actively targeted nanomedicines. In: Drug Delivery with Targeted Nanoparticles. 1st ed. Singapore: Jenny Stanford Publishing; 2021. p. 17

[45] Cai X, Jin M, Yao L, *et al.* Physicochemical properties, pharmacokinetics, toxicology and application of nanocarriers. J Mater Chem B Mater Biol Med 2023; 11(4): 716-33. [http://dx.doi.org/10.1039/D2TB02001G] [PMID: 36594785]

[46] AbouSamra MM. Liposomal nano-carriers mediated targeting of liver disorders: mechanisms and applications. J Liposome Res 2024; 34(4): 728-43. [http://dx.doi.org/10.1080/08982104.2024.2377085] [PMID: 38988127]

[47] Majumder J, Minko T. Multifunctional and stimuli-responsive nanocarriers for targeted therapeutic delivery. Expert Opin Drug Deliv 2021; 18(2): 205-27. [http://dx.doi.org/10.1080/17425247.2021.1828339] [PMID: 32969740]

[48] Luo S, Lv Z, Yang Q, Chang R, Wu J. Research progress on stimulus-responsive polymer nanocarriers for cancer treatment. Pharmaceutics 2023; 15(7): 1928. [http://dx.doi.org/10.3390/pharmaceutics15071928] [PMID: 37514114]

[49] Pelaz B, del Pino P, Maffre P, *et al.* Surface functionalization of nanoparticles with polyethylene glycol: effects on protein adsorption and cellular uptake. In: Bio-Nano Interfaces. Singapore: Jenny Stanford Publishing; 2024. p. 861□894.

[50] Haripriyaa M, Suthindhiran K. Pharmacokinetics of nanoparticles: current knowledge, future directions and its implications in drug delivery. Future J Pharm Sci 2023; 9(1): 113. [http://dx.doi.org/10.1186/s43094-023-00569-y]

[51] Li Q, Wen C, Yang J, *et al.* Zwitterionic biomaterials. Chem Rev 2022; 122(23): 17073-154. [http://dx.doi.org/10.1021/acs.chemrev.2c00344] [PMID: 36201481]

[52] Shishir MRI, Gowd V, Suo H, *et al.* Advances in smart delivery of food bioactive compounds using stimuli□responsive carriers: Responsive mechanism, contemporary challenges, and prospects. Compr Rev Food Sci Food Saf 2021; 20(6): 5449-88. [http://dx.doi.org/10.1111/1541-4337.12851] [PMID: 34668321]

[53] Vasvani S, Bardhan R, Uthaman S, Park I-K. pH-responsive polymer prodrug micelles for anti-cancer therapy. In: Smart Systems in Biotechnology. Boca Raton: CRC Press. 2024; pp. 201-24.

[54] Meng X, Shen Y, Zhao H, Lu X, Wang Z, Zhao Y. Redox-manipulating nanocarriers for anticancer drug delivery: a systematic review. J Nanobiotechnology 2024; 22(1): 587. [http://dx.doi.org/10.1186/s12951-024-02859-w] [PMID: 39342211]

[55] Kong X, Zheng T, Wang Z, *et al.* Remote actuation and on-demand activation of biomaterials pre-incorporated with physical cues for bone repair. Theranostics 2024; 14(11): 4438-61.

[http://dx.doi.org/10.7150/thno.97610] [PMID: 39113795]

[56] Song J, Vikulina AS, Parakhonskiy BV, Skirtach AG. Hierarchy of hybrid materials. Part-II: The place of organics-*on*-inorganics in it, their composition and applications. Front Chem 2023; 11: 1078840. [http://dx.doi.org/10.3389/fchem.2023.1078840] [PMID: 36762189]

[57] Slezak A, Chang K, Hossainy S, *et al.* Therapeutic synthetic and natural materials for immunoengineering. Chem Soc Rev 2024; 53(4): 1789-822. [http://dx.doi.org/10.1039/D3CS00805C] [PMID: 38170619]

[58] Marques L, Costa B, Pereira M, *et al.* Advancing precision medicine: a review of innovative in silico approaches for drug development, clinical pharmacology and personalized healthcare. Pharmaceutics 2024; 16(3): 332. [http://dx.doi.org/10.3390/pharmaceutics16030332] [PMID: 38543226]

[59] Tesoro L, Hernandez I, Saura M, Badimón L, Zaragoza C. Novel cutting edge nano-strategies to address old long-standing complications in cardiovascular diseases. A comprehensive review. Eur J Clin Invest 2024; 54(7): e14208. [http://dx.doi.org/10.1111/eci.14208] [PMID: 38622800]

[60] Singh S, Sharma N, Shukla S, *et al.* Understanding the potential role of nanotechnology in liver fibrosis: a paradigm in therapeutics. Molecules 2023; 28(6): 2811. [http://dx.doi.org/10.3390/molecules28062811] [PMID: 36985782]

[61] Chopra H, Dey PS, Das D, *et al.* Curcumin nanoparticles as promising therapeutic agents for drug targets. Molecules 2021; 26(16): 4998. [http://dx.doi.org/10.3390/molecules26164998] [PMID: 34443593]

[62] Maryam T, Rana NF, Alshahrani SM, *et al.* Silymarin encapsulated liposomal formulation: an effective treatment modality against copper toxicity associated liver dysfunction and neurobehavioral abnormalities in wistar rats. Molecules 2023; 28(3): 1514. [http://dx.doi.org/10.3390/molecules28031514] [PMID: 36771180]

[63] Zhou JE, Sun L, Liu L, *et al.* Hepatic macrophage targeted siRNA lipid nanoparticles treat non-alcoholic steatohepatitis. J Control Release 2022; 343: 175-86. [http://dx.doi.org/10.1016/j.jconrel.2022.01.038] [PMID: 35092721]

[64] Cruz DRD, Zheng A, Debele T, Larson P, Dion GR, Park YC. Drug delivery systems for wound healing treatment of upper airway injury. Expert Opin Drug Deliv 2024; 21(4): 573-91. [http://dx.doi.org/10.1080/17425247.2024.2340653] [PMID: 38588553]

[65] Moghadasi S, Elveny M, Rahman HS, *et al.* RETRACTED ARTICLE: A paradigm shift in cell-free approach: the emerging role of MSCs-derived exosomes in regenerative medicine. J Transl Med 2021; 19(1): 302. [http://dx.doi.org/10.1186/s12967-021-02980-6] [PMID: 34253242]

[66] Cheng Q, Li R, He Y, Zhu Y, Kang Y, Ji X. Genetically engineered cellular nanovesicles: Theories, design and perspective. Adv Funct Mater 2024; 34(46): 2407842. [http://dx.doi.org/10.1002/adfm.202407842]

[67] Ramírez-Cortés F, Ménová P. Hepatocyte targeting *via* the asialoglycoprotein receptor. RSC Medicinal Chemistry. 2025. [http://dx.doi.org/10.1039/D4MD00652F]

[68] Mallick AM, Tripathi A, Mishra S, *et al.* Emerging approaches for enabling RNAi therapeutics. Chem Asian J 2022; 17(16): e202200451. [http://dx.doi.org/10.1002/asia.202200451] [PMID: 35689534]

[69] Tang R, Li R, Li H, *et al.* Design of hepatic targeted drug delivery systems for natural products: insights into nomenclature revision of nonalcoholic fatty liver disease. ACS Nano 2021; 15(11): 17016-46. [http://dx.doi.org/10.1021/acsnano.1c02158] [PMID: 34705426]

[70] Paradiso A, Volpi M, Rinoldi C, *et al. In vitro* functional models for human liver diseases and drug screening: beyond animal testing. Biomater Sci 2023; 11(9): 2988-3015. [http://dx.doi.org/10.1039/D1BM01872H] [PMID: 36468579]

[71] Krishnaswamy S. Phytopharmaceutical biotechnology: integration of botany, pharmacology and plant biotechnology to deliver the best therapeutic potential of herbs. In: Concepts in Pharmaceutical Biotechnology and Drug Development. Cham: Springer; 2024. p. 437□464

[72] Abou Assi R, Abdulbaqi IM, Siok Yee C. The evaluation of drug delivery nanocarrier development and pharmacological briefing for metabolic-associated fatty liver disease (MAFLD): an update. Pharmaceuticals (Basel) 2021; 14(3): 215. [http://dx.doi.org/10.3390/ph14030215] [PMID: 33806527]

[73] Addissouky TA, Ali MMA, El Tantawy El Sayed I, *et al.* Preclinical promise and clinical challenges for innovative therapies targeting liver fibrogenesis. Arch Gastroenterol Res 2023; 4(1): 14-23. [http://dx.doi.org/10.33696/Gastroenterology.4.044]

[74] Mohammadi AT, Far YK, Mohammadaein H, *et al.* Unveiling the invisible: A journey through the landscape of disease. Nobel Sciences 2024.

[75] Khurana A, Hartmann P. Gut microbiome-specific nanoparticle-based therapeutics for liver diseases. World J Gastroenterol 2025; 31(27): 109105. [http://dx.doi.org/10.3748/wjg.v31.i27.109105] [PMID: 40741099]

[76] Qosa H, de Oliveira CHMC, Cizza G, *et al.* Pharmacokinetics, safety, and tolerability of BMS□986263, a lipid nanoparticle containing HSP47 siRNA, in participants with hepatic impairment. Clin Transl Sci 2023; 16(10): 1791-802. [http://dx.doi.org/10.1111/cts.13581] [PMID: 37654022]

[77] Pimenta C, Bettiol V, Alencar-Silva T, *et al.* Advanced therapies and regulatory framework in different areas of the globe: past, present, and future. Clin Ther 2021; 43(5): e103-38. [http://dx.doi.org/10.1016/j.clinthera.2021.02.006] [PMID: 33892966]

[78] Tripathi D, Pandey P, Sharma S, Rai AK, Prabhu B H M. Advances in nanomaterials for precision drug delivery: Insights into pharmacokinetics and toxicity. Bioimpacts 2024; 15(1): 30573. [http://dx.doi.org/10.34172/bi.30573] [PMID: 40256227]

[79] Demetzos C. Nanosimilars: a scientific or a regulatory debate? AAPS J 2024; 26: 74. [http://dx.doi.org/10.1208/s12248-024-00942-6]

[80] Zhang W, Taheri-Ledari R, Ganjali F, *et al.* Effects of morphology and size of nanoscale drug carriers on cellular uptake and internalization process: a review. RSC Advances 2022; 13(1): 80-114. [http://dx.doi.org/10.1039/D2RA06888E] [PMID: 36605676]

[81] Chávez-López L, Carballo-López GI, del Carmen Lugo-Ibarra K, Castro-Ceseña AB. A comprehensive framework for managing metabolic dysfunction-associated steatotic liver disease: analyzing novel risk factors and advances in nanotechnology-based treatments and diagnosis. RSC Medicinal Chemistry 2024.

[82] Medlinskiene K, Tomlinson J, Marques I, Richardson S, Stirling K, Petty D. Barriers and facilitators to the uptake of new medicines into clinical practice: a systematic review. BMC Health Serv Res 2021; 21(1): 1198. [http://dx.doi.org/10.1186/s12913-021-07196-4] [PMID: 34740338]

[83] Hamdy NM, Basalious EB, El-Sisi MG, *et al.* Advancements in current one-size-fits-all therapies compared to future treatment innovations for better improved chemotherapeutic outcomes: a step-toward personalized medicine. Curr Med Res Opin 2024; 40(11): 1943-61. [http://dx.doi.org/10.1080/03007995.2024.2416985] [PMID: 39412377]

[84] Mitchell MJ, Billingsley MM, Haley RM, Wechsler ME, Peppas NA, Langer R. Engineering precision nanoparticles for drug delivery. Nat Rev Drug Discov 2021; 20(2): 101-24. [http://dx.doi.org/10.1038/s41573-020-0090-8] [PMID: 33277608]

[85] Xue Y, Gao Y, Meng F, Luo L. Recent progress of nanotechnology-based theranostic systems in cancer treatments. Cancer Biol Med 2021; 18(2): 336-51.
[http://dx.doi.org/10.20892/j.issn.2095-3941.2020.0510] [PMID: 33861527]

[86] Wang J, Zhao Y, Nie G. Intelligent nanomaterials for cancer therapy: recent progresses and future possibilities. Medical Review 2023; 3(4): 321-42.
[http://dx.doi.org/10.1515/mr-2023-0028] [PMID: 38235406]

[87] Kenchegowda M, Rahamathulla M, Hani U, *et al.* Smart nanocarriers as an emerging platform for cancer therapy: A review. Molecules 2021; 27(1): 146.
[http://dx.doi.org/10.3390/molecules27010146] [PMID: 35011376]

[88] Flessa CM, Kyrou I, Nasiri-Ansari N, Kaltsas G, Kassi E, Randeva HS. Endoplasmic reticulum stress in nonalcoholic (metabolic associated) fatty liver disease (NAFLD/MAFLD). J Cell Biochem 2022; 123(10): 1585-606.
[http://dx.doi.org/10.1002/jcb.30247] [PMID: 35490371]

[89] Wang Y, Deng T, Liu X, *et al.* Smart nanoplatforms responding to the tumor microenvironment for precise drug delivery in cancer therapy. Int J Nanomedicine 2024; 19: 6253-77.
[http://dx.doi.org/10.2147/IJN.S459710] [PMID: 38911497]

[90] Caddeo A, Romeo S. Precision medicine and nucleotide-based therapeutics to treat steatotic liver disease. Clin Mol Hepatol 2025; 31 (Suppl.): S76-93.
[http://dx.doi.org/10.3350/cmh.2024.0438] [PMID: 39103998]

CHAPTER 15

Emerging Trends and Future Perspectives for Fatty Liver Disease Management

Vinod Kumar Gauttam[1], **Kavita Munjal**[2,*], **Arushi**[3], **Sheelu Singh**[4] and **Kunal Nepali**[5]

[1] *SGT College of Pharmacy, SGT University, Gurugram, Haryana, India*

[2] *Amity Institute of Pharmacy, Amity University, Noida, Uttar Pradesh, India*

[3] *RIMS Split Campus, Motherhood University, Roorkee, Uttarakhand, India*

[4] *IES Institute of Pharmacy, IES University, Bhopal, Madhya Pradesh, India*

[5] *School of Pharmacy, Taipei Medical University, Taipei, Taiwan*

Abstract: The term "fatty liver" describes the buildup of triglycerides in the hepatocytes, which can result in steatohepatitis and is linked to a number of illnesses, including type 2 diabetes, elevated oxidative stress, inflammation, obesity, heart disease, and liver disease, especially metabolic dysfunction associated with fatty liver disease. This may then develop into cirrhosis and ultimately a higher chance of hepatocellular carcinoma (HCC) development. Fatty liver disease appears in two main types: alcoholic liver disease and non alcoholic liver disease, which may develop into cirrhosis, fibrosis, and hepatocellular cancer. Although liver biopsies are the gold standard for assessing fat and determining the extent of fibrosis, they are invasive and cannot be used in large patient groups. Traditional methods, such as ultrasound, are more subjective and yield qualitative evaluations of fat. Furthermore, its medical significance needs to be re-evaluated, as it may be challenging to detect inflated hepatocytes with limited biopsied specimens. Body fluid indicators and less invasive imaging techniques are required because repeated liver biopsies to evaluate histological NAFLD activity for therapy response are also unfeasible. The significance of advanced fibrosis as a factor influencing the outcome of non-alcoholic fatty liver disease has been highlighted by recent longitudinal observational studies. A number of clinical trials are underway to develop a first-in-class medication, despite the significant heterogeneity of NAFLD with respect to underlying disease, patient age, and fibrosis stage. To address unmet medical needs, this chapter provides an overview of the current state and future prospects of fatty liver disease research.

Keywords: Fatty liver, Fibrosis, Hepatocytes, Hepatocellular cancer.

[*] **Corresponding author Kavita Munjal:** Amity Institute of Pharmacy, Amity University, Noida, Uttar Pradesh - 201301, India; E-mail: kavitamunjal914@gmail.com

Anjali Sharma, Devkant Sharma, Ajmer Singh Grewal, Geeta Deswal & Ganga Reddy Velma (Eds.)

INTRODUCTION

Overview of Fatty Liver Disease

The term "fatty liver" refers to the accumulation of triglycerides in hepatocytes, which can lead to steatohepatitis [1]. Subsequent development of liver cirrhosis and hepatocellular carcinoma (HCC) may occur. Fatty liver disease appears in two main types: non-alcoholic fatty liver disease (NAFLD), which is primarily associated with insulin resistance and metabolic syndrome, and alcoholic fatty liver disease, which is induced by chronic alcohol consumption. The frequency of NAFLD in India has been shown to range from 9 to 53%, making fatty liver a major global epidemic. Given India's enormous population, fatty liver can have a detrimental effect on the country's limited resources and place a significant strain on the healthcare system [2]. The frequency of NAFLD in India has been shown to range from 9 to 53%, making fatty liver a major global epidemic. Given India's enormous population, fatty liver can have a detrimental effect on the country's limited resources and place a significant strain on the healthcare system [3]. The liver can store fat for several reasons, as shown in Fig. (**1**).

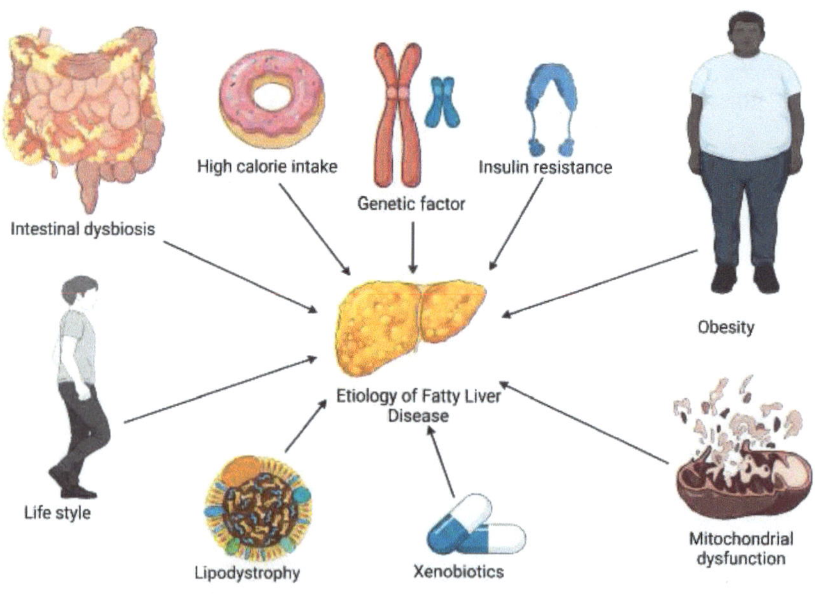

Fig. (1). Etiology of fatty liver disease.

Stellate cells can be activated by oxidative stress in hepatocytes, leading to inflammation and collagen synthesis. In the 19th century, pathologists began to understand the importance of higher fat deposition in the liver. Numerous extensive studies conducted by American and European pathologists over the 20th century have shown links between cirrhosis and hepatic steatosis and alcohol, diabetes, and obesity [4]. The 1980s Mayo Clinic study is credited with introducing the term "NASH" into the fatty liver disease nomenclature, even though it was not the first to use the term. In the study on 20 individuals with liver biopsies, Ludwig *et al*. found that 90% of them were obese, 65% were female, 25% had diabetes and/or hyperlipidemia, and 15% had hypertension. Over the next ten years, the concept of NAFLD gained acceptance, in large part due to pathologists' contributions to clinico-pathologic studies [5]. According to these studies, 2.8% of the U.S. population had "unexplained" elevations in liver tests. In the latter study, an elevated body mass index (BMI) accounted for 68% of these instances [6]. These findings highlight the usefulness of tissue evaluation in identifying non-fatty entities, such as diabetic hepatosclerosis. Significant steatosis is not observed in either of these conditions [7]. This chapter covers the types, pathophysiology, and treatment of fatty liver disease.

Types of Fatty Liver Diseases

There are various types of fatty liver disease [8]. Some of them are mentioned in Fig. (**2**), and their detailed introduction is discussed as follows:

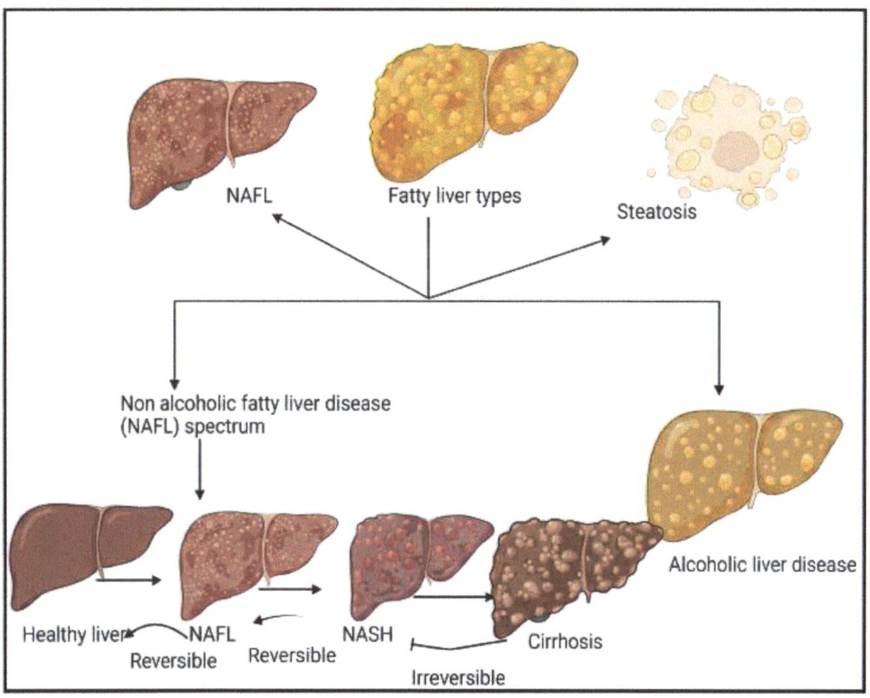

Fig. (2). Types of fatty liver disease.

Simple Fatty Liver Disease:

A federal organisation describes simple fatty liver as having fat in the liver without seriously harming the liver cells [9].

NAFL Disease:

NAFLD refers to a set of liver illnesses that affect nondrinkers, including cirrhosis, NASH, and hepatic steatosis. NAFLD affects all age groups and ethnicities, making it the second most significant cause of mortality in the general population. Currently, the high prevalence and unsatisfactory clinical outcomes lead to a significant economic burden on many countries. Unfortunately, there is currently no effective therapy for the illness [10].

Steatosis

It occurs when an excess amount of fat builds up inside the liver [11].

Alcoholic Fatty Liver Disease:

Alcoholic liver refers to the buildup of fats in the liver caused by alcohol intake [12].

PATHOPHYSIOLOGY OF HEPATIC STEATOSIS

Hepatic steatosis is a hallmark of fatty liver disease; other symptoms may include varying degrees of hepatocyte death, inflammation, and, in some cases, fibrosis. Hepatic lipid buildup in the context of obesity is caused by a number of reasons. First, gaining weight is linked to a noticeable increase in adipose tissue, which causes adipocyte malfunction and ultimately death. When adipose tissue malfunctions, cytokines that promote insulin resistance are upregulated, leading to local inflammation. Insulin resistance impairs adipocytes' ability to store fat, leading to the release of free fatty acids into the circulation and their absorption by other organs, such as the liver [13].

Obesity-related adipose tissue dysfunction leads the liver to produce more circulating free fatty acids, and insulin compensates for systemic insulin resistance. The transporters fatty acid transport protein 5 (FATP5; also known as bile acyl-CoA synthetase) and CD, both of which are increased in obesity, facilitate hepatocyte uptake of these fatty acids [14]. Hepatocyte fatty acid buildup stimulates triglyceride production. This mechanism generates diacylglycerol intermediates that inhibit hepatic insulin signalling by activating protein kinase Cε. Insulin resistance in hepatocytes enhances glucose synthesis, elevating blood sugar levels and stimulating further compensatory insulin production. Dietary nutrients contribute to hepatic steatosis by promoting triglyceride production. Dietary sugars are converted to fatty acids through de novo lipogenesis (DNL), and these fatty acids are subsequently taken up by the liver and adipose tissue. Dietary carbohydrates and fats accumulate in the liver [15].

NAFLD Involves the Gut-Liver Axis

Interactions between the liver and the intestines are increasingly identified as significant factors in NAFLD [16]. Changes in the gut microbiota that increase nutritional extraction from food have been linked to obesity, a significant risk factor for non-alcoholic fatty liver disease. Although no single microbiome profile is associated with NAFLD, the intestinal microbiota of individuals with the disease differs significantly from that of healthy individuals. Intestinal dysbiosis can exacerbate liver disease by weakening the intestinal barrier, allowing the passage of bacteria or bacterial products [17]. Beneficial nutrients, such as choline, which are necessary for hepatic lipid regulation, can be eliminated at the luminal level due to dysbiosis [18]. First, increased fatty acid metabolism places stress on hepatocyte mitochondria, leading to mitochondrial uncoupling, reactive oxygen species (ROS) production, and JNK (Jun N-terminal Kinase) activation. The initiation of the feed-forward loop involving reactive oxygen species (ROS) generation and c-Jun N-terminal kinase (JNK) activation results in cell death, mitochondrial damage, and reduced ATP synthesis [19].

Fibrosis and Inflammation in Fatty Livers

One of the main characteristics of NASH is immune system activation. The traditional hepatic inflammatory effectors in NASH, including macrophages, Kupffer cells, and natural killer T cells, are linked to the progression of liver disease [20]. These compounds also activate TLRs and inflammasomes in target immune cells, resulting in the production of a variety of cytokines [21].

Hepatic Fibrosis as a Bad Prognosis for NASH

The activation of hepatic stellate cells leads to fibrogenesis. Stellate cells may also be triggered by oxidative stress; in people with diabetes, CYBB-encoded advanced glycation end products activate NADPH oxidase 2 (NOX2), leading to ROS production [22]. The role of inflamed hepatocytes in hepatic fibrosis is a key factor to be taken into account in NASH. Sonic Hedgehog is produced by enlarged hepatocytes and functions as a tissue fibrosis–promoting protein. Sonic Hedgehog is now being studied to determine whether it induces fibrosis directly through its effects on stellate cells [23].

Genetics

A substantial portion of the population is susceptible to progressive NAFLD, defined as the development of NASH with severe fibrosis or cirrhosis, driven by insulin resistance and excess lipid accumulation [24]. However, only a small percentage of NAFLD patients develop more severe conditions, such as HCC. Although the causes of this are still not fully understood, NAFLD is best considered a complex disease, with modest interindividual differences influencing its development and progression [25]. These variations include both host genetic and environmental factors, which together shape the disease phenotype and influence its progression. While environmental determinants have a significant impact on NAFLD development, genetic factors also contribute and, more critically, may determine individual susceptibility to severe disease [26].

The Study of Epigenetics

The biology of NAFLD is beginning to recognize the significance of epigenetic factors, which have enabled the integration of gene expression data with internal and external metabolic information [27]. The transcriptional machinery of hepatocytes is reprogrammed by epigenetic changes resulting from inflammation, oxidative stress, and adaptation to a lipotoxic environment [28]. These epigenetic modifications may help explain why individuals with the same genetic background (for instance, carriers of the PNPLA3 I148M risk allele [29]) respond differently to comparable insults (such as fat overload) in terms of the extent of histological damage and/or recovery [30].

RNAs that Do Not Code

Numerous studies on liver disease have examined microRNAs (miRNAs), and there is consistent evidence of their involvement in NAFLD [31]. Numerous miRNAs, such as miR-122, miR-192, miR-375, and miR-34a109–111, have been linked to the severity of NAFLD, liver damage, and lipid metabolism. miR-122 is particularly significant in the pathogenesis of NAFLD, since its expression is significantly higher in healthy livers [32]. Its network of regulated genes plays a role in hepatocarcinogenesis, liver inflammation, and cholesterol metabolism [33]. An *in vitro* study found that miR-122 regulates hepatic stellate cell collagen synthesis, suggesting a critical role in liver fibrogenesis [34].

EMERGING TRENDS IN THE MANAGEMENT OF FATTY LIVER DISEASE

Personalized Medicines

with Reference to the Patient's Sex

Estrogen's impact on the onset and progression of NAFLD has not been well elucidated; however, it is generally accepted that estrogens help maintain liver health. NAFLD is more common among postmenopausal women, according to several studies. Additionally, the prevalence of NAFLD is lower in premenopausal women, higher in postmenopausal women, and greatest in men. While anti-estrogen medications like tamoxifen (a selective ER modulator) and ovariectomy increase the prevalence of NAFLD, hormone replacement therapy lowers it in postmenopausal women. Consequently, postmenopausal women should be treated with hormone replacement therapy [35]. Patients with adult growth hormone (GH) deficiency, who have a higher prevalence of NAFLD, illustrate the influence of GH on the development of the disease. Treatment of these individuals with GH replacement treatment demonstrates significant progress in liver diseases [36]. For individuals with NAFLD who have reduced GH levels, GH treatment may be helpful. However, as the data remain controversial [37], further research is needed to fully understand the relationship among GH, IGF-1, and NAFLD. Lean-NAFLD patients need to be treated with extra care [38]. Weight loss is not a treatment option for these people because they are not obese. They may still benefit from diet and exercise, so this, in addition to medication therapy, ought to be investigated further [39].

With the Help of Computer Models

Numerous variables contribute to the complexity of NAFLD, as previously mentioned, and these factors are not necessarily closely related [40]. The knowledge with regards to the disease mechanism, evolution, and treatment opportunities is also not exhaustive [41].. Although biomarkers are increasingly identified, their clinical application has not kept pace. In such situations, computational models can be particularly valuable. Several computational models have been developed to simulate the structure and function of multiple organs, including the liver, as well as biological interactions at different levels, such as those among proteins, RNA, DNA, medications, and other metabolites [42]. One objective is to model approximately 90% of human anatomy computationally by 2038. The liver, in particular, is the most complex organ in terms of metabolism. Numerous computational models aim to replicate hepatic physiological functions to predict key metabolic pathways that drive disease. These initiatives include the models described by Cvitanović *et al.*, which provide further information on the therapeutic applications of hepatic computational models and review progress toward developing distinct liver models for men and women [43]. Simulations using validated computational models can predict the outcomes of therapies with various drugs, thereby suggesting the most effective individualized treatment for each patient [44].

With Reference to Drug Metabolism

Numerous metabolic processes in the liver are mediated by the CYP proteins, a superfamily of enzymes that are altered in diseases, such as fatty liver disease. As previously stated, the liver's CYP genes exhibit significant sexual dimorphism in expression [45], making them crucial considerations for individualized therapy. Table **1** lists the main CYPs whose expression varies in NAFLD. A large number of them metabolize medications used to treat NAFLD or its complications [46]. In addition to altered CYP levels in pathological NAFLD, single nucleotide polymorphisms (SNPs) in CYP genes, of which more than 2,000 have been identified to date, play a significant role in drug metabolism. Numerous SNPs alter the efficiency of medication metabolism by influencing the activity of CYP enzymes. Since several medications are now used to treat NAFLD and related comorbidities [47], modifications in mRNA levels, enzyme activity, or SNPs in CYP enzymes may change how a medication affects the course of treatment for NAFLD. Treatment for patients with NALFD should take into account each patient's unique SNP variant and altered CYP levels, thereby significantly enhancing treatment outcomes [48].

Table 1. Synthetic drugs currently under phase 3 clinical trial for fatty liver disease management.

Sr. No.	Drug Name	Utilization	Reference
1.	Obeticholic Acid	Liver inflammation and fibrosis treatment	[88]
2.	Resmetirom	Selective THR-Beta agonist	[89]
3.	Semaglutide	GLP-1 analog	[90]
4.	Lanifibranor	PPAR-alpha, gamma, and delta agonist	[91]
5.	NATiV3	NASH and fibrosis treatment	[92]
6.	MAESTRO-NAFLD1	Liver inflammation	[93]

Imaging Biomarker

To diagnose NAFLD, pathologic fat must be present in at least 5% of the liver. Currently, fatty liver is often detected incidentally or through evaluation of elevated liver enzymes. Traditional ultrasound and similar imaging modalities may fail to identify the subgroup of patients who require attention and intervention [49].

Liver Fat Indicators Based on Ultrasound

VCTE, which is sold under the brand name FibroScan, can be used to obtain the CAP concurrently with an LSM. Additionally, CAP and VCTE are acquired simultaneously [50]. Notwithstanding these advantages, CAP has many drawbacks, including the influence of probe selection, the determination of the ideal cut point, and the implementation of validity requirements. In a meta-analysis of individual patient data evaluating the diagnostic accuracy of the controlled attenuation parameter (CAP) using liver biopsy as the reference standard, Karlas *et al.* identified 248 dB/m as the optimal cut-off for diagnosing hepatic steatosis [51]. Crucially, most of the study's participants had liver diseases other than NAFLD, and later research showed greater ideal cutpoints in NAFLD groups that were well-characterized. Although CAP may be able to differentiate between mild and moderate-to-severe steatosis, its ability to distinguish between moderate and severe steatosis is unreliable [52].

Liver Fat Indicators Based on Magnetic Resonance Spectroscopy

To differentiate between fat and water signal fractions, magnetic resonance spectroscopy (MRS) evaluates proton signals as a function of their resonance frequency. MRS is considered the most precise noninvasive technique for measuring liver fat, as it can detect even trace amounts. However, MRS has certain limitations that restrict its widespread use, including the need for specialized expertise to perform and interpret the scans and potential sampling errors due to its limited spatial coverage [53]. Magnetic resonance imaging–proton density fat fraction (MRI-PDFF) has been validated in several studies and is more accurate than liver biopsy for detecting changes in hepatic fat in longitudinal assessments. Using liver biopsy steatosis grade as the reference, head-to-head studies have shown that MRI-PDFF outperforms controlled attenuation parameter (CAP) in diagnostic accuracy [54]. Currently, CAP is primarily used to diagnose fatty liver in clinical studies and may be useful for monitoring responses to interventions. Before MRI-PDFF can be widely implemented in clinical practice, further research is needed to establish the cost-effectiveness and prognostic significance of excessive liver fat measured by this method [55].

Lifestyle Interventions

For most NAFLD patients, diet and exercise are the cornerstones of therapy. Losing weight has advantages, and the amount of weight dropped strongly correlates with the level of liver histological improvement. A 10% reduction in body weight was found to be linked to histological improvement in a prospective evaluation of a nutritional intervention in individuals with biopsy-confirmed nonalcoholic steatohepatitis [56]. In a study on 154 patients, weight reduction was also observed to have an impact. The patients were randomized to receive either general weight-loss counseling for 1 year or a dietitian-reinforced lifestyle intervention comprising dietary advice and mandatory moderate-intensity activity 3 times a week. Compared to just 20% of the control group, 64% of the intervention group showed resolution of NAFLD (as determined by magnetic resonance spectroscopy) [57].

These actions of agents on the liver have multiple mechanisms, including reductions in endotoxin translocation, promotion of SCFA production for their anti-inflammatory properties, regulation of bile acid metabolism, and, finally, effects on lipid metabolism [58]. Different models and trials have demonstrated their capacity to suppress hepatic steatosis, reduce elevations in liver enzymes, and at least influence hepatic fibrosis. It is important to note that these agents are more effective in combination than alone, and their monotherapy is less effective than combination approaches with lifestyle modification [59].

PRACTICAL USAGE: CASES IN VARIOUS PATIENTS

To put theory into practice, the following scenarios can be considered. The initial treatment for a patient with overweight, a sedentary lifestyle, and elevated liver enzymes would involve a structured hypocaloric diet with a daily caloric deficit of 500–750 kcal, combined with a Mediterranean-style dietary pattern. It is advised to walk or ride a bicycle for 30-60 minutes most days and to do resistance training 2 times a week. A synbiotic supplement containing *Lactobacillus* and *Bifidobacterium* strains, along with a prebiotic (FOS), can be used to improve gut microbiota diversity, minimize inflammation, and promote weight loss [60]. Conversely, in the case of a lean person with NAFLD, the emphasis is not on weight reduction but on diet quality and insulin sensitivity. In this case, it is important to reduce sugar and refined carbohydrates, increase omega-3 intake, and ensure sufficient fiber intake. Exercise is also recommended, and dietary fiber and fermented foods containing live cultures (such as yogurt and traditional fermented vegetables) could be beneficial for microbiome support [61]. Even with limited resources and without advanced diagnostics or supplements, significant changes are possible. Liver fat can be reduced by making fundamental dietary changes, *e.g.*, replacing white rice with millets, adding legumes and local greens, avoiding sweet beverages, and encouraging home-cooked meals. Long-term benefits may be sustained by encouraging walking or manual labor, using behavioral nudges *via* mobile phone reminders, or joining community support groups [62].

Examples and Trial Data

Dietary and Physical Activity Interventions

Reduction of liver fat in NASH can be achieved through exercise alone. Exercise reduced hepatic triglyceride content (as measured by proton magnetic resonance spectroscopy, HTGC) by approximately 16% after 12 weeks in patients with nonalcoholic steatohepatitis [63], and also decreased visceral fat and plasma triglycerides relative to controls in a randomized controlled trial [63].

Exercise Training and Liver Fat

A meta-analysis of 14 studies and 551 participants showed that exercise training increased the likelihood that an individual would achieve 30% reduction in liver fat, as measured by MRI, even without a clinically significant weight loss, compared with non-exercise controls. The cutoff dose was approximately 750 MET-minutes per week [64].

Intrahepatic fat Reductions through Dietary (Mediterranean / Green Mediterranean) means

The "DIRECT PLUS" trial: A three-year randomized trial in individuals with abdominal obesity compared three diets: a standard healthy guidelines diet, a Mediterranean diet, and a variant of the green-Mediterranean diet supplemented with polyphenols and low in red and processed meats. The green-MED diet reduced liver fat by approximately 39%, compared with 20% in the standard Mediterranean group and 12% in the control diet group. These effects remained significant even after adjusting for weight loss. According to a systematic review and meta-analysis, both Mediterranean and low-fat diets reduced ALT, AST, hepatic steatosis, fatty liver indices, and related measures. The composition of the diet is important, although in short-term studies, both diet types were equally effective across a variety of outcomes [65].

Combinations Diet + Exercise + Fibre in Pre-diabetic/NAFLD:

In a randomized controlled trial of prediabetic patients with NAFLD in Shanghai, China, participants were allocated to one of four groups: aerobic exercise (2–3 times per week), a fiber-enriched diet, a combination of both, or a control group, over 8–9 months. Diet or exercise alone led to a decrease of approximately 24–25% in liver fat content (HFC), while the combined diet and exercise intervention resulted in a reduction of about 48% compared with the control group [66].

Combining Gut-liver and Lifestyle Approaches to Achieve Optimal Results:

A combination of lifestyle change and microbiota-based treatment is probably the best approach to the control of liver fat, particularly when it comes to NAFLD. Although dietary and physical exercise are the basis, probiotics, prebiotics, or synbiotics may be useful to improve results, as they help balance gut-liver axis dysfunction, lower systemic inflammation, and improve metabolism. Notably, the interventions are complementary. A fiber-rich diet, *e.g.*, does not just lower calorie density but also serves as a prebiotic, feeding beneficial microbes that generate anti-inflammatory metabolites, such as SCFAs. Likewise, exercise enhances insulin sensitivity and may have subtle effects on microbiota composition [67]. Liver fat reduction is a complex problem that clinicians and patients should address as a multidimensional issue, considering dietary quality, caloric balance, physical activity, and gut health simultaneously. Individualized approaches, culturally oriented nutrition, and continuous encouragement are critical to the long-term change. As more and more evidence supports the gut-liver relationship, the addition of microbiome-based approaches to mainstream NAFLD management can be seen as a step toward a more effective, holistic approach to liver health [68].

Clinical Trial and Meta-Analysis Evidence

There is an ever-growing body of clinical literature confirming the use of probiotics and synbiotics as adjunctive treatments for NAFLD. Thousands of patients participating in meta-analyses of randomized controlled trials (RCTs) demonstrated a significant reduction in key liver enzymes, including alanine aminotransferase (ALT), aspartate aminotransferase (AST), and gamma-glutamyl transferase (GGT). In one meta-analysis involving over 12,000 patients, probiotic and synbiotic supplements demonstrated more favorable outcomes, not only in reductions in liver enzymes but also in liver ultrasound findings, indicating resolution of steatosis. Moreover, minimal differences in liver stiffness and fibrosis over short periods were demonstrated by elastography; nevertheless, the study was short, and no data were available on long-term outcomes [69, 70].

Additionally, along with liver-specific effects, they often provoke positive changes in metabolic parameters, triglycerides, LDL-cholesterol, fasting insulin, and inflammation markers TNF-α and IL-6. The significance of systemic effects lies in the fact that NAFLD is strongly associated with the metabolic syndrome, and the management of the metabolic disorder provides the key to sustainable NAFLD therapy. However, owing to the diversity of the trials, such as the selection of applied strains and probiotic dosages, patients, and treatment duration, generalized recommendations could hardly be made. However, despite the aforementioned considerations, there are many reasons to believe that the application of microbiota-targeted therapies for the treatment of NAFLD in its initial stages could be well justified [71, 72].

The Gut-Liver Axis and Its Role in Liver Fat Accumulation

The gut-liver axis is the two-way communication between the liver and the gastrointestinal tract, typically *via* the portal vein, through which gut-derived substances flow directly to the liver [73]. Over the past few years, the axis has become an important contributor to the pathogenesis of non-alcoholic fatty liver disease (NAFLD), particularly through mechanisms involving the gut microbiome. In a healthy state, the gut microbiota can maintain intestinal barrier integrity and facilitate host metabolism by producing beneficial metabolites, such as short-chain fatty acids (SCFAs) [74]. Nevertheless, when one experiences dysbiosis, or an imbalance in the gut microbiota, the integrity of the gut barrier is impaired, leading to enhanced intestinal permeability, commonly known as a leaky gut. This enables endotoxins, including lipopolysaccharide (LPS), to be translocated to the portal circulation and enter the liver, where they trigger inflammatory responses, oxidative stress, and insulin resistance, factors that lead to hepatic steatosis and progression to non-alcoholic steatohepatitis (NASH) and fibrosis. Thus, interventions that focus on replenishing the gut microbiota balance have attracted attention as promising therapeutic solutions for liver fat control [75].

Probiotics, Prebiotics, and Synbiotics in Reducing Fat in the Liver

Probiotics are live microorganisms that, when used at appropriate doses, confer health benefits to the host. Some common strains are species of *Lactobacillus, Bifidobacterium*, and *Streptococcus*, each with specific roles in restoring microbial balance in the gut, decreasing inflammation, and improving gut barrier function. Prebiotics, in turn, are non-digestible food substances, such as inulin, oligofructose, and fructooligosaccharides (FOS), that have a selective effect on beneficial bacteria in the colon. Combining probiotics with prebiotics is called a synbiotic and is intended not only to support the survival and activity of the given probiotics but also to support the native beneficial microbes [76].

The effects that the agents have on the liver are multifactorial. They decrease endotoxin translocation, stimulate the synthesis of SCFAs with anti-inflammatory effects, regulate bile acid metabolism, and can also affect lipid metabolism in the liver. A number of experimental models and clinical studies indicate that hepatic steatosis can be suppressed by specific microbiome modulation. It was found that liver enzymes can be decreased, and that at least the progression of fibrosis can be slowed. Notably, the therapies are less effective when applied alone but are more effective when combined with lifestyle interventions [77].

Probiotics, Synbiotics, and Microbiome Interventions

Trial on synbiotic yogurt in adults with NAFLD:

In a 24-week randomized controlled trial involving 102 NAFLD patients (mean BMI = 31 kg/m^2), participants were assigned to one of three groups: synbiotic yogurt (containing *Bifidobacterium animalis* and inulin), conventional yogurt with lifestyle advice, or control (lifestyle advice only). The synbiotic group showed significantly greater improvements in steatosis grades (assessed by ultrasound) and reductions in liver enzymes (ALT, AST), alkaline phosphatase (ALP), gamma-glutamyl transferase (GGT), and other markers compared with the other groups [78].

Synbiotic Supplementation in Lean NAFLD

A pilot RCT involving 50 lean/normal-BMI NAFLD patients comparing 28 weeks of synbiotic supplementation to a placebo (along with conventional lifestyle guidance) demonstrated the superiority of the synbiotic group in reducing hepatic steatosis and fibrosis, and improving fasting glucose, triglycerides, and inflammatory markers [79].

Synbiotics for NAFLD: A Meta-analysis Review:

A meta-analysis of approximately 10 RCTs (634 patients) that incorporated systematic review revealed a significant reduction in ALT, AST, GGT, total cholesterol, and LDL, an improvement of HDL, a reduction in liver stiffness measure, and a control of attenuation parameter (a measure of steatosis) in NAFLD patients with synbiotic supplementation [80].

Probiotics in Children/adolescents:

In obese children with NAFLD (ages not specified, but presumably around 12 months), a 12-week randomized intervention with a combination of *Lactobacillus acidophilus, Bifidobacterium lactis, B. bifidum, L. rhamnosus,* and other probiotics resulted in reductions in ALT and AST, total cholesterol, LDL, triglycerides, and waist circumference, although no significant effect on BMI was observed. These findings demonstrated that beneficial metabolic and hepatic effects can occur prior to significant weight changes [81].

Meta-analyses of Probiotics and Synbiotics:

In another meta-analysis of 15 RCTs, including approximately 782 patients, probiotics and synbiotics were found to have a significant positive effect on liver steatosis, liver enzymes, lipid profile, and insulin resistance; however, the magnitude of these effects and the specific outcomes that improved varied across studies [82].

Digital Health Technologies

Models for internet-enabled remote management based on mobile devices must take into account how well digital services can be tailored to certain user groups. Firstly, the prevalence of NAFLD is increasing among older adults due to poor metabolism, intestinal microbiology disorders, diabetes, and hyperlipidemia [83]. It is important to note that, compared with younger individuals, older adults often have lower learning capacity and are less likely to adopt network-related information gadgets [84]. Similarly, it is impossible to overlook the large number of pediatric patients with concomitant NAFLD [85]. When creating Digital Therapeutics (DTx), the role of family members must be fully considered, as these patients may not be able to use electronic devices freely. Second, there is growing evidence that internet usage habits differ by gender, and that this difference also extends to the health care DTx offers. Generally, women utilize social networking sites more than men, while men spend more time online for leisure and games. For DTx programs and devices to be properly designed and developed, gender characteristics must be taken into account [86]. Third, simpler, more user-friendly programs or devices may be more accessible in low-income areas, as patients may have limited access to the internet and to equipment for remote internet administration. The efficacy and safety of DTx can be enhanced through customized feedback and prompt intervention adjustments informed by thorough, real-time data monitoring [87 - 90]. Prior research has acknowledged the potential of using technology to monitor physical activity. Monitoring nutritional parameters is even more challenging. Therefore, researchers should explore ways to enhance both the accuracy and user-friendliness of food quantification methods [87, 91 - 93].

NEW DRUG DEVELOPMENT AND CLINICAL TRIALS

Although the road to NASH treatments has been long and costly, the field has gained important insights from lessons learnt along the way. Some examples of the drugs approved in clinical trials for fatty liver disease management are listed in Table **1** and **2**.

Table 2. Currently undergoing trials of herbal medicines for fatty liver management.

Herb/Compound	Clinical Trial Phase	Results	References
Picroliv (Picrorhiza kurroa)	Phase 3	Developed by the Central Drug Research Institute (CDRI) in India. Approved for Phase 3 clinical trials for the treatment of NAFLD.	[94]
Heptex® (Phyllanthus niruri and Silybum marianum)	Phase 2	Completed Phase 2 trials; Phase 3 trials are anticipated based on Phase 2 results.	[95]
Jian-Pi Huo-Xue Granule (Traditional Chinese Medicine)	Phase 2	Undergoing a randomized, double-blind, placebo-controlled Phase 2 trial for the treatment of NAFLD.	[96]

FUTURE PERSPECTIVES ON FATTY LIVER DISEASE MANAGEMENT

Even with all the major progresses made in the pathophysiology of fatty liver disease, the existing methods of diagnosing and treating the disease are still disjointed and inadequate to match the increasing prevalence of the disease in the global population. The future research directions should therefore go beyond minor improvements and adopt revolutionary technologies that can change the way diseases are controlled [97]. The integration of artificial intelligence (AI) and machine learning (ML) into imaging and diagnostic pathways is one of the most promising fields. Existing conventional imaging techniques, including ultrasound, elastography, CT, and MRI, already provide useful information about hepatic steatosis and fibrosis but are often compromised by operator variability and non-standardized scoring [98]. Algorithms using AI and ML can combine multimodal imaging data with laboratory and clinical data to produce consistent, understandable risk scores that accurately stratify patients between simple steatosis and severe fibrosis. Notably, explainable AI models can build clinician trust and expedite regulatory uptake by highlighting the imaging areas or features on which predictions are made. It is expected that the anti-long-term objective will be the establishment of multi-center, well-labeled datasets that can be used to connect imaging with histology and longitudinal outcomes, and that will subsequently serve as the basis for clinically validated, generalizable AI tools. When these systems are implemented, they can be used in primary care as triage assistance to identify high-risk individuals, enabling early intervention and reducing the need for invasive liver biopsy. Smart nanocarriers can be used not only to deliver therapeutics (small molecules, siRNA, CRISPR-based constructs) to distinct cell populations of the liver but also to deliver imaging agents that can provide real-time biodistribution/target-binding feedback. Activatable probes can remain inactive until disease-specific enzymes or pH conditions in the fibrotic niche trigger the unexpected release of their therapeutic payload, allowing visualization of pathological activity and therapeutic delivery. This enables adaptive treatment schemes in which therapy is adjusted in real time based on molecular or imaging feedback. The potential of hepatocyte-targeted lipid nanoparticles and stellate cell-targeted carriers to regulate steatosis and fibrosis has already been demonstrated by early preclinical research, and the next step is to conduct first-in-human microdosing trials to assess safety and biodistribution. The synthesis of these two emerging paradigms seems to be the most significant paradigmatic shift. The analytics application enabled by AI can be used on top of the theranostic imaging inputs to form a closed-loop system in which the diagnosis, treatment, and follow-up of fatty liver disease are analysed and synthesised. For example, theranostic nanoparticles can be continuously analyzed using AI to predict drug release dynamics and early biological responses, which directly inform real-time dose adjustments. Such adaptive systems would reduce global therapeutic performance and unnecessary exposure, enhancing safety and cost-effectiveness. Clinically robust models may further accelerate generalizable learning by leveraging federated learning methods that enable training on distributed imaging datasets without violating patient privacy. To achieve this, it is necessary to focus on enabling infrastructure. Similar funding in health economics and implementation science will ensure that ultra-technologies, including edge-AI-controlled ultrasound, are available in low-resource environments rather than limited to tertiary centers. Besides, hepatologists, radiologists, data scientists, nanomaterials engineers, regulators, and patient advocates must all work closely to reconcile so that technological potential is recapitulated into factual clinical requirements. Hence, approaches to addressing heterogeneity in data, algorithmic bias, nanoparticle immunogenicity, and regulatory complexity will need to be implemented deliberately and in a coordinated way, and all of these can be overcome through active multidisciplinary mechanisms.

Going forward, the future of management of fatty liver diseases will reach the level of diagnosing personalized and precise care, specifically, the flexible strategies through precise, real-time monitoring. AI-enhanced imaging will enable early detection of diverse risks and their mitigation; theranostic nanomedicines will provide targeted, personalized treatment for diverse cancers; and their combination will enable closed-loop therapeutic ecosystems that continuously learn and maximize care. Although significant efforts are still needed in the area of data standardization and validation of safety as well as fair treatment, the combination of these technologies promises to alter the course of fatty liver disease, from a silent epidemic to a disease that can be addressed effectively through the use of precision medicine and, perhaps, reversed.

CONCLUSION

Liver biopsy is still the gold standard for determining the severity of nonalcoholic fatty liver disease (NAFLD), even though it is the most prevalent chronic liver disease in the world. Non-invasive identification and monitoring of this group is a significant unmet need, especially in light of the anticipated rise in the burden of advanced liver disease caused by NAFLD and new treatment options. As of now, imaging biomarkers for liver fat measurement and NAFLD diagnosis are reliable, and MRI-PDFF could even be more instructive than liver biopsies. Currently, there are not many imaging markers available to diagnose NASH. Elastography offers exceptional diagnostic precision in the early phases of fibrosis with MRE and can consistently detect advanced fibrosis. To guide the treatment of patients with NAFLD, strategies to integrate multiple biomarker platforms in specific use cases with defined cutoff criteria would be required.

LIST OF ABBREVIATIONS

ALFD Alcoholic fatty liver disease

CAP Controlled attenuation parameter

EBMI Elevated Body Mass Index (EBMI)

FLD Fatty liver disease (FLD)

HCC Hepatocellular carcinoma

LSM Liver Stiffness measurement

MRS Magnetic resonance spectroscopy

NAFLD Nonalcoholic fatty liver disease

NASH Nonalcoholic steatohepatitis

VCTE Vibration–controlled transient elastography

REFERENCES

[1] Neuschwander-Tetri BA. Hepatic lipotoxicity and the pathogenesis of nonalcoholic steatohepatitis. Hepatology 2010; 52(2): 774-88.
[http://dx.doi.org/10.1002/hep.23719] [PMID: 20683968]

[2] Khare T, Liu K, Chilambe LO, Khare S. NAFLD and NAFLD related HCC: Emerging treatments and clinical trials. Int J Mol Sci 2025; 26(1): 306.
[http://dx.doi.org/10.3390/ijms26010306] [PMID: 39796162]

[3] Singh SP, Madke T, Chand P. Global epidemiology of hepatocellular carcinoma. J Clin Exp Hepatol 2025; 15(2): 102446.
[http://dx.doi.org/10.1016/j.jceh.2024.102446] [PMID: 39659901]

[4] Zhang Y, Jin D, Zhu H, Lin M, Peng X. Hepatocytes and hepatic stellate cells carry different levels of DNA damage due to their sensitivity to oxidative stress in chronic hepatitis B. J Viral Hepat 2025; 32(3): e70017.
[http://dx.doi.org/10.1111/jvh.70017] [PMID: 39991880]

[5] Polyzos SA, Mantzoros CS. Metabolic dysfunction-associated steatotic liver disease: Recent turning

points for its diagnosis and management. Metabolism 2024; 157: 155936. [http://dx.doi.org/10.1016/j.metabol.2024.155936] [PMID: 38763229]

[6] Cohen JC, Horton JD, Hobbs HH. Human fatty liver disease: old questions and new insights. Science 2011; 332(6037): 1519-23. [http://dx.doi.org/10.1126/science.1204265] [PMID: 21700865]

[7] Ahmadizar F, Younossi ZM. Exploring biomarkers in nonalcoholic fatty liver disease among individuals with type 2 diabetes mellitus. J Clin Gastroenterol 2025; 59(1): 36-46. [http://dx.doi.org/10.1097/MCG.0000000000002079] [PMID: 39352015]

[8] Díaz LA, Arab JP, Louvet A, Bataller R, Arrese M. The intersection between alcohol-related liver disease and nonalcoholic fatty liver disease. Nat Rev Gastroenterol Hepatol 2023; 20(12): 764-83. [http://dx.doi.org/10.1038/s41575-023-00822-y] [PMID: 37582985]

[9] Yun-xiao LI, Wei SU, Jing DO, *et al.* Correlation between metabolic dysfunction-associated fatty liver disease and liver fibrosis based on Fibrotouch. Hainan Yixueyuan Xuebao 2023; 29(22)

[10] Huang X, Yu R, Tan X, *et al.* Comparison of NAFLD, MAFLD, and MASLD prevalence and clinical characteristics in Asia adults. J Clin Exp Hepatol 2025; 15(1): 102420. [http://dx.doi.org/10.1016/j.jceh.2024.102420] [PMID: 39564428]

[11] Grander C, Grabherr F, Tilg H. Non-alcoholic fatty liver disease: pathophysiological concepts and treatment options. Cardiovasc Res 2023; 119(9): 1787-98. [http://dx.doi.org/10.1093/cvr/cvad095] [PMID: 37364164]

[12] Mitra S, De A, Chowdhury A. Epidemiology of non-alcoholic and alcoholic fatty liver diseases. Transl Gastroenterol Hepatol 2020; 5: 16. [http://dx.doi.org/10.21037/tgh.2019.09.08] [PMID: 32258520]

[13] Polyzos SA, Kountouras J, Mantzoros CS. Obesity and nonalcoholic fatty liver disease: From pathophysiology to therapeutics. Metabolism 2019; 92: 82-97. [http://dx.doi.org/10.1016/j.metabol.2018.11.014] [PMID: 30502373]

[14] Munjal K, Chopra H, Gauttam V K, Vashist C, Kushwaha B, Kamal M A. Phytochemicals against cancer: Exploring plant-based compounds. Nature's Arsenal Against Cancer: Harnessing the Power of Natural Compounds for Treatment and Prevention. 2024; pp. 83-95.

[15] Haas JT, Francque S, Staels B. Pathophysiology and mechanisms of nonalcoholic fatty liver disease. Annu Rev Physiol 2016; 78(1): 181-205. [http://dx.doi.org/10.1146/annurev-physiol-021115-105331] [PMID: 26667070]

[16] Kirpich IA, Marsano LS, McClain CJ. Gut–liver axis, nutrition, and non-alcoholic fatty liver disease. Clin Biochem 2015; 48(13-14): 923-30. [http://dx.doi.org/10.1016/j.clinbiochem.2015.06.023] [PMID: 26151226]

[17] Paolella G, Mandato C, Pierri L, Poeta M, Di Stasi M, Vajro P. Gut-liver axis and probiotics: Their role in non-alcoholic fatty liver disease. World J Gastroenterol 2014; 20(42): 15518-31. [http://dx.doi.org/10.3748/wjg.v20.i42.15518] [PMID: 25400436]

[18] Miele L, Marrone G, Lauritano C, *et al.* Gut-liver axis and microbiota in NAFLD: insight pathophysiology for novel therapeutic target. Curr Pharm Des 2013; 19(29): 5314-24. [http://dx.doi.org/10.2174/1381612811319290011] [PMID: 23432669]

[19] Compare D, Coccoli P, Rocco A, *et al.* Gut–liver axis: The impact of gut microbiota on non alcoholic fatty liver disease. Nutr Metab Cardiovasc Dis 2012; 22(6): 471-6. [http://dx.doi.org/10.1016/j.numecd.2012.02.007] [PMID: 22546554]

[20] Lieber CS. Alcoholic fatty liver: its pathogenesis and mechanism of progression to inflammation and fibrosis. Alcohol 2004; 34(1): 9-19. [http://dx.doi.org/10.1016/j.alcohol.2004.07.008] [PMID: 15670660]

[21] Hammerich L, Tacke F. Hepatic inflammatory responses in liver fibrosis. Nat Rev Gastroenterol

Hepatol 2023; 20(10): 633-46.
[http://dx.doi.org/10.1038/s41575-023-00807-x] [PMID: 37400694]

[22] Akkız H, Gieseler RK, Canbay A. Liver fibrosis: from basic science towards clinical progress, focusing on the central role of hepatic stellate cells. Int J Mol Sci 2024; 25(14): 7873.
[http://dx.doi.org/10.3390/ijms25147873] [PMID: 39063116]

[23] Stål P. Liver fibrosis in non-alcoholic fatty liver disease - diagnostic challenge with prognostic significance. World J Gastroenterol 2015; 21(39): 11077-87.
[http://dx.doi.org/10.3748/wjg.v21.i39.11077] [PMID: 26494963]

[24] Lee E, Korf H, Vidal-Puig A. An adipocentric perspective on the development and progression of non-alcoholic fatty liver disease. J Hepatol 2023; 78(5): 1048-62.
[http://dx.doi.org/10.1016/j.jhep.2023.01.024] [PMID: 36740049]

[25] Dongiovanni P, Valenti L. Genetics of nonalcoholic fatty liver disease. Metabolism 2016; 65(8): 1026-37.
[http://dx.doi.org/10.1016/j.metabol.2015.08.018] [PMID: 26409295]

[26] Severson TJ, Besur S, Bonkovsky HL. Genetic factors that affect nonalcoholic fatty liver disease: A systematic clinical review. World J Gastroenterol 2016; 22(29): 6742-56.
[http://dx.doi.org/10.3748/wjg.v22.i29.6742] [PMID: 27547017]

[27] Del Campo J, Gallego-Durán R, Gallego P, Grande L. Genetic and epigenetic regulation in nonalcoholic fatty liver disease (NAFLD). Int J Mol Sci 2018; 19(3): 911.
[http://dx.doi.org/10.3390/ijms19030911] [PMID: 29562725]

[28] Njei B, Al-Ajlouni YA, Ugwendum D, Abdu M, Forjindam A, Mohamed MF. Genetic and epigenetic determinants of non-alcoholic fatty liver disease (NAFLD) in lean individuals: a systematic review. Transl Gastroenterol Hepatol 2024; 9: 11.
[http://dx.doi.org/10.21037/tgh-23-31] [PMID: 38317742]

[29] Choudhary NS, Duseja A. Genetic and epigenetic disease modifiers: non-alcoholic fatty liver disease (NAFLD) and alcoholic liver disease (ALD). Transl Gastroenterol Hepatol 2021; 6: 2.
[http://dx.doi.org/10.21037/tgh.2019.09.06] [PMID: 33409397]

[30] Wu YL, Lin ZJ, Li CC, *et al.* Epigenetic regulation in metabolic diseases: mechanisms and advances in clinical study. Signal Transduct Target Ther 2023; 8(1): 98.
[http://dx.doi.org/10.1038/s41392-023-01333-7] [PMID: 36864020]

[31] Ilieva M, Dao J, Miller HE, *et al.* Systematic analysis of long non-coding RNA genes in nonalcoholic fatty liver disease. Noncoding RNA 2022; 8(4): 56.
[http://dx.doi.org/10.3390/ncrna8040056] [PMID: 35893239]

[32] Zhao XY, Xiong X, Liu T, *et al.* Long noncoding RNA licensing of obesity-linked hepatic lipogenesis and NAFLD pathogenesis. Nat Commun 2018; 9(1): 2986.
[http://dx.doi.org/10.1038/s41467-018-05383-2] [PMID: 30061575]

[33] Webster NJG. Alternative RNA splicing in the pathogenesis of liver disease. Front Endocrinol (Lausanne) 2017; 8: 133.
[http://dx.doi.org/10.3389/fendo.2017.00133] [PMID: 28680417]

[34] Zhao Y, Wu J, Liangpunsakul S, Wang L. Long non-coding RNA in liver metabolism and disease: Current status. Liver Res 2017; 1(3): 163-7.
[http://dx.doi.org/10.1016/j.livres.2017.09.001] [PMID: 29576888]

[35] Lonardo A, Arab JP, Arrese M. Perspectives on precision medicine approaches to NAFLD diagnosis and management. Adv Ther 2021; 38(5): 2130-58.
[http://dx.doi.org/10.1007/s12325-021-01690-1] [PMID: 33829368]

[36] Jamalinia M, Lonardo A, Weiskirchen R. Sex and gender differences in liver fibrosis: pathomechanisms and clinical outcomes. Fibrosis 2024; 2(4): 10006.
[http://dx.doi.org/10.70322/fibrosis.2024.10006]

[37] Lonardo A, Ballestri S. Perspectives of nonalcoholic fatty liver disease research: a personal point of view. Explor Med 2020; 1(3): 85-107.
[http://dx.doi.org/10.37349/emed.2020.00007]

[38] Ábel T, Benczúr B, Csobod ÉC. Sex differences in pathogenesis and treatment of dyslipidemia in patients with type 2 diabetes and steatotic liver disease. Front Med (Lausanne) 2024; 11: 1458025.
[http://dx.doi.org/10.3389/fmed.2024.1458025] [PMID: 39376658]

[39] Zhou H, Chen H, Lu H, *et al.* Sex differences in mortality and liver□related events in non□alcoholic fatty liver disease: A systematic review and meta□analysis. Liver Int 2024; 44(7): 1600-9.
[http://dx.doi.org/10.1111/liv.15910] [PMID: 38506430]

[40] Gerussi A, Scaravaglio M, Cristoferi L, *et al.* Artificial intelligence for precision medicine in autoimmune liver disease. Front Immunol 2022; 13: 966329.
[http://dx.doi.org/10.3389/fimmu.2022.966329] [PMID: 36439097]

[41] Wu CC, Yeh WC, Hsu WD, *et al.* Prediction of fatty liver disease using machine learning algorithms. Comput Methods Programs Biomed 2019; 170: 23-9.
[http://dx.doi.org/10.1016/j.cmpb.2018.12.032] [PMID: 30712601]

[42] Mukherjee S, Thapliyal K, Maurya A, Chaudhary N, Sudeshna S. AI in bioinformatics and genomics. 2024 International Conference on Intelligent & Innovative Practices in Engineering & Management (IIPEM). IEEE. 2024; pp. 1-8.

[43] Cvitanović Tomaš T, Urlep Ž, Moškon M, Mraz M, Rozman D. LiverSex computational model: sexual aspects in hepatic metabolism and abnormalities. Front Physiol 2018; 9: 360.
[http://dx.doi.org/10.3389/fphys.2018.00360] [PMID: 29706895]

[44] Ghosh S, Zhao X, Alim M, Brudno M, Bhat M. Artificial intelligence applied to 'omics data in liver disease: towards a personalised approach for diagnosis, prognosis and treatment. Gut 2025; 74(2): 295-311.
[http://dx.doi.org/10.1136/gutjnl-2023-331740] [PMID: 39174307]

[45] Sharpton SR, Schnabl B, Knight R, Loomba R. Current concepts, opportunities, and challenges of gut microbiome-based personalized medicine in nonalcoholic fatty liver disease. Cell Metab 2021; 33(1): 21-32.
[http://dx.doi.org/10.1016/j.cmet.2020.11.010] [PMID: 33296678]

[46] Al Hashmi K, Giglio RV, Pantea Stoian A, *et al.* Metabolic dysfunction-associated fatty liver disease: current therapeutic strategies. Front Nutr 2024; 11: 1355732.
[http://dx.doi.org/10.3389/fnut.2024.1355732] [PMID: 38567250]

[47] Zgheib NK, Branch RA. Drug metabolism and liver disease: a drug–gene–environment interaction. Drug Metab Rev 2017; 49(1): 35-55.
[http://dx.doi.org/10.1080/03602532.2016.1271807] [PMID: 27957864]

[48] Everett JR, Loo RL, Pullen FS. Pharmacometabonomics and personalized medicine. Ann Clin Biochem 2013; 50(6): 523-45.
[http://dx.doi.org/10.1177/0004563213497929] [PMID: 23888060]

[49] Yu JH, Lee HA, Kim SU. Noninvasive imaging biomarkers for liver fibrosis in nonalcoholic fatty liver disease: current and future. Clin Mol Hepatol 2023; 29 (Suppl.): S136-49.
[http://dx.doi.org/10.3350/cmh.2022.0436] [PMID: 36503205]

[50] Acharya UR, Faust O, Molinari F, Sree SV, Junnarkar SP, Sudarshan V. Ultrasound-based tissue characterization and classification of fatty liver disease: A screening and diagnostic paradigm. Knowl Base Syst 2015; 75: 66-77.
[http://dx.doi.org/10.1016/j.knosys.2014.11.021]

[51] Ballestri S, Nascimbeni F, Baldelli E, *et al.* Ultrasonographic fatty liver indicator detects mild steatosis and correlates with metabolic/histological parameters in various liver diseases. Metabolism 2017; 72: 57-65.

[http://dx.doi.org/10.1016/j.metabol.2017.04.003] [PMID: 28641784]

[52] Radmard AR, Rahmanian MS, Abrishami A, *et al.* Assessment of abdominal fat distribution in non-alcoholic fatty liver disease by magnetic resonance imaging: a population-based study. Arch Iran Med 2016; 19(10): 693-9.

[53] Jang W, Song JS. Non-invasive imaging methods to evaluate non-alcoholic fatty liver disease with fat quantification: a review. Diagnostics (Basel) 2023; 13(11): 1852.
[http://dx.doi.org/10.3390/diagnostics13111852] [PMID: 37296703]

[54] Koch M, Borggrefe J, Barbaresko J, *et al.* Dietary patterns associated with magnetic resonance imaging–determined liver fat content in a general population study. Am J Clin Nutr 2014; 99(2): 369-77.
[http://dx.doi.org/10.3945/ajcn.113.070219] [PMID: 24305680]

[55] Pavlides M, Banerjee R, Sellwood J, *et al.* Multiparametric magnetic resonance imaging predicts clinical outcomes in patients with chronic liver disease. J Hepatol 2016; 64(2): 308-15.
[http://dx.doi.org/10.1016/j.jhep.2015.10.009] [PMID: 26471505]

[56] Thoma C, Day CP, Trenell MI. Lifestyle interventions for the treatment of non-alcoholic fatty liver disease in adults: A systematic review. J Hepatol 2012; 56(1): 255-66.
[http://dx.doi.org/10.1016/j.jhep.2011.06.010] [PMID: 21723839]

[57] Younossi ZM, Zelber-Sagi S, Henry L, Gerber LH. Lifestyle interventions in nonalcoholic fatty liver disease. Nat Rev Gastroenterol Hepatol 2023; 20(11): 708-22.
[http://dx.doi.org/10.1038/s41575-023-00800-4] [PMID: 37402873]

[58] Kaufmann B, Seyfried N, Hartmann D, Hartmann P. Probiotics, prebiotics, and synbiotics in nonalcoholic fatty liver disease and alcohol-associated liver disease. Am J Physiol Gastrointest Liver Physiol 2023; 325(1): G42-61.
[http://dx.doi.org/10.1152/ajpgi.00017.2023] [PMID: 37129252]

[59] Wang CY, Chen WL, Cheng-Chung Wei J. Link between inflammatory bowel disease and risk of chronic kidney disease. Clin Gastroenterol Hepatol 2021; 19(9): 1993-4.
[http://dx.doi.org/10.1016/j.cgh.2020.10.040] [PMID: 33248103]

[60] Alharbi M, Chiurazzi M, Nasti G, *et al.* Caloric restriction (CR) plus high-nitrate beetroot juice does not amplify CR-Induced metabolic adaptation and improves vascular and cognitive functions in overweight adults: a 14-Day pilot randomised Trial. Nutrients 2023; 15(4): 890.
[http://dx.doi.org/10.3390/nu15040890] [PMID: 36839248]

[61] Tan AT, Meng F, Jin J, *et al.* Immunological alterations after immunotherapy with short lived HBV□TCR T cells associates with long□term treatment response in HBV□HCC. Hepatol Commun 2022; 6(4): 841-54.
[http://dx.doi.org/10.1002/hep4.1857] [PMID: 34935312]

[62] Dubey S, Deshpande S, Krishna L, Zadey S. Evolution of Government-funded health insurance for universal health coverage in India. Lancet Reg Health Southeast Asia 2023; 13
[http://dx.doi.org/10.1016/j.lansea.2023.100177] [http://dx.doi.org/10.1016/j.lansea.2023.100180]

[63] Virk AK, Atun R. Towards universal health coverage in India: a historical examination of the genesis of Rashtriya Swasthya Bima Yojana—the health insurance scheme for low-income groups. Public Health 2015; 129(6): 810-7.

[64] Hu S, Cao C, Poddar M, *et al.* Hepatocyte β□catenin loss is compensated by Insulin□mTORC1 activation to promote liver regeneration. Hepatology 2023; 77(5): 1593-611.
[http://dx.doi.org/10.1002/hep.32680] [PMID: 35862186]

[65] Yaskolka Meir A, Rinott E, Tsaban G, *et al.* Effect of green-Mediterranean diet on intrahepatic fat: the DIRECT PLUS randomised controlled trial. Gut 2021; 70(11): 2085-95.
[http://dx.doi.org/10.1136/gutjnl-2020-323106] [PMID: 33461965]

[66] Lee MW, Raman SS, Asvadi NH, *et al.* Radiofrequency ablation of hepatocellular carcinoma as bridge

therapy to liver transplantation: A 10□year intention□to□treat analysis. Hepatology 2017; 65(6): 1979-90.
[http://dx.doi.org/10.1002/hep.29098] [PMID: 28170115]

[67] Maiwall R, Rao Pasupuleti SS, Hidam AK, *et al.* A randomised-controlled trial (TARGET-C) of high *vs.* low target mean arterial pressure in patients with cirrhosis and septic shock. J Hepatol 2023; 79(2): 349-61.
[http://dx.doi.org/10.1016/j.jhep.2023.04.006] [PMID: 37088310]

[68] Hyun JY, Kim SK, Yoon SJ, *et al.* Microbiome-based metabolic therapeutic approaches in alcoholic liver disease. Int J Mol Sci 2022; 23(15): 8749.
[http://dx.doi.org/10.3390/ijms23158749] [PMID: 35955885]

[69] Fromenty B, Roden M. Mitochondrial alterations in fatty liver diseases. J Hepatol 2023; 78(2): 415-29.
[http://dx.doi.org/10.1016/j.jhep.2022.09.020] [PMID: 36209983]

[70] Liu L, Li P, Liu Y, Zhang Y. Efficacy of probiotics and synbiotics in patients with nonalcoholic fatty liver disease: A meta-analysis. Dig Dis Sci 2019; 64(12): 3402-12.
[http://dx.doi.org/10.1007/s10620-019-05699-z] [PMID: 31203554]

[71] Schönenberger KA, Saxer C, Neyer PJ, *et al.* Aluminum and other chemical elements in parenteral nutrition components and all-in-one admixtures. Clin Nutr 2023; 42(12): 2475-83.
[http://dx.doi.org/10.1016/j.clnu.2023.10.012] [PMID: 38411019]

[72] Sharpton SR, Maraj B, Harding-Theobald E, Vittinghoff E, Terrault NA. Gut microbiome–targeted therapies in nonalcoholic fatty liver disease: a systematic review, meta-analysis, and meta-regression. Am J Clin Nutr 2019; 110(1): 139-49.
[http://dx.doi.org/10.1093/ajcn/nqz042] [PMID: 31124558]

[73] Tripathi A, Debelius J, Brenner DA, *et al.* The gut–liver axis and the intersection with the microbiome. Nat Rev Gastroenterol Hepatol 2018; 15(7): 397-411.
[http://dx.doi.org/10.1038/s41575-018-0011-z] [PMID: 29748586]

[74] Fernandez-Cantos MV, Garcia-Morena D, Iannone V, El-Nezami H, Kolehmainen M, Kuipers OP. Role of microbiota and related metabolites in gastrointestinal tract barrier function in NAFLD. Tissue Barriers 2021; 9(3): 1879719.
[http://dx.doi.org/10.1080/21688370.2021.1879719] [PMID: 34280073]

[75] Le Roy T, Llopis M, Lepage P, *et al.* Intestinal microbiota determines development of non-alcoholic fatty liver disease in mice. Gut 2013; 62(12): 1787-94.
[http://dx.doi.org/10.1136/gutjnl-2012-303816] [PMID: 23197411]

[76] Markowiak P, Śliżewska K. Effects of probiotics, prebiotics, and synbiotics on human health. Nutrients 2017; 9(9): 1021.
[http://dx.doi.org/10.3390/nu9091021] [PMID: 28914794]

[77] Koning M, Herrema H, Nieuwdorp M, Meijnikman A S. Targeting nonalcoholic fatty liver disease *via* gut microbiome-centered therapies. Gut Microbes 2023; 15(1): 2226922.
[http://dx.doi.org/10.1080/19490976.2023.2226922]

[78] Eslamparast T, Poustchi H, Zamani F, Sharafkhah M, Malekzadeh R, Hekmatdoost A. Synbiotic supplementation in nonalcoholic fatty liver disease: a randomized, double-blind, placebo-controlled pilot study. Am J Clin Nutr 2014; 99(3): 535-42.
[http://dx.doi.org/10.3945/ajcn.113.068890] [PMID: 24401715]

[79] Alghamdi W, Mosli M, Alqahtani SA. Gut microbiota in MAFLD: therapeutic and diagnostic implications. Ther Adv Endocrinol Metab 2024; 15: 20420188241242937.
[http://dx.doi.org/10.1177/20420188241242937] [PMID: 38628492]

[80] Zhao L, Zhang F, Ding X, *et al.* Gut bacteria selectively promoted by dietary fibers alleviate type 2 diabetes. Science 2018; 359(6380): 1151-6.
[http://dx.doi.org/10.1126/science.aao5774] [PMID: 29590046]

[81] Gkiourtzis N, Kalopitas G, Vadarlis A, *et al.* The benefit of probiotics in pediatric nonalcoholic fatty liver disease. J Pediatr Gastroenterol Nutr 2022; 75(3): e31-7. [http://dx.doi.org/10.1097/MPG.0000000000003537] [PMID: 35758473]

[82] Cao C, Shi M, Wang X, Yao Y, Zeng R. Effects of probiotics on non-alcoholic fatty liver disease: a review of human clinical trials. Front Nutr 2023; 10: 1155306. [http://dx.doi.org/10.3389/fnut.2023.1155306] [PMID: 37457967]

[83] Björnsdottir S, Ulfsdottir H, Gudmundsson EF, *et al.* User engagement, acceptability, and clinical markers in a digital health program for nonalcoholic fatty liver disease: Prospective, single-arm feasibility study. JMIR Cardio 2024; 8: e52576. [http://dx.doi.org/10.2196/52576] [PMID: 38152892]

[84] Hallsworth K, McPherson S, Anstee QM, Flynn D, Haigh L, Avery L. Digital intervention with lifestyle coach support to target dietary and physical activity behaviors of adults with nonalcoholic fatty liver disease: systematic development process of VITALISE using intervention mapping. J Med Internet Res 2021; 23(1): e20491. [http://dx.doi.org/10.2196/20491] [PMID: 33448929]

[85] Haye A, Ansari MA, Saini A, *et al.* Polyherbal formulation improves glucose-lipid metabolism and prevent hepatotoxicity in streptozotocin-induced diabetic rats: Plausible role of IRS-PI3K-Akt-GLUT2 signaling. Sci Rep 2022; 18(77)

[86] Kazankov K, Novelli S, Chatterjee DA, *et al.* Evaluation of CirrhoCare® – a digital health solution for home management of individuals with cirrhosis. J Hepatol 2023; 78(1): 123-32. [http://dx.doi.org/10.1016/j.jhep.2022.08.034] [PMID: 36087864]

[87] Han Z, Yang M, Bi L, *et al.* Quantitative imaging using [^{18}F]F-TZ3108 to assess metabolic-associated fatty liver disease progression and low-carbohydrate diet efficacy. Nucl Med Biol 2025; 144-145: 108997. [http://dx.doi.org/10.1016/j.nucmedbio.2025.108997] [PMID: 39923314]

[88] Chen VL, Morgan TR, Rotman Y. Resmetirom therapy for metabolic dysfunction-associated steatotic liver disease: October 2024 updates to AASLD Practice Guidance. Hepatology 2025; 81(1): 312-20. [http://dx.doi.org/10.1097/HEP.0000000000001112] [PMID: 39422487]

[89] Ditzenberger GL, Lake JE, Kitch DW, *et al.* Effects of semaglutide on muscle structure and function in the SLIM LIVER study. Clin Infect Dis 2025; 80(2): 389-96. [http://dx.doi.org/10.1093/cid/ciae384] [PMID: 39046173]

[90] Rautou PE, Chotkoe S, Biquard L, *et al.* Altered liver sinusoidal endothelial cells in MASLD and their evolution following lanifibranor treatment. JHEP Rep 2025; 101366. [http://dx.doi.org/10.1016/j.jhepr.2025.101366]

[91] Eeda V, Patil NY, Joshi AD, Awasthi V. Advancements in metabolic□associated steatotic liver disease research: Diagnostics, small molecule developments, and future directions. Hepatol Res 2024; 54(3): 222-34. [http://dx.doi.org/10.1111/hepr.14008] [PMID: 38149861]

[92] Guirguis E, Dougherty J, Thornby K, Grace Y, Mack K. Resmetirom: The first food and drug administration–approved medication for nonalcoholic steatohepatitis (NASH). Ann Pharmacother 2025; 59(2): 162-73. [http://dx.doi.org/10.1177/10600280241259528] [PMID: 38887011]

[93] Gauttam VK, Munjal K, Chopra H, Ahmad A, Rana MK, Kamal MA. A mechanistic review on therapeutic potential of medicinal plants and their pharmacologically active molecules for targeting metabolic syndrome. Curr Pharm Biotechnol 2024; 30(1): 10-30. [http://dx.doi.org/10.2174/0113816128274446231220113957] [PMID: 38155468]

[94] Correspondent HT. Clinical trial of CDRI's plant-based drug for fatty liver soon. Hindustan Times 2022.

[95] Shaker MK, Hassany M, Eysa B, Adel A, Zidan A, Mohamed S. The activity of a herbal medicinal product of Phyllanthus niruri and Silybum marianum powdered extracts (Heptex®) in patients with apparent risk factors for nonalcoholic steatohepatitis: a phase II, multicentered, randomized, double-blind, placebo-controlled clinical trial. BMC Complement Med Ther 2025; 25(1): 8. [http://dx.doi.org/10.1186/s12906-024-04692-y] [PMID: 39789561]

[96] Sun Y, Chen G, Chen S, Wang Y, Hu Y, Zhao Y. Efficacy and safety of Jian-Pi Huo-Xue granule for non-alcoholic fatty liver disease: study protocol for a randomized, double-blind, placebo-controlled trial. Trials 2022; 23(1): 455. [http://dx.doi.org/10.1186/s13063-022-06393-8] [PMID: 35655225]

[97] Paulino PJ, Cuthrell KM, Tzenios N. Non-alcoholic fatty liver disease; disease burden, management, and future perspectives. International Research Journal of Gastroenterology and Hepatology 2024; 7: 1-3.

[98] Rani I, Munjal K, Singla RK, Gautam RK. Artificial intelligence and machine learning–based new drug discovery process with molecular modelling. Trends for Pharmaceutical Drug Discovery and Development. 2023; pp. 19-35.

SUBJECT INDEX

A

Abundance 162, 195
  increased 195
  lower 162
Acetone 107
Acidic environments 112, 249
Active Targeting 70, 89, 105, 242
Alcoholic liver disease (ALD) 148, 149, 212, 232, 324

B

Biochemical analyses 197
Biodegradability 64, 66, 76, 88, 102, 114, 130, 201, 244, 267, 274
Bloodstream 49, 110, 114, 115, 116, 219, 220, 238, 239, 240, 248, 250

C

Calcium pump 214
Carcinomas 86, 145, 241
Cardiovascular disease 29, 60, 128, 212
Cell signalling 252
Chronic immunosuppression 178
Clinical trials 51, 52, 101, 150, 151, 154, 159, 165, 167, 282, 308, 309, 338, 339
Composition 15, 33, 155, 166, 193, 221, 255, 290, 334
  chemical 221
  hepatic fatty acid 290
  microbial 166
Conjugated linoleic acid (CLA) 253
Cytotoxic 49, 268, 304

D

Dendrimers 44, 45, 46, 67, 127, 128, 131, 132, 133, 135, 136, 137, 268, 274, 301
Deoxyhemoglobin 185
Diabetes mellitus 3, 154, 218, 233, 297
Digital therapeutics (DTx) 338
Drug accumulation 273
Dyslipidaemia 146, 150
E-coupled systems 72
Empirical observation 47
Emulsification 109
Encapsulate lipophilic drugs 86, 92
Endocytosis 135, 183, 221, 243, 246, 250, 255

F

Fatty acids 2, 5, 104, 111, 150, 214, 252, 285, 327, 328, 336
Fatty liver 1, 2, 4, 26, 27, 100, 128, 195, 197, 324, 325, 327, 328, 331, 332
  alcoholic 4, 100
Formulations 16, 49, 110, 111, 113, 114, 115, 154, 157, 158, 200, 272, 273, 275, 285, 303, 306
  cationic 49
  conventional 16
Free fatty acids (FFAs) 5, 7, 29, 104, 148, 213, 214, 327

G

Gamma-oxidation 214
Gene editing 74, 158, 166
Gene expression 159
Gold nanoparticles 63, 66, 179, 191, 201, 219, 235, 299, 301

H

Heart disease 25, 32, 324
Hemolysis 268, 270, 274
Hepatic binding 221
Hepatic fibrosis (HF) 5, 15, 44, 99, 101, 157, 199, 200, 236, 328, 333
High-fat diet (HFD) 92, 111, 191, 194, 253, 289, 307

Anjali Sharma, Devkant Sharma, Ajmer Singh Grewal, Geeta Deswal & Ganga Reddy Velma (Eds.)

I

Imaging Biomarker 331, 341
Immunoglobulins 90, 243
Insulin sensitivity 31, 32, 152, 153, 154, 156, 161, 163, 214, 217, 218, 333, 335

K

Keto-carotenoid 113
Ketogenic diets 161
Key liver enzymes 335
Key metabolites 185
Kupffer cells (KCs) 6, 48, 89, 90, 103, 104, 105, 115, 116, 189, 190, 241, 242, 297, 304

L

Lipid metabolism 72, 74, 150, 151, 156, 157, 215, 218, 304, 308, 329, 333, 336
Lipid nanocapsules 91
Lipid nanoparticles 75, 159, 340
  effective 159
  hepatocyte-targeted 340
  retinoid-conjugated 75
Lipophilic drugs 13, 62, 64, 73, 88, 106, 108, 253, 254
Liver biopsy 9, 10, 11, 28, 30, 31, 34, 50, 51, 61, 324, 326, 332, 341
Liver cirrhosis 41, 145, 194, 237, 282, 325
Liver enzymes 27, 28, 31, 100, 161, 165, 212, 331, 333, 335, 336, 337, 338
  elevated 27, 28, 212, 331, 333
Liver injury 2, 29, 139, 148, 186, 196, 198, 299
  chronic 148
Lymph nodes 238, 239
  local 238
  regional 239
Lymphocytes 110, 240

M

Macrophages 6, 48, 90, 112, 130, 190, 239, 240, 241, 244, 249, 284, 304, 306, 328
  alveolar 239
  hepatic 244, 284
  liver-resident 6, 190
  local 241
  resident 249
  splenic 304
Metabolic disorders 29, 31, 32, 71, 75, 114, 146, 149, 178, 183, 212, 231, 232, 282, 286
  associated 212
  liver-related 114

N

Nano-emulsions 131
Nano lipid carriers 68
Nanomaterials 130, 219, 220, 221, 222, 224, 266, 269, 270, 273, 281
Nanomedicines 17, 40, 42, 76, 77, 101, 102, 105, 218, 219, 266, 281, 305, 310, 315
  generic 310
  lipid-based 102
Nonalcoholic fatty liver disease 3, 4, 40, 43, 59, 60, 66, 100, 108, 186, 192
Nucleic acids 42, 43, 69, 101, 106, 110, 113, 219, 241, 299, 301

O

Oleic acid 92, 289
Oligofructose 336
Oxidation 60, 93, 186, 193, 298
  dysfunctional 298
  impairing lipid 60
Oxidative stress 5, 6, 7, 14, 15, 16, 17, 28, 29, 148, 149, 150, 151, 254, 270

P

Pathophysiology 1, 4, 29, 47, 50, 51, 146, 147, 235, 237, 298, 300, 326, 327
Pathways 52, 128, 148, 157, 158, 159, 186, 212, 250, 251, 252, 237, 238, 249, 312, 339
  biological 237
  cellular stress 312
  diagnostic 339
  endocytic 249, 250, 252
  endocytotic 251
Peptides 42, 91, 105, 198, 219, 231, 242, 269, 273, 306

Protein binding 48, 243
Proteomics 51, 266, 313
Public health 34, 194

Q

Qualitative research 234
Quantum Dots (QDs) 45, 68, 107, 179, 191, 192, 194, 201, 274, 282

R

Radiation 180, 186, 195
  detected electromagnetic 195
  ionizing 180, 186
  scattering dielectric 195
Randomized controlled trials (RCTs) 335, 337, 338
Reticuloendothelial processes 132
Routine LFTs 31

S

Sick cells 105
Side effects 11, 13, 18, 113, 114, 129, 130, 137, 145, 150, 157, 158
Single nucleotide polymorphisms (SNPs) 331
Steatosis 2, 4, 5, 10, 11, 26, 27, 31, 32, 146, 180, 187, 213, 232, 298
Systemic toxicity 17, 70, 75, 235, 244, 273, 275, 299, 300, 302, 306

T

Targeted drug delivery 66, 67, 88, 93, 130, 132, 137, 235, 238, 241, 248, 249, 255
Therapeutic approaches 87, 101, 158, 159, 167, 267, 285, 299
Therapeutic interventions 73, 79, 87, 313
Thermogenesis 155
Thiazolidinediones 11, 87, 150, 234
Thin film hydration 88
Thyroid-stimulating hormone (TSH) 213
Toxicity 51, 52, 76, 77, 136, 137, 200, 201, 202, 215, 265, 266, 268, 269, 270, 271, 273, 304
  cellular 76
  chronic 270, 271, 304
  lipid 215
Transferrin 243
Triglycerides 2, 31, 104, 139, 159, 213, 214, 324, 325, 335, 337
Tyrosine kinase inhibitors (TKIs) 113

U

Ultrasonography 2, 10, 212
Ursodeoxycholic acid 217

V

Vaccines 43, 106, 110, 210, 308
  mRNA 308
  traditional 110
Venipuncture 194
Vitamin 4, 11, 15, 16, 72, 87, 99, 103, 105, 150, 151, 216
  antioxidant 87
  fat-soluble 103
Vivo research 49

W

Water solubility 46, 64, 114, 127, 279
  high 64, 127
  low 297

X

X-ray 185, 199
Xenobiotic-metabolizing capabilities 244

Z

Zwitterionic 78, 306

www.ingramcontent.com/pod-product-compliance
Lightning Source LLC
LaVergne TN
LVHW070945210926
848482LV00002B/99

* 9 7 9 8 8 9 8 8 1 5 6 9 1 *